LIBRARY

D0590299

WITHDRAWN
FROM THE LIBRARY OF
UNIVERSITY OF ULSTER

100392094

Principles of
Biomedical
Instrumentation and
Measurement

Principles of Biomedical Instrumentation and Measurement

Richard Aston

Pennsylvania State University
Wilkes-Barre

Merrill, an imprint of
Macmillan Publishing Company
New York

Maxwell Macmillan Canada, Inc.
Toronto

Maxwell Macmillan International Publishing Company
New York Oxford Singapore Sydney

100 392 094
610.28
AST
x+

Cover Art: Steve Botts
This book was set in English Times.

Administrative Editor: David Garza
Production Coordinator: JoEllen Gohr
Cover Designer: Russ Maselli

Copyright © 1990 by Macmillan Publishing Company, a division of Macmillan, Inc. "Merrill" is an imprint of Macmillan Publishing Company.

All rights reserved. No part of this book may be reproduced in any form, electronic or mechanical, including photocopy, recording, or any information storage and retrieval system, without permission in writing from the Publisher.

Printed in the United States of America

Macmillan Publishing Company
866 Third Avenue, New York, New York 10022

Macmillan Publishing Company is
part of the Maxwell Communication
Group of Companies.

Maxwell Macmillan Canada, Inc.
1200 Eglinton Avenue East
Suite 200
Don Mills, Ontario M3C 3N1

Library of Congress Catalog Card Number: 89-62576
International Standard Book Number: 0-675-20943-9

PRINT 3 4 5 6 7 8   YEAR 4 5 6 7 8 9

To my biomed students

Merrill's International Series in Electrical and Electronics Technology

ADAMSON *Applied Pascal for Technology*, 20771-1
Structured BASIC Applied to Technology, 20772-X
Structured C for Technology, 20993-5
Structured C for Technology (w/disks), 21289-8

ANTONAKOS *The 68000 Microprocessor: Hardware and Software, Principles and Applications*, 21043-7

ASSER/
STIGLIANO/
BAHRENBURG *Microcomputer Servicing: Practical Systems and Troubleshooting*, 20907-2
Microcomputer Theory and Servicing, 20659-6
Lab Manual to accompany Microcomputer Theory and Servicing, 21109-3

ASTON *Principles of Biomedical Instrumentation and Measurement*, 20943-9

BATESON *Introduction to Control System Technology, Third Edition*, 21010-0

BEACH/JUSTICE *DC/AC Circuit Essentials*, 20193-4

BERLIN *Experiments in Electronic Devices, Second Edition*, 20881-5
The Illustrated Electronics Dictionary, 20451-8

BERLIN/GETZ *Experiments in Instrumentation and Measurement*, 20450-X
Fundamentals of Operational Amplifiers and Linear Integrated Circuits, 21002-X
Principles of Electronic Instrumentation and Measurement, 20449-6

BOGART *Electronic Devices and Circuits, Second Edition*, 21150-6

BOGART/BROWN *Experiments in Electronic Devices and Circuits, Second Edition*, 21151-4

BOYLESTAD *DC/AC: The Basics*, 20918-8
Introductory Circuit Analysis, Sixth Edition, 21181-6

BOYLESTAD/
KOUSOUROU *Experiments in Circuit Analysis, Sixth Edition*, 21182-4
Experiments in DC/AC Basics, 21131-X

BREY *8086/8088 Microprocessor: Architecture, Programming, and Interfacing*, 20443-7
Microprocessors and Peripherals: Hardware, Software, Interfacing, and Applications, Second Edition, 20884-X

BROBERG *Lab Manual to accompany Electronic Communication Techniques, Second Edition*, 21257-X

BUCHLA *Digital Experiments: Emphasizing Systems and Design, Second Edition*, 21180-8
Experiments in Electric Circuits Fundamentals, 20836-X
Experiments in Electronics Fundamentals: Circuits, Devices and Applications, 20736-3

COX *Digital Experiments: Emphasizing Troubleshooting, Second Edition*, 21196-4

DELKER *Experiments in 8085 Microprocessor Programming and Interfacing*, 20663-4

FLOYD *Digital Fundamentals, Fourth Edition*, 21217-0
Electric Circuits Fundamentals, 20756-8

FLOYD (cont.)	*Electronic Devices, Second Edition,* 20883-1
	Electronics Fundamentals: Circuits, Devices and Applications, 20714-2
	Essentials of Electronic Devices, 20062-8
	Principles of Electric Circuits, Third Edition, 21062-3
	Principles of Electric Circuits, Electron Flow Version, Second Edition, 21292-8
GAONKAR	*Microprocessor Architecture, Programming, and Applications with the 8085/8080A, Second Edition,* 20675-8
	The Z80 Microprocessor: Architecture, Interfacing, Programming, and Design, 20540-9
GILLIES	*Instrumentation and Measurement for Electronic Technicians,* 20432-1
HUMPHRIES	*Motors and Controls,* 20235-3
KULATHINAL	*Transform Analysis and Electronic Networks with Applications,* 20765-7
LAMIT/LLOYD	*Drafting for Electronics,* 20200-0
LAMIT/WAHLER/ HIGGINS	*Workbook in Drafting for Electronics,* 20417-8
MARUGGI	*Technical Graphics: Electronics Worktext,* 20311-2
McINTYRE	*Study Guide to accompany Electronic Devices, Second Edition,* 21145-X
	Study Guide to accompany Electronics Fundamentals, 20676-6
MILLER	*The 68000 Microprocessor: Architecture, Programming, and Applications,* 20522-0
MONACO	*Introduction to Microwave Technology,* 21030-5
	Laboratory Activities in Microwave Technology, 21031-3
NASHELSKY/ BOYLESTAD	*BASIC Applied to Circuit Analysis,* 20161-6
QUINN	*The 6800 Microprocessor,* 20515-8
REIS	*Electronic Project Design and Fabrication,* 20791-6
ROSENBLATT/ FRIEDMAN	*Direct and Alternating Current Machinery, Second Edition,* 20160-8
SCHOENBECK	*Electronic Communications: Modulation and Transmission,* 20473-9
SCHWARTZ	*Survey of Electronics, Third Edition,* 20162-4
SORAK	*Linear Integrated Circuits: Laboratory Experiments,* 20661-8
STANLEY, B. H.	*Experiments in Electric Circuits, Third Edition,* 21088-7
STANLEY, W. D.	*Operational Amplifiers with Linear Integrated Circuits, Second Edition,* 20660-X
TOCCI	*Electronic Devices: Conventional Flow Version, Third Edition,* 20063-6
	Fundamentals of Electronic Devices, Third Edition, 9887-4
	Fundamentals of Pulse and Digital Circuits, Third Edition, 20033-4
	Introduction to Electric Circuit Analysis, Second Edition, 20002-4
WEBB	*Programmable Controllers: Principles and Applications,* 20452-6
WEBB/ GRESHOCK	*Industrial Control Electronics,* 20897-1
YOUNG	*Electronic Communication Techniques, Second Edition,* 21045-3
ZANGER	*Fiber Optics: Communications and Other Applications,* 20944-7

Preface

The primary objective of this text is to provide the instructional materials that a student needs to understand widely used medical equipment. The emphasis is on those types of equipment used for patient care in the hospital. Another goal is to develop the student's ability to think analytically about problems that arise with complex medical equipment. Thus the text also emphasizes the development of troubleshooting skills useful to clinical engineers (CEs) and biomedical equipment technologists and technicians (BMETs). These skills are developed in such a way as to be useful as part of the design process.

The text is divided into three parts. Part I, "Basics," presents the fundamental ideas that are, for the most part, prerequisite to the subsequent parts. These fundamentals include the basics of biopotentials, hospital equipment safety, physiological transducers, differential amplifiers, instrumentation, amplifiers, and the approach to troubleshooting.

In Part II, "Patient-Care Equipment," we describe equipment likely to be used with the patient in the hospital. Examples include electrocardiographs, electroencephalographs, defibrillators, pacemakers, electrosurgical and laser surgical units, catheters, and respirators. In each case, a different aspect of electronics is also presented, particularly important to the device under discussion, but relevant to other medical equipment as well.

Part III, "Specialized Medical Equipment," deals with larger-scale equipment, such as imaging devices, x-ray and ultrasonic equipment, and clinical laboratory instruments. These types of equipment might be found in special centers outside the hospital.

The discussions in Parts II and III are generally independent of each other, but both often require the background in Part I. Therefore it is possible to pick and choose chapters from these parts of the text as is convenient, without breaking the continuity of the presentation. For example, an introductory course in biomedical instrumentation can use Part I and several selected topics from Parts II and III.

It is assumed that all users of the text will have a background in electronic circuit theory, such as is typically given to first-year students in electronic technology programs. The text is written for a second- or third-year course in such a program, depending upon the requirements of the program. Naturally, some sections are more specialized, and perhaps more difficult, than others. In general, the chapters are structured so that descriptive material is presented first, with the more complex materials at the end of the chapter. This makes it easy to skip some more detailed discussions, in the interest of time, without breaking the continuity of the text.

The text presents enough differential-amplifier–based linear electronics that a student will be able to understand basic medical equipment circuits. However, the text is designed also to serve the needs of students who already have sufficient background in these topics and who need a shorter, more descriptive course. Such a course may emphasize those topics that are unique to the biomedical field, such as biopotentials, equipment safety, equipment block diagrams, patient-equipment interface connections, and troubleshooting. For example, the instructor could delete a large portion of the discussion of electronics in the text by skipping Chapter 5 on differential amplifiers and the latter sections of Chapter 6 on the electrocardiograph, Chapter 7 on the electroencephalograph, Chapter 9 on the pacemaker unit, and Chapter 10 on the electrosurgical unit, since the descriptive material is presented in the earlier sections of these chapters.

If the student does not already have sufficient background in linear electronics, the other sections of the text can be used. It is valuable to use all of this material, however, even if the student has studied linear electronics, to reinforce those topics important in medical instruments or to expand the student's knowledge.

ACKNOWLEDGMENTS

This text would not have been possible without the previous work done by those mentioned in the bibliography. Many medical equipment manufacturers have been helpful in providing photographs and information. Specific assistance with the appendix was given by Marcia H. Aston in medical terminology and Seth Krogoll on BASIC programs. Constance J. Dorula helped with the illustrations. Many reviewers have contributed to the book with their comments, including Cheryl Ebel, John Loney, James O. Wear, John Ephriam, J. D. Schlatter, and David Harrington. The students of the Pennsylvania State University, Wilkes-Barre Campus, and a pioneering former biomed teacher there, John Gesink, deserve thanks. Merrill editors who helped prepare this text were Stephen Helba, Becky Savage, and David Garza.

Contents

Part I Basics

1 A Perspective on Medical Instrumentation   3

1.1 Definition of a Medical Instrument   3
1.2 Historical Considerations   5
     The Invention of the Thermometer   6
     The Stethoscope and Hearing Enhancement   6
     Sight Enhancement   7
     Chemical Instrumentation and the Senses   9
     Twentieth-Century Developments   10
1.3 The Role of Electronic Circuit Theory   19
     a.c. Circuits   21
     Voltage Division   28
     Current Division   29
     Gain Function Analysis   30
     BJT Equivalent Circuit   32
References   34
Exercises   34

2 The Origin of Biopotentials, Electrocardiograms, and Electrical Shock   37

2.1 Fundamental Laws for Current in Biological Tissue   37
     Fick's Law   39
     Particle Drift   40
     Single-Cell Membrane Potential   40
     Resting Potential in a Cell   42
     Action Potential and Muscle Contraction   44
2.2 Biopotentials in the Heart   45
2.3 The Electrocardiogram   46
2.4 Electrical Shock   49
     High-Frequency Effects   53
     Microshock and Macroshock   55
References   56
Exercises   56

**3   Hospital Equipment Safety and
Organization, and a Logical Approach
to Troubleshooting**   **59**

3.1   Electrical Hazards of Medical Instruments   59
      Macroshock Hazards   62
      Microshock Hazards   64
3.2   Devices to Protect Against Electrical Hazards   68
      Ground Fault Interrupter   68
      Isolation Transformer   69
      Line Isolation Monitor   70
      Receptacle Tester   70
      Electrical Safety Analyzer Equipment   72
3.3   An Equipment Safety Program   72
      Hospital Regulations   73
      Inspections of Equipment   74
      Emergency Power Systems   75
      Oxygen Safety   77
      Safety in the Operating Room   77
      Hazards of Gases   79
      Pressure Chambers   81
3.4   Preventive Maintenance   82
3.5   A Logical Approach to Troubleshooting   83
References   86
Exercises   87

**4   Medical Instrument Transducers and
Component-Level Troubleshooting**   **89**

4.1   Electrode Transducers   89
      The Surface Electrode   90
      Half-Cell Potential and Equivalent Circuit
          Elements   94
4.2   Thermal Transducers   100
4.3   The Wheatstone Bridge   107
      Sensitivity of a Wheatstone Bridge   111
4.4   Strain Gauges   113
      The Strain Gauge in a Wheatstone Bridge   118
      Sensitivity of a Strain Gauge   120
4.5   The Differential Capacitive Transducer   121
4.6   Inductive Transducers   126

4.7 Troubleshooting at the Component Level   127
References   128
Exercises   129

5   Biopotential Amplifiers   135

5.1 A Transistor Differential Amplifier   137
       Inverting and Noninverting Amplifiers   140
5.2 Operational Amplifier Analysis   143
       Operational Amplifier Voltage and
             Current Sources   147
       Operational Amplifiers in Tandem   149
       High-Input-Impedance Amplifiers with
             Controlled Gain   152
       Differential Amplifier with Controlled Gain   154
       Buffer Amplifier for a Diff Amp   157
5.3 Biopotential Measurement Interference   158
       Common-Mode Rejection in a Diff Amp   161
5.4 Troubleshooting Medical Instrumentation
       Amplifiers   163
References   164
Exercises   165

Part II   Patient-Care Equipment

**6   The Electrocardiograph and
       Unit-Level Troubleshooting   177**

6.1 The ECG   177
       The ECG Block Diagram   180
6.2 ECG Lead Connections   185
       Augmented ECG Lead Connections   190
       Chest Lead Connection   191
6.3 Common-Mode Voltage Reduction   198
6.4 Push-Pull Power Amplifiers   201
       Maximum Power Transfer   206
       A Push-Pull Amplifier with Crossover
             Compensation   209
       Power Amplifier with Offset Control   210
6.5 Power Supplies   211
       Power Supply Regulation   214

6.6   Unit-Level Troubleshooting: ECGs   215
Circuit-Board Swapping   216
References   217
Exercises   217

7   The Electroencephalograph and Filtering   223

7.1   The EEG   223
EEG Electrodes   223
An EEG Block Diagram   227
Electroencephalograms   230
EEGs in Diagnosis   231
7.2   Filters   233
First-Order Filters   236
Higher-Order Active Filters   240
Second-Order Low-Pass Filters   241
Second-Order High-Pass Filters   244
Third-Order Low-Pass Filters   247
Band-Reject Filters   251
7.3   Troubleshooting an EEG   254
References   255
Exercises   255

8   The Defibrillator and Step Response   261

8.1   The Defibrillator   261
Example Defibrillators   264
8.2   Defibrillator Energy Delivery   267
8.3   Analysis of the Defibrillator
Voltage Waveform   270
The Lown Voltage Waveform of a Defibrillator   271
Case I (Underdamped)   273
Case II (Overdamped)   275
8.4   Troubleshooting Defibrillators   277
References   278
Exercises   278

9   The Pacemaker — A Digital Pulse Oscillator   283

9.1   Properties of the Pacemaker   284
Pacemaker Batteries   286
Illustrative Pacemaker Characteristics   288
9.2   Programmable Pacemakers   291

9.3 Digital Pulse Oscillators 294
A Comparator Circuit 294
A Threshold Detector Analysis 297
Square-Wave Generator 299
Monostable Multivibrator 304
Positive-Edge Triggered Multivibrator 306
An Illustrative Pacemaker Circuit 307
References 309
Exercises 310

10 Electrosurgical Units and Laser Surgery 313
10.1 The Basic ESU 313
Active Electrodes 315
The Active Electrode Resistance 316
The Return Electrode 318
A Block Diagram 321
10.2 Sinusoidal Oscillators 323
10.3 An ESU Power Amplifier 327
10.4 Troubleshooting an ESU 330
10.5 Laser Surgical Devices 333
The CO_2 Laser 333
The Argon Laser Surgical Unit 335
The Nd:YAG Laser 336
References 337
Exercises 337

11 Catheters and Blood Pressure Monitoring 341
11.1 Circulation System Measurements 341
Pumping Action of the Heart 341
Arterial Pressure Measurement 344
Invasive Blood Pressure Measurement 346
Fluid Resistance 347
Instrumentation for Direct Pressure
Measurement 348
Pressure Transducer Calibration 349
Pressure Measurements in the Heart 351
11.2 Catheter Measurements 355
The Equivalent Circuit of a Catheter 356
Fluid Inertance 356
Compliance 357

The Fluid-Electrical Analogy   358
The Catheter Equivalent Circuit   359
The Physical Formulas for Catheter Components   359
Frequency Response of a Catheter with
    a Diagram   360
Tuning a Catheter   363
Pinches, Bubbles, and Leaks in a Catheter   363
References   368
Exercises   368

**12   Respiratory Equipment and Pulmonary
       Function Monitoring   371**

12.1 Therapeutic and Diagnostic Equipment   371
12.2 The Ventilator   374
     Ventilator Modes of Operation   374
12.3 A Spirometer   381
12.4 Pneumotachograph Airflow Measurement   383
     The Integrator Circuit   385
     Pneumotachograph Volume Measurements   386
12.5 The Plethysmograph   389
     Measurement of Total Lung Capacity   390
12.6 Troubleshooting Pneumatic Equipment   392
References   393
Exercises   393

**13   The Central Station Monitor,
       Microprocessor-Based Equipment,
       and System-Level Troubleshooting   395**

13.1 Machine Language   396
13.2 Microprocessor Block Diagram   398
     The CPU   399
     The Memory Chip   402
     Input/Output Units   403
13.3 A Microprocessor-Based Monitor   405
     Central Station Monitoring   410
     Troubleshooting Microprocessor-Based
         Equipment   413
     Self-Test   415
     A Logical Approach to Troubleshooting   416
References   417
Exercises   417

Part III Specialized Medical Equipment

14 Clinical Laboratory Equipment   423

14.1 Chemical Electrodes   423
The pH Electrode   424
14.2 A Blood Gas Analyzer   425
The $^PCO_2$ Electrode   426
The $^PO_2$ Electrode   427
Noninvasive Blood Gas Monitoring   429
14.3 Photometers and Colorimeters   431
Diffraction Gratings   431
Flame Photometers   433
14.4 Blood Cell Counter   437
Optical Methods of Cell Counting   442
References   443
Exercises   443

15 Medical X-Ray Equipment   445

15.1 X-Rays   445
The X-Ray Tube   446
The Nature of X-Rays   449
X-Ray Absorption   452
Tissue Contrast   455
15.2 X-Ray Equipment Block Diagram   456
The X-Ray Tube   458
The Collimator   461
The Bucky Grid   463
The X-Ray Detector   463
The Power Supply   464
15.3 Fluoroscopic System   467
15.4 X-Ray CT Scanners   469
15.5 Nuclear Medicine Imaging   473
Radioisotopes and Radiopharmaceuticals   474
Radiation Detectors   474
The Photomultiplier Tube   478
Gamma-Ray Camera   478
15.6 Radiation Dose   481
References   487
Exercises   487

16   Ultrasonic Equipment   **489**

16.1 Therapeutic and Diagnostic Equipment   489
     Therapeutic Ultrasonic Equipment   489
     Piezoelectric Transducers   491
     Ultrasonic Imaging Equipment   491
     The Display Unit   493
     Scanning-Type Displays   493
16.2 Ultrasonic Waves   496
     Wave Reflections   500
     Analysis of a Typical Ultrasonic Reflection   503
     Ultrasonic Power   504
     Attenuation in Ultrasonic Waves   505
16.3 Ultrasonic Blood Flow Equipment   506
     An Analysis of the Doppler Effect   506
     An Analysis of Transit Time   509
     References   510
     Exercises   510

Appendix A   Computer Programs   **515**

Appendix B   Laplace Transforms   **526**

B.1 The Laplace Method   526
     The Step Source   526
     Laplace Equivalent Impedances   527
     Circuit Analysis of Laplace Equivalent Elements   529
     Laplace Transform Tables   531
     RC Circuit Step Response   532

Appendix C   Medical Terminology   **537**

C.1 Common Prefixes   537
C.2 Common Suffixes   538
C.3 The Terminology of General Anatomy   539
C.4 Terminology of Circulation   541
C.5 Terminology of Respiration   542
C.6 Terminology of the Nervous System   542
C.7 Terminology of Sensory Organs   543

Index   **545**

PART I
Basics

1. A Perspective on Medical Instrumentation

2. The Origin of Biopotentials, Electrocardiograms, and Electrical Shock

3. Hospital Equipment Safety and Organization, and a Logical Approach to Troubleshooting

4. Medical Instrument Transducers and Component-Level Troubleshooting

5. Biopotential Amplifiers

1 A Perspective on Medical Instrumentation

1.1 DEFINITION OF A MEDICAL INSTRUMENT

The physical forms taken by most examples of medical devices, such as instruments, tools, and machines, are illustrated by the block diagram in Figure 1.1. Each switch position sets the instrument up in one of the physical forms as an instrument for measurement, for monitoring, for diagnosis of disease, for therapy of patients, or for surgery. Most medical instruments fall into one of these categories.

A medical instrument performs a specific function on a biological system. The function may be the exact measurement of physiological param-

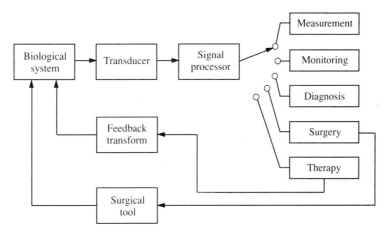

FIGURE 1.1
A block diagram of a generalized medical instrument.

eters—pressure, flow, voltage, current, chemical pH, volume, weight, temperature—and rates of change of these parameters. In physiological systems, because the parameters often have small magnitudes or are otherwise difficult to process, a transducer (illustrated in Figure 1.1) is necessary to transform the physiological signal into a form that can be read by the signal processor. The transducer may, for example, amplify voltages or pressures, select an appropriate parameter for measurement, provide a transitional medium, or effect an impedance match of the biological system to the signal processor.

In physiological systems, measurable parameters cover a wide range. Voltages range from 1 microvolt (μV) to several millivolts (mV) and up to thousands of volts (V) of static charge. Frequencies range from d.c. to 20 kilohertz (kHz). The dynamic range of sound amplitudes is 100 decibels (dB) and above. Pressures range from 0.1 millimeter of mercury (mmHg) to approximately 1000 mmHg. Fluid flow rates rise to 25 liters per minute (liters/min) and air flow up to 600 liters/min. The need to maintain physiological stability and control feedback is illustrated by the relatively narrow temperature range in the human body, 90 to 104 degrees Fahrenheit (°F).

The output of a transducer should be a signal compatible with the signal processor illustrated in the figure. This output may be a force or flow rate sufficient to move a gauge, a voltage or current that can deflect a meter needle, a sound capable of being amplified above ambient noise so it can be measured, or an ionic concentration requiring further processing. For many signal processors (for example, those having digital components), the compatible signal is binary, typically either +5 or 0 V. Only upon appropriately processed signals can the arithmetic and logical functions of microprocessors and digital circuits be performed.

The type of signal processing depends upon the function of the instrument—measurement, monitoring, diagnosis, therapy, or surgery. The function is selected by a switch in the figure.

A common example of a *measuring* instrument is the thermometer. The transducer is the glass bulb and scale; the signal processor and monitor are the observer who records the measurement. Other examples of measuring devices are sphygmomanometers, electroencephalographs, and electrocardiographs. A *monitoring* instrument represents a higher level of complexity in that it includes a memory, which can take the form of a paper strip recorder, a storage oscilloscope, or a computer memory, which holds information for later use. An even higher level of sophistication is usually required for machine *diagnosis*. The diagnostic function may be performed by an instrument as simple as an alarm that warns of an excessive heart rate, or as complex as a mainframe computer that processes symptoms and prescribes a health care program.

In order for a medical instrument to be used in the performance of *therapy*, it must feed back a signal or force to the biological system, as indicated by the position of the feedback transform in Figure 1.1. Therapy is applied by a crutch, for example, allowing a leg to heal while the patient remains ambulatory. More complex therapy may be applied by a biofeedback instrument such as a speech therapy device capable of deriving the information-bearing elements from speech and applying them to another sense such as sight or touch. Other therapeutic instrumentation may operate independently of physiological parameters in the system to which the therapy is applied. An example is an ultrasonic massager operated by a physical therapist. This is closely related to another category of instruments used in *surgery* and surgical procedures, namely *invasive* units, which penetrate the skin of the patient. These include electrosurgical knives, hypodermic needles, and lasers.

The medical instruments illustrated in Figure 1.1 are those that may be used in connection with the patient. Another category is assigned to laboratory instruments used to investigate and assess biological fluids and tissue. The measurement of pH is fundamental to the operation of many of these instruments, as are techniques for investigating particles in fluids.

1.2 HISTORICAL CONSIDERATIONS

The fundamental purpose of tools is to enhance the capabilities of human beings by helping them to lift more weight, to move faster and more comfortably, to communicate over greater distances, and to use the five senses more effectively. Throughout history, as technology was developed, the number of human functions extended by the use of tools increased. Most recently, the introduction of computers has extended even our ability to think, particularly in calculating, analyzing, and storing large amounts of information.

Consider, for example, the sense of touch. The ancient Greeks used the technique of "laying on of hands" to determine the size of organs, the nature of wounds, and the extent of bodily growths; the technique is still used today. Modern instruments that extend the sense of touch include devices for massage, such as electrical current stimulators, automatic vibrators, and ultrasonic therapy equipment. In the Tadoma method of speech therapy, the therapist places a hand on the speaker's face during speech training to feel where the sounds are placed. An electronic tactile vocoder can be used to extend the therapist's ability to locate these placements by amplifying these acoustic cues and transferring them to other, more convenient cutaneous body sites.

One specific bit of information obtained by the sense of touch is a relative measure of body temperature. In this function, the thermometer extends the sense of touch, serving to quantify a measurement that had previously been only approximate.

The Invention of the Thermometer

In 1603, the Italian scientist Galileo showed that a closed glass tube inserted in a container of water could be arranged so that the height of the water sucked into the tube by a partial vacuum varied with the temperature. In 1625, Santorio Santonio, a Slavic physician, constructed a similar device, which he used to measure the temperature in the human body. The problem with the instrument (Figure 1.2a) was that the height of the water was also affected by the atmospheric pressure. This problem was solved a quarter of a century later when Ferdinand II, Grand Duke of Tuscany, sealed the water in a closed vessel to eliminate the effect of atmospheric pressure. The essentially modern thermometer shown in Figure 1.2(b) was introduced by the Dutch instrument maker Gabriel D. Fahrenheit, who in the eighteenth century replaced the water with mercury and improved the instrument's accuracy. This thermometer is still widely used, although more recently liquid crystal thermometers have been adopted for special applications.

The Stethoscope and Hearing Enhancement

From the time of the ancient Greeks, physicians have used their hearing for diagnosis, such as in placing the ear against the chest or back to listen for

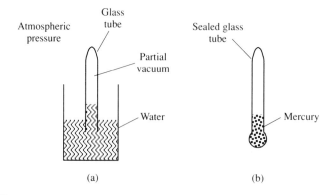

(a)   (b)

FIGURE 1.2
Thermometer development.

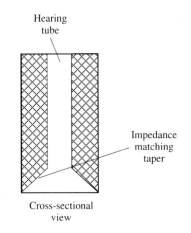

FIGURE 1.3
A stethoscope.

the sounds of breathing and the heart. An early enhancement of this sense was achieved by the use of a "hearing tube," or stethoscope.

The stethoscope is a refinement of the hearing tube, attributed to Rene T. H. Laennec, a French physician who probably used it as much to avoid touching the bodies of his patients with his ear as to improve his ability to hear heart and breathing sounds. His device, a simple hollow tube, was reported in 1819 in his treatise, "On Mediate Auscultation." He evidently designed it to amplify sound, since it contained a taper (Figure 1.3) that served to improve the coupling of chest to ear by the impedance matching principle.

Further improvement was achieved with the binaural stethoscope, designed by the American George P. Cammann in 1851. This stethoscope had an assortment of flanges or tapers that could be used in different areas of the body. This addition improved the device because acoustic impedance varies among patients and among sites of the body. A binaural, differential stethoscope was invented by S. Scott Alison in the 1860s. These improvements increased the number of variables in the instrument that the physician had to adjust. Such flexibility tends to introduce confusion, so it is little wonder that the physician today still uses Cammann's simple device. A 100-year-old stethoscope appears in Figure 1.4.

Sight Enhancement

As a device to enhance the sense of sight, the candle was used for a remarkably long time, from the prehistoric age until the nineteenth century, when it was replaced by the incandescent lamp. Also, to enhance vision, glass

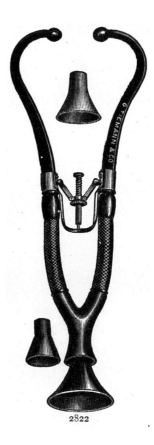

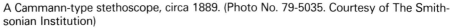

FIGURE 1.4
A Cammann-type stethoscope, circa 1889. (Photo No. 79-5035. Courtesy of The Smithsonian Institution)

magnifiers were used in the ancient world for reading. The lens that developed from them was systematically studied by the English scientist Isaac Newton in 1666. As a medical application, lenses are most often used in eyeglasses and contact lenses.

The ophthalmoscope invented in the mid-nineteenth century by the German scientist Hermann von Helmholtz is an example of an instrument that enables the examiner to look into body cavities, such as the ear, eye, and nose, *noninvasively*—that is, without cutting the skin. The ophthalmoscope is particularly significant because it is one of the earliest examples of instruments that present images of internal organs, and in this sense is a forerunner of x-ray.

The translucent glass in the sketch of the Helmholtz ophthalmoscope (Figure 1.5) directs a fraction of light into the subject's eye, from which another fraction is reflected into the observer's eye. The observer can then

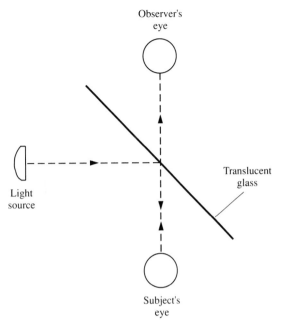

Observer's
eye

Translucent
glass

Light
source

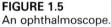

Subject's
eye

FIGURE 1.5
An ophthalmoscope.

see the retina of the subject. Without the translucent glass, the observer's head would cast a shadow over the subject's cornea, making it appear black and opaque.

In a similar development in 1855, Manuel Garcia used a mirror in the back of the throat to observe vibrations of the vocal cords.

A breakthrough in the enhancement of sight came in 1895 with the discovery of x-ray by the German physicist Wilhelm Roentgen, who was experimenting with cathode rays. In a darkened room one day, Roentgen noticed that paper saturated with barium platinocyanide began to glow even though it was well out of range of the cathode rays. Subsequent experiments showed that denser materials placed against the paper cast a shadow on the paper. By these observations the x-ray tube was developed. In December 1895, these observations were reported at the Physio-Medical Society of Wurzberg, and the device became a diagnostic tool that has remained useful to the present day. One of these early x-ray machines is shown in Figure 1.6.

Chemical Instrumentation and the Senses

The senses of taste and smell are used in medicine to diagnose body fluids. Medieval physicians reported that the urine of diabetics had a sweet taste. In 1776 Matthew Dobson, an English physician, noticed that the residue ob-

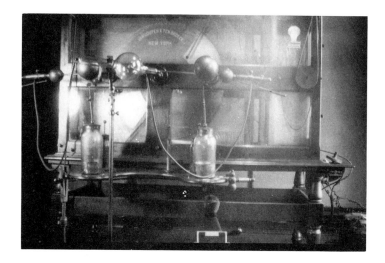

FIGURE 1.6
A turn-of-the-century x-ray machine composed of a Crookes tube and a Van Houten &
Tenbroeck static machine. (Photo No. 33977. Courtesy of The Smithsonian Institution)

tained by evaporating urine sometimes smelled and tasted like sugar. In 1797
the English physician John Rollo and the Scottish anatomist William Cruikshank reported their analysis of the residue, an early example of the application of chemical analysis to medical practice.

The analysis of blood was greatly improved in 1877 when the English-
man William Gowers announced his invention of the "haemacytometer,"
a device consisting of one-tenth-millimeter squares ruled at the bottom of
an indentation in a glass slide. Using a microscope, the observer could then
count the red blood cells in the blood. To increase the accuracy of the count,
in 1899 Magnus Blix and Sven Hedin of Sweden developed a centrifuge,
known as the hematocrit, to separate red blood cells from the blood by centrifugal force.

As the techniques involving chemical analysis became increasingly complicated, physicians relinquished the task to specialists who developed the
clinical laboratory. In 1885, the German Hugo von Zeimssen established
one of the first clinical laboratories. Well-known hospitals such as Massa-
chusetts General Hospital established on-site laboratories beginning at the
turn of the century.

Twentieth-Century Developments

The major impetus for the development of medical instrumentation in the
twentieth century was electronics. Beginning in 1903 with the invention of

the electrocardiograph (ECG) by the Dutch physiologist Willem Einthoven, these developments continue today with such devices as magnetic resonance imagers (MRI) and lasers used in clinical applications. Einthoven's device, illustrated in Figure 1.7, used a wire suspended between the poles of a magnet. Motion of the wire due to body currents between the two arms, generated by the heart, was measured by recording light reflected off a mirror supported by the wire. As electronic amplifiers were developed, improvements in the ECG followed. Recording of ECG traces on paper chart recorders was introduced in the 1940s. Four modern forms of the ECG are illustrated in Figure 1.8.

A fundamental breakthrough was made by M. Cremer in 1906 with the introduction of the pH electrode for quantifying the acid/base content of biological solutions. This device measured the membrane potential changes resulting from changes in ionic content and activity. Its invention led to a series of devices for measuring the blood gases, including a device that measures the partial pressure of oxygen and carbon dioxide.

Advances in electronics also made possible the invention of the electroencephalograph (EEG) in 1924. The German psychiatrist Hans Berger used a galvanometer to measure currents from metal strips attached to the scalp and found that these currents resulted from brain activity. Berger's

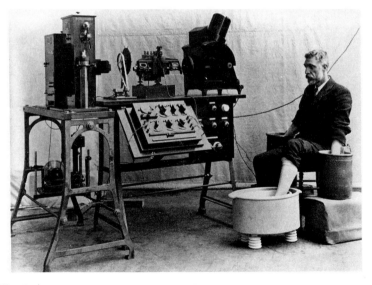

FIGURE 1.7
The original Cambridge electrocardiograph (1912), built for Sir Thomas Lewis and produced under agreement with Prof. Willem Einthoven, the father of electrocardiography. (Courtesy of Cambridge Instruments, Inc.)

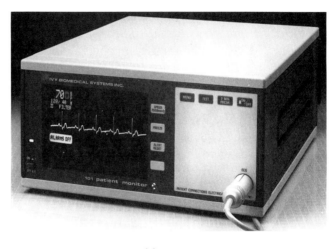

(a)

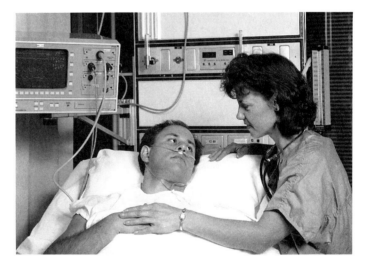

(b)

FIGURE 1.8
Four modern forms of the ECG: (a) a neonatal monitor for infants. (Courtesy of Biomedical Systems Inc.) (b) A monitor for ECG — among other parameters, such as temperature and pressure — shown connected to a patient. (Courtesy of Marquette Electronics, Inc.) (c) An ECG monitor connected to a patient during a stress test. (Courtesy of Sullivan & Brownell, Inc.) (d) A monitoring system in which hardware, software, and parameter functions are separated into individual plug-in modules. (Courtesy of Hewlett-Packard Company)

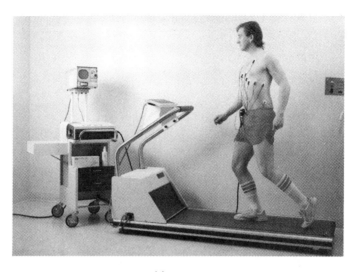

(c)

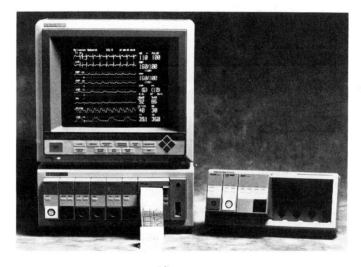

(d)

FIGURE 1.8 (continued)

systematic investigations laid the foundation for studies of the correlation between brain waves, sleep, and epilepsy.

Spark gap transmitters for radio communication provided the components for the clinically useful electrosurgical unit (ESU) introduced in 1928 by W. T. Bovie and the American surgeon Harvey Cushing. The ESU demonstrated that surgery could be done with less blood loss, but its use was limited by the danger of explosion of the flammable anesthetics in use at the time. The radio frequency energy vaporized the cells when applied by a metal electrode, and it tended to cauterize blood vessels to reduce bleeding. Widespread use of the ESU was encouraged by the introduction of nonflammable anesthetics in the 1950s.

The development of automatic mechanisms in the early twentieth century led to new mechanical and pneumatic instruments as well. Mechanical assistance to respiration came about in 1928 with the introduction of the iron lung for patients with respiratory paralysis. The patient was sealed in this device from the neck down, and a negative pressure was applied by the iron lung to draw air into the lungs. The positive pressure respirator used to assist breathing by pushing air into the lungs became clinically practical in the mid-1940s. A modern positive pressure respirator is shown in Figure 1.9.

The clinical application of nuclear radiation was introduced in 1936 by the American physicist John Lawrence, who artificially produced radionuclides in a cyclotron and used them in the treatment of leukemia, thus beginning the field of nuclear medicine. A gamma camera for recording

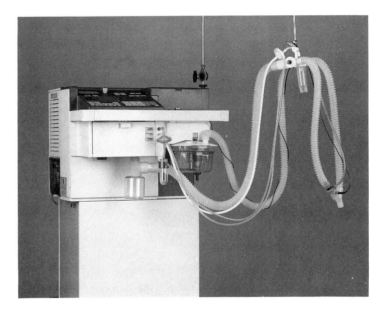

FIGURE 1.9
A modern positive pressure respirator that operates either from a hospital-line air supply or from an internal air compressor. (Courtesy of Puritan-Bennett, Inc.)

nuclear medicine images is illustrated in Figure 1.10. The exerciser is used to induce stress reactions in the patient.

Clinical application of electrical heart defibrillation began in 1956, when P. M. Zoll led a group of investigators who succeeded in reversing a heart fibrillation, a form of heart attack, by application of a.c. currents through the chest wall. The reliability of the defibrillator was significantly improved when B. Lown introduced the d.c. defibrillator in 1962. This device applied a d.c. current from a discharging capacitor through the chest wall into the heart to stop heart fibrillations. This type of defibrillator is illustrated in Figure 1.11.

In 1957, C. Walton Lillehei paced a heart during surgery by attaching wires to it and applying pulses of current spaced at a normal heart rate. This external pacemaker could be applied only during surgery. A most significant breakthrough in heart pacing was made by William Chardack and Wilson Greatbatch in 1960, when they developed the implantable pacemaker. A pacemaker of this type is illustrated in Figure 1.12.

The pacemaker was an early heart "spare part," which preceded artificial valves and ultimately the artificial heart, first implanted into Barney Clark by W. C. DeVries and R. Jarvik in 1984.

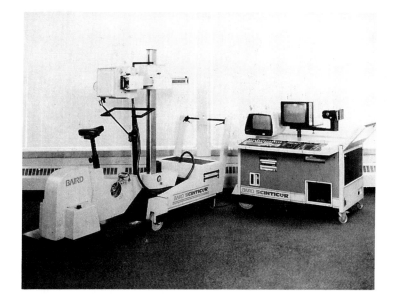

FIGURE 1.10
A gamma camera for recording nuclear medicine images. The rotary-pedal exerciser is used to induce stress reactions in the patient. (Courtesy of Baird Corporation)

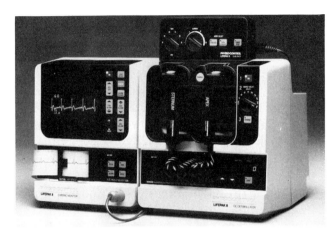

FIGURE 1.11
A d.c. defibrillator with a diagnostic ECG monitor. (Courtesy of Physio-Control Inc.)

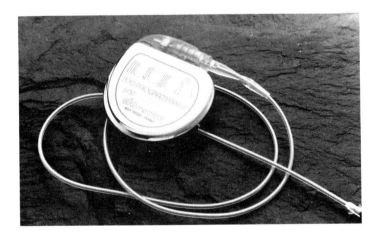

FIGURE 1.12
An implantable pacemaker. (Courtesy of Ela Medical, Inc.)

Another type of prosthesis, artificial tubes for replacing sections of arteries, was introduced in 1954, and its development led to the artificial kidney. Although hemodialysis, a process for removing impurities from blood, was first achieved in 1944, a clinically useful device was not developed until 1960, when B. H. Scribner led a group who developed a technique for continuous hemodialysis. The equipment used in this technique is called the artificial kidney because it compensates for a failed kidney.

In 1970, the technique for measuring the blood pressure, temperature, and flow rate in the heart and lungs was significantly advanced with the introduction of a balloon-tipped catheter by Harold J. Swan and William Ganz. The catheter is threaded through the veins into the heart; the balloon on the tip is then inflated, and blood flow carries the catheter into the lung. Advances in materials then led to the invention of the intra-aortic balloon pump by W. J. Kolft and J. Lawson in 1975. This device increases blood pressure and assists in blood flow. The balloon is implanted into the aorta and inflated in step with the heart-pumping action to assist the blood flow of patients with weak hearts. A balloon inflatable catheter used for opening blocked blood vessels is illustrated in Figure 1.13. The balloon is placed in an occluded vessel and inflated to open the passage so that it will stay open after the balloon is withdrawn.

The ultrasonic principles developed during World War II for the sonar used in undersea navigation have found medical applications. To measure blood flow, for example, an ultrasound transducer emits sound waves that are reflected by the moving blood cells and particles. If the blood is ap-

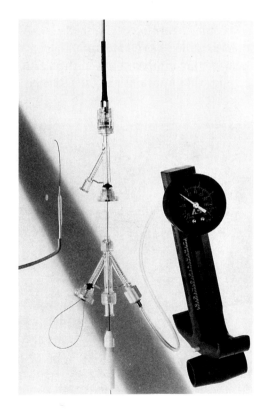

FIGURE 1.13
A dilation catheter for opening occluded vessels. (Courtesy of Advanced Cardiovascular Systems)

proaching the transducer, the sound will rise in pitch as a chirp. The difference in frequency over the duration of the chirp indicates the velocity, or rate of blood flow.

World War II sonar also provided the components of an ultrasonic imaging device tested for clinical application in 1957 by O. H. Houry and W. R. Bliss. This instrument measures sonar-type reflections from internal organs in order to construct an image of structures including heart valves and the midline of the brain. A modern ultrasound scanner is shown in Figure 1.14. Ultrasound has an advantage over x-ray because it does not produce the negative side effects x-rays do with their carcinogenic ionizing radiation. However, ultrasonic images are not as good as x-rays in some cases, so x-ray still has its niche.

Probably the most important advance in imaging of internal body structures since the invention of x-ray is the computer tomography (CT) scanner. The CT scanner was invented in 1970 by Allan Cormack and Geoffrey Hounsfield, who discovered that by computing the amount of x-ray absorbed at the intersections of columns and rows of a matrix of regions in tissue, they could determine the dimensions of those regions. By this technique they were able to produce an image of a slice through the body. The development of the minicomputer in the 1970s made it feasible to build imaging machines that automatically performed the necessary computations.

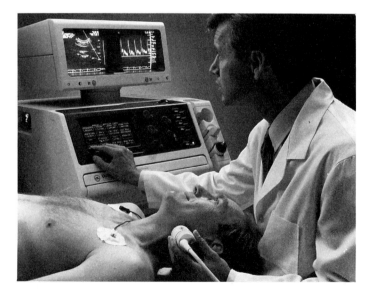

FIGURE 1.14
Equipment for obtaining ultrasonic images of internal organs. The transducer is held against the patient by the attendant. (Courtesy of Advanced Technology Laboratories)

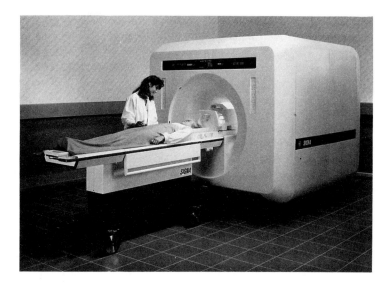

FIGURE 1.15
An MRI showing a patient in position for scanning. (Courtesy of General Electric Corporation)

Developments in the microprocessor and the minicomputer have improved many medical instruments. In the case of the CT scanner, the computer is an essential component, since the computations that produce the image would take far too much time if they had to be done by hand.

Further improvement of the imaging of internal organs, especially of soft tissues, was achieved with the commercial introduction of the magnetic resonance imager (MRI) in 1982. This device measures the frequency and duration of a nuclear magnetic resonance of protons. To get the image, the patient is placed in a strong magnetic field and radiated with a pulse of radio frequency (RF) energy. The frequency and duration of the ringing of the proton after the RF field is shut off provides the data from which the image is computed. An MRI is shown in Figure 1.15.

The advantages of the MRI over x-ray are that it makes better images of some soft tissue and does not emit ionizing radiation. Its disadvantage is that it does not respond to bone and therefore cannot be used to diagnose bone injuries. A van-mounted MRI is illustrated in Figure 1.16.

1.3 THE ROLE OF ELECTRONIC CIRCUIT THEORY

The brief history of medical instrumentation presented in the previous section is intended to help you develop a perspective, or overview, of medi-

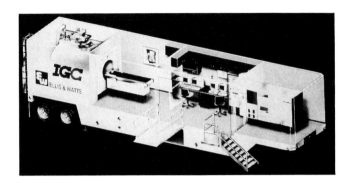

FIGURE 1.16
A mobile MRI unit. [Courtesy of Intermagnets General Corporation (IGC)]

cal instrumentation and to increase your basic understanding of it. To deal with instrumentation in detail, it is necessary to analyze it. The fundamental skill required by an engineer or service professional is the ability to analyze, to figure things out, to determine how a piece of equipment is supposed to work. This skill is essential both for engineering design and for trouble-shooting of equipment.

Probably the most comprehensive expression of the engineering analysis procedure is electronic circuit theory. This theory applies to electronic circuits, of course, but it also applies to fluid systems, pneumatic systems, and mechanical machines, all of which are present in medical equipment. Strict analogies can be made to allow you to apply what you learn in circuit theory to those types of systems. To learn engineering analysis, it is helpful to study electrical circuits and electronics. Systems using these components are often the most complex and contain the largest number of components. If you become skilled in electrical and electronic circuit analysis, dealing with pneumatics, mechanics, and fluids — of which many medical instruments are composed — will be much easier.

The variables in an electronic system are voltage and current. Physiological potentials arising from the heart, such as the electrocardiogram (ECG), are periodic and may be represented by sinusoidal signals. The general mathematical form of a voltage sinusoid is

$$v_1 = V_1 \cos(\omega t + \theta)$$

This voltage is defined by its frequency ω (in radians per second), its phase angle θ (in radians), and its peak magnitude V_1. In instrumentation such a signal is operated upon by elements such as resistors, R (in ohms, Ω), capacitors, C (in farads, F), and inductors, L (in henrys, H). Applications of these elements give rise to complicated current and voltage relations, some of which are described by differential equations that are usually unwieldy and difficult to solve. Fortunately, however, mathematical methods have been developed to transform differential equations into algebraic equations containing complex numbers. The process for solution of such equations is called *a.c. circuit theory*, and it uses phasors.

Electrical circuits are structures composed of resistors, R, inductors, L, and capacitors, C. The connections between these elements are called *nodes*. The voltage and current variables are created by ideal sources. An *ideal voltage source*, illustrated in Figure 1.17, maintains the voltage, v_S, across the nodes, regardless of the current passing through it. In effect, it has an internal impedance of zero.

The *ideal current source* maintains a current i_S regardless of the voltage across it. Its internal impedance approaches infinity.

a.c. Circuits

Alternating current circuit theory is based on the phasor expressions for sinusoidal steady state voltages and currents. A *phasor* is a complex-number representation of a circuit quantity, consisting of a real part, [Re], and an imaginary part, [Im]. Phasors are manipulated mathematically by complex-number algebra.

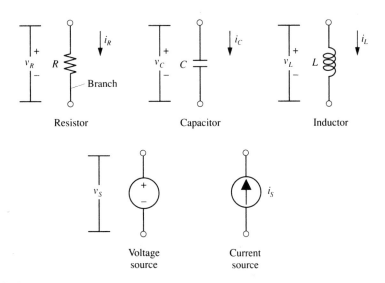

FIGURE 1.17
The time domain representation of electrical circuit components.

A set of phasor domain relationships that define R, L, and C for sinusoidal steady state is as follows:

$$V_R = (R)I_R \tag{1.1}$$

$$V_L = (j\omega L)I_L \tag{1.2}$$

$$V_C = \left(\frac{1}{j\omega C}\right)I_C \tag{1.3}$$

where j is the imaginary number $\sqrt{-1}$ used in complex-number algebra, and ω is the radian frequency. These relationships are basic to a.c. circuit theory. The quantities in parentheses are called *resistance* (R), *inductive reactance* $(j\omega L)$, and *capacitive reactance* $(1/j\omega C)$. Here the symbols R, L, and C have the same meaning as previously indicated. Equations (1.1) through (1.3) are expressions of Ohm's law in the phasor domain.

Each of these equations has the following form, generally known as Ohm's law:

$$V = ZI \tag{1.4}$$

where V is the phasor voltage, I the phasor current, and Z the impedance. These phasor quantities, V, I, and Z, are complex numbers containing real and imaginary parts. The impedance of a resistor in a series with a capacitor, for example, is given by

$$Z = R + \frac{1}{j\omega C}$$

expressed in rectangular form. The expression in polar form has the symbol

$$Z = |Z| \angle \theta$$

where $|Z|$ is the magnitude of the impedance and θ is the phase angle. Conversion between the rectangular form and the polar form is easily done with the aid of a hand-held scientific calculator. (It is assumed that most students have such calculators and will not have to do the conversions by hand.) An extensive listing of keystroke programs specifically written for the circuits analyzed in this text is given in Appendix A and can be used with commonly available calculators.

The impedance of a resistor, a capacitor, and an inductor connected in series is

$$Z = R + j\omega L + \frac{1}{j\omega C}$$

$$Z = R + j\left(\omega L - \frac{1}{\omega C}\right)$$

Since modern scientific programmable calculators accept and manipulate complex numbers directly, the effort required in calculations using impedance is minimal. The use of a calculator with these capabilities is strongly encouraged as an aid to performing calculations on medical instrument circuits. For example, plotting a complex impedance versus frequency is often practically impossible without a programmable calculator.

One of the most widely used and most effective techniques for troubleshooting defective equipment involves voltage measurement at test points. Comparison of measured voltages with predicted voltages may reveal discrepancies that can be used as clues to locate defective parts or components.

Troubleshooting Tip

Signal tracing may be done by measuring the voltage at a node and comparing it with the voltage calculated for it. Differences aid in locating troubles.

To predict the voltage at one point in a circuit due to a known voltage elsewhere, it is often necessary to use circuit analysis. Circuit analysis in the phasor domain is the process by which one finds a circuit variable, such as listed in Table 1.1 in terms of the network component values or variables. In a fixed network, the variables R, L, and C are often constant, while the radian frequency $\omega = 2\pi f$, where frequency, f, measured in hertz, is variable. The current through a circuit branch, or the voltage across the branch, is often computed as a function of frequency.

In Figure 1.18, each branch illustrates either a phasor source or impedance. Positive, conventional current travels in the direction of the current arrow, and the positive voltage terminal is shown by the plus (+) sign. Capacitive reactance and inductive reactance are represented by imaginary numbers.

TABLE 1.1
Phasor Domain Components and Variables

Variables (units)	Components	(units)
V (volts)	R, Resistance	(ohms)
I (amps)	$j\omega L$, Inductive reactance	(vars)
	$\dfrac{1}{j\omega C}$, Capacitive reactance	(vars)

Phasor voltages across element branches and phasor currents entering (or leaving) the nodes are governed by Kirchhoff's laws.

Kirchhoff's current law (KCL): The complex-number sum of phasor currents *entering* a node equals zero. An equivalent statement of this law is: The complex number sum of phasor currents *leaving* a node equals zero. In Figure 1.19(a), each of the currents is defined as leaving the node. KCL then implies that

$$I_1 + I_2 + I_3 + I_4 + I_5 = 0$$

Kirchhoff's voltage law (KVL): The complex-number sum of phasor voltages drops, or alternatively rises, around any closed loop of branches trav-

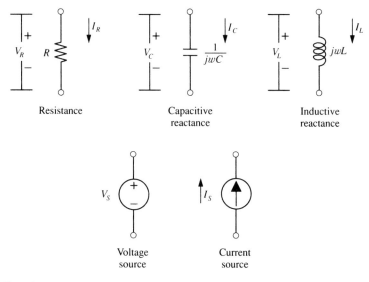

Resistance   Capacitive   Inductive
                  reactance   reactance

Voltage   Current
source   source

FIGURE 1.18
Electrical circuit components in the phasor domain.

eled in the same direction is zero. In Figure 1.19(b), applying KVL as current travels in the clockwise direction through the closed loop implies that

$$V_1 + V_2 + V_3 + V_4 + V_5 - V_S = 0$$

The plus (+) sign before V_1 through V_5 indicates that they are voltage drops. The minus (−) sign on V_S indicates that voltage rises occur as current travels through the branch going in the clockwise direction.

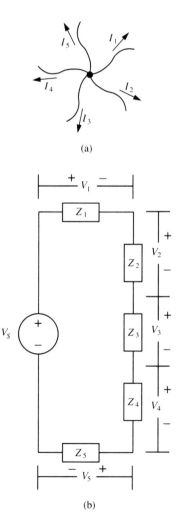

(a)

(b)

FIGURE 1.19
(a) An illustration of KCL. (b) An illustration of KVL.

EXAMPLE 1.1   Apply Kirchhoff's current law to Figure 1.20 and derive an equation for the node voltage drop V_3 from node 3 to the reference ground in terms of the given quantities V_1, V_2, I_1, I_2, and I_3.

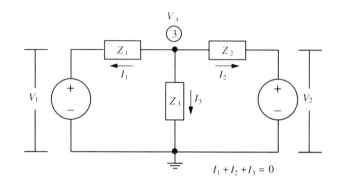

FIGURE 1.20

SOLUTION   The currents I_1, I_2, and I_3 are defined as leaving node 3. KCL then gives

$$I_1 + I_2 + I_3 = 0$$

Ohm's law applied to the branch containing Z_1 gives

$$I_1 = \frac{V_3 - V_1}{Z_1}$$

Likewise,

$$I_2 = \frac{V_3 - V_2}{Z_2}$$

and

$$I_3 = \frac{V_3 - 0}{Z_3}$$

Putting the three preceding equations into the first equation yields

$$\frac{V_3 - V_1}{Z_1} + \frac{V_3 - V_2}{Z_2} + \frac{V_3 - 0}{Z_3} = 0$$

This equation can be solved for V_3, yielding

$$V_3 = \frac{Z_1 Z_2 Z_3}{Z_1 Z_2 + Z_2 Z_3 + Z_1 Z_3} \left(\frac{V_1}{Z_1} + \frac{V_2}{Z_2} \right)$$

Each of the quantities in this equation is a complex number, which in polar form has a magnitude and a phase.

EXAMPLE 1.2   Apply Ohm's law and KCL to Figure 1.21 and obtain equations for the node voltages V_1 and V_2.

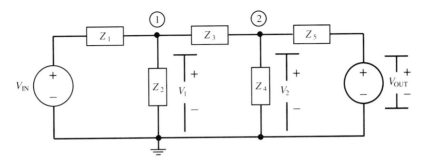

FIGURE 1.21

SOLUTION   KCL is applied to node 1 by defining three currents leaving it. In each case, Ohm's law is used to write the currents in terms of node voltage as

$$\frac{V_1 - V_{IN}}{Z_1} + \frac{V_1 - V_2}{Z_3} + \frac{V_1}{Z_2} = 0$$

A second equation is obtained by defining three different currents leaving node 2 and applying Ohm's law to each branch. KCL then gives

$$\frac{V_2 - V_1}{Z_3} + \frac{V_2}{Z_4} + \frac{V_2 - V_{OUT}}{Z_5} = 0$$

If V_{IN}, V_{OUT}, and all of the circuit impedances are known quantities, the previous two equations can be solved simultaneously to find the node voltages V_1 and V_2. This would then be sufficient information to compute all branch currents by application of Ohm's law.

Voltage Division

Ohm's law and Kirchhoff's current and voltage laws are sufficient to enable one to compute the voltages and current in any R, L, C circuit. However, it is often convenient to use the voltage division principle as derived from Figure 1.22. Applying KVL then gives

$$V_{IN} = IZ_1 + IZ_2$$

Then, Ohm's law applied to Z_2 gives

$$I = \frac{V_{OUT}}{Z_2}$$

This current substituted into the first equation yields

$$V_{IN} = V_{OUT}\left(\frac{Z_1}{Z_2} + \frac{Z_2}{Z_2}\right)$$

Solving this for V_{OUT} gives

$$V_{OUT} = \frac{Z_2}{Z_1 + Z_2}\,V_{IN} \tag{1.6}$$

Equation 1.6 is an expression of the voltage division principle for impedances connected in series. An easy way to remember this widely used formula

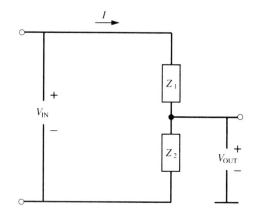

FIGURE 1.22
A voltage divider.

for voltage division is to think of the output voltage as being proportional to the load impedance over the sum of the impedances in series.

Current Division

The current division principle is derived from Figure 1.23. Here,

$$I_{IN} = \frac{V}{Z_2} + \frac{V}{Z_1}$$

and

$$V = I_{OUT} Z_1$$

Eliminating the voltage V between these two equations gives

$$I_{IN} = I_{OUT}\left(\frac{Z_1}{Z_2} + \frac{Z_1}{Z_1}\right)$$

Rearranging this gives the expression for the division of current between two impedances in parallel:

$$I_{OUT} = \frac{Z_2}{Z_1 + Z_2} I_{IN} \tag{1.7}$$

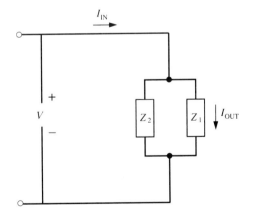

FIGURE 1.23
A current divider.

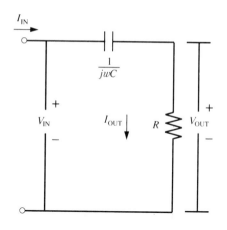

FIGURE 1.24

An easy way to remember this widely used formula is to think of the current as being proportional to the opposite over the sum of the impedances in parallel.

Gain Function Analysis

The gain functions for voltage or current are defined from Figure 1.24. The *voltage gain A_V* equals the ratio of output voltage V_{OUT} to input voltage V_{IN} computed as a function of R's, L's, C's, and frequency f:

$$A_V = \frac{V_{\text{OUT}}}{V_{\text{IN}}}$$

Likewise, the *current gain A_I* is defined as the ratio of the output current to the input current, or

$$A_I = \frac{I_{\text{OUT}}}{I_{\text{IN}}}$$

Calculation of either gain function, A_V or A_I, is accomplished by application of Kirchhoff's laws and Ohm's law to the circuit network.

EXAMPLE 1.3 Compute the voltage gain function A_V for the circuit of Figure 1.24 as a function of frequency f. Consider R, L, and C values to be given numbers.

SOLUTION Applying the voltage division principle to Figure 1.24 yields

$$V_{OUT} = \frac{R}{R + \dfrac{1}{j\omega C}} V_{IN}$$

Therefore,

$$A_V = \frac{V_{OUT}}{V_{IN}} = \frac{R}{R + \dfrac{1}{j\omega C}}$$

or

$$A_V = \frac{1}{1 - j\,\dfrac{1}{2\pi f R C}} \qquad \text{(1.8)}$$

It is clear that A_V is a function of f, R, and C alone.

EXAMPLE 1.4 Take the values $C = 1\ \mu F$ and $R = 100\ k\Omega$ and plot A_V versus frequency.

SOLUTION Putting these values in Equation (1.8) yields

$$A_V = \frac{1}{1 - j\,\dfrac{1}{2\pi f(10^{-6})(10^5)}}$$

$$= \frac{1}{1 - j\,\dfrac{1.59}{f}}$$

Putting this in polar form, we have

$$A_V = \frac{1}{\sqrt{1 + \left[\dfrac{1.59}{f}\right]^2}}\ \angle\theta$$

where $\theta = \tan^{-1}(1.59/f)$. Thus, the magnitude $|A_V|$ and angle θ may be computed to form the plot in Figure 1.25.

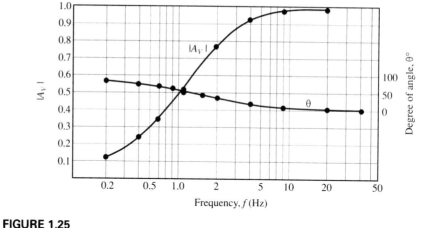

FIGURE 1.25
The calculation for Example 1.4.

BJT Equivalent Circuit

In addition to R, L, and C elements, electronic circuits contain various *pn-junction* semiconductor devices, including semiconductor diodes, bipolar junction transistors (BJTs), and integrated circuits. For use in electronic circuit analysis, the BJT can be represented as an equivalent circuit, consisting of R, L, and C elements and an ideal current or voltage source.

Bipolar junction transistors consist of three layers of semiconductor material doped with impurities that make them either *p*-type or *n*-type. The circuit symbols for the BJT (Figure 1.26) represent two types: the *PNP* and the *NPN* transistors. In Figure 1.26(a), I_B is the base current entering the base node B, I_C is the collector current entering the collector node C, and I_E is the emitter current leaving the emitter node E of the *NPN* transistor.

The characteristics of the transistor are described by the collector-to-emitter voltage, V_{CE} versus I_C. The curve plotting this voltage is shown in Figure 1.27. Each of the family of curves is measured at a different value of base current: I_B, labeled I_{B0}, I_{B1}, I_{B2}, and so on. In d.c. analysis of the transistor element, an important parameter usually specified by the manufacturer is the d.c. current gain, β_{dc}, defined as

$$\beta_{dc} = \frac{I_C}{I_B} \qquad (1.9)$$

Applying Kirchhoff's current law to Figure 1.26(a) yields

$$I_E = I_C + I_B$$

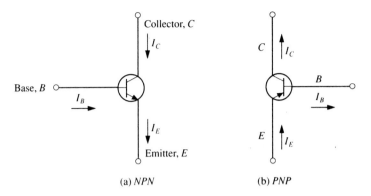

(a) *NPN*   (b) *PNP*

FIGURE 1.26
(a) *NPN* and (b) *PNP* transistor circuit symbols.

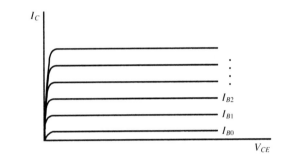

FIGURE 1.27
The voltage-current characteristics of a BJT.

Combining these equations yields

$$I_E = (1 + \beta_{dc})I_B$$

Furthermore, when $\beta_{dc} \gg 1$, we have

$$I_E \approx \beta_{dc}I_B = I_C \tag{1.10}$$

Since the transistor is designed as a current gain device, the approximation $\beta_{dc} \gg 1$ often holds.

Because of the principle of superposition in electronic circuit theory, the analysis of the circuit due to the d.c. bias supply can be done separately from the analysis resulting from a.c. signal voltage. The a.c. analysis is per-

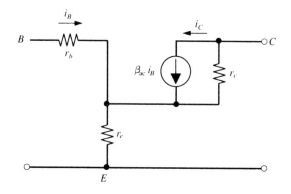

FIGURE 1.28
A small signal a.c. equivalent circuit of a BJT.

formed using the small a.c. signal equivalent circuit given in Figure 1.28. In Figure 1.28 the equivalent circuit parameters are defined as follows:

$\beta_{ac} = i_C/i_B$ is the a.c. current gain
r_e is the emitter resistance to a.c. currents
r_b is the base resistance to a.c. currents
r_c is the collector resistance to a.c. currents.

The lowercase "r" is used to indicate an a.c. equivalent circuit element. Capital "R" designates the values of resistors in this text.

REFERENCES

Bronzino, J. D. *Biomedical Engineering and Instrumentation.* Boston: Prindle, Weber & Schmidt, 1986.

Reiser, Stanley Joel. *Medicine and the Reign of Technology.* Cambridge, UK: Cambridge University Press, 1978.

Washburn, Sherwood. "Tools and Human Evolution." In *Scientific Technology & Social Change*, edited by G. I. Rochlin. San Francisco: W. H. Freeman, 1974.

EXERCISES

1. Name an early investigator or inventor of the following instruments, and give the approximate date of introduction according to the text.
   pH electrode
   Stethoscope

d.c. defibrillator
Balloon-tipped catheter
Implantable pacemaker
Electrocardiograph
Thermometer
Continuous hemodialysis
Mercury thermometer
Ophthalmoscope
Binaural stethoscope
Haemacytometer
Electroencephalograph
Artificial heart
Artificial radionuclides

2. List the important devices that advanced the art of internal imaging of human organs.

3. Name an early medical device that extended each of the senses of a diagnosing physician.

4. Draw a block diagram that represents a general monitor for human physiological parameters.

5. Draw a block diagram that represents a therapeutic medical instrument.

6. Make a chronological chart depicting the development of major medical instruments from the earliest times to the present.

7. In Example 1.1, fill in the details in the derivation of the equation for V_3 in terms of V_1, V_2, Z_1, Z_2, and Z_3.

8. In Figure 1.21, let $V_{IN} = 3$, $V_{OUT} = 2$, $Z_1 = 1$, $Z_2 = 2$, $Z_3 = 2$, $Z_4 = 3$, and $Z_5 = 2$, and calculate the voltages V_1 and V_2.

9. In Figure 1.23, $Z_1 = 5$, $Z_2 = 3$, and $V = 6$. Compute I_{IN} and I_{OUT}.

10. In Figure 1.23, $Z_1 = 1 + j3$, $Z_2 = 2 + j1$, and $V = 5 \angle 0°$. Compute I_{IN} and I_{OUT}.

11. In Figure 1.24 the frequency $f = 60$ Hz, the capacitance $C = 200$ μF, and the resistance $R = 20$ Ω. If $V_{IN} = 20 \angle 0°$ V, find the magnitude and phase of V_{OUT}.

12. In Figure 1.22, $Z_1 = 5$, $Z_2 = 3$, and $V_{IN} = 6$ V. Compute V_{OUT}.

13. In Figure 1.22, the component producing Z_1 is a 20-Ω resistor. The component producing Z_2 is a 200-μF capacitor. $V_{IN} = 20 \angle 0°$ V, and frequency $f = 60$ Hz. Find the magnitude and phase of V_{OUT}.

2 The Origin of Biopotentials, Electrocardiograms, and Electrical Shock

The *biopotential* was scientifically investigated as early as 1786 by Luigi Galvani, an Italian physiologist and physicist. His studies led to the invention of the voltaic cell by another Italian physicist, Count Alessandro Volta. The process in the body that produces biopotentials is very similar to the process that produces the voltage in a conventional battery; hence the following definition: A biopotential is an electrical voltage caused by a current flow of ions through biological tissue.

The study of biopotentials is fundamental to the understanding of medical instrumentation. Several of the major types of equipment, including electrocardiographs and electroencephalographs, measure biopotentials from the surface of the body. Physicians use the data obtained from these instruments to assess the health of their patients. Patients having biopotentials monitored are shown in Figure 2.1.

All professionals who work with medical instrumentation must understand the safety hazards associated with biopotentials. The primary hazard is electrical shock. Certain occurrences, called microshock, can cause a fatality at current levels as low as 20 microamps (μA). Corresponding dangerous voltages are on the order of millivolts (mV).

2.1 FUNDAMENTAL LAWS FOR CURRENT IN BIOLOGICAL TISSUE

The single cell is the unit from which living systems are built. Its complexity is illustrated by the fact that within its membrane hundreds of chemical reactions take place, many of which are not understood. You can observe a

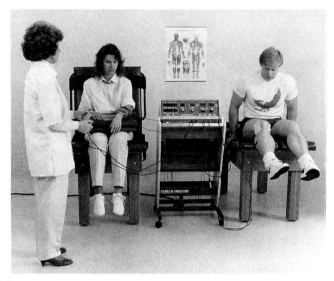

FIGURE 2.1
Patients connected to instrumentation through biopotential electrodes. (Courtesy of Cybex, a division of Lumex, Inc.)

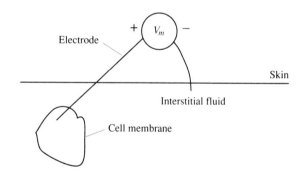

FIGURE 2.2
A circuit for measuring cell membrane potential.

membrane potential, V_m, in living cells by inserting a microtip wire or conductor-filled glass electrode into a cell, as shown in Figure 2.2. The value of V_m measured is usually about -90 mV.

The potential appearing across the cell membrane is the basis for the biopotentials measured on the body, including the electrocardiogram (ECG), electroencephalogram (EEG), electrooculogram, electroretinogram, and electromyogram (EMG). Notice here that the suffix "gram," as in electrocardiogram, designates the potential itself, whereas the suffix "graph," as in electrocardiograph, designates the instrument that measures or records the potential.

Whereas the particle producing electrical events in passive circuits is the free electron, the particle producing electrical events in biological tissue is the ion in an electrolyte solution. The rules governing these ionic events are (1) Fick's law for diffusion, (2) the drift equation, and (3) the Einstein relation.

Fick's Law

Fick's law for diffusion states that if there is a high concentration $[C]$ of particles in one region that are free to move, they will flow in a direction to equalize the concentration $[C]$ throughout the region. Fick's law for diffusion holds for the diffusion of perfume molecules throughout a room, electrons in a doped semiconductor, or ions in an electrolyte. In one dimension, Fick's law is expressed as

$$J = -D \frac{d[C]}{dx} \tag{2.1}$$

for positive ions. The minus sign is dropped for negative ions. The current density, J, expressed in amperes per unit area, is caused by the concentration gradient. As illustrated in Figure 2.3, $[C]$ is the concentration of ions as a function of the distance, x, in units of moles per liter (mol/liter). (Recall that a mole is an amount of the substance in grams equal to the sum of the atomic weights of its constituent atoms.) D is the diffusion constant, x is the position, and $[C]$ is a positive number.

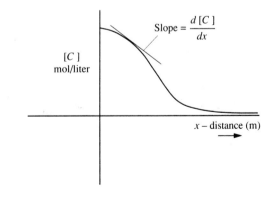

FIGURE 2.3
An ionic concentration as a function of position.

In Figure 2.3 the slope $d[C]$ for $x > 0$ is negative; the ionic current flow is in the positive x direction, as indicated in Equation (2.1). A typical system of units is: $[C]$ in moles per liter (mol/liter); x, meters (m); J, amperes per meter squared (A/m^2); and D, liter amperes per mole meter [(liter $\cdot$ A)/(mol $\cdot$ m)].

Particle Drift

In addition to the diffusion force acting on ions, there is a force due to electric fields acting as well. Charged particles such as ions in an electric field will move under the forces of electrical attraction and repulsion. The resulting ionic flow is called the *drift current*. Drift current is proportional to the voltage drop, V, the ion valence, Z, and the concentration, $[C]$. Z is equal to the number of charges on the ion. The proportionality constant is called the mobility, μ. That is, the current density due to particle drift is given by

$$J_{\text{drift}} = -\mu Z \frac{dV}{dx} [C] \qquad (2.2)$$

where μ is the mobility expressed in liter amperes per volt meter mole [(liter $\cdot$ A)/(V $\cdot$ m $\cdot$ mol)]; Z is valence; $E = -dV/dx$ is the electric field intensity in volts per meter (V/m); and $[C]$ is the concentration of ions taken as a positive number in moles per liter (mol/liter). The two physical constants, mobility μ and the diffusion coefficient D, are related to each other by the *Einstein relationship* usually derived in the theory of solid-state *pn*-junction diodes. (See Sze, 1981.) The Einstein relationship is

$$\frac{D}{\mu} = \frac{kT}{q} \qquad (2.3)$$

where k is Boltzmann's constant, q is the charge, and T is the absolute temperature.

Equations (2.1) through (2.3) can be used to derive the membrane potential in biological cells. (See Bahill, 1981.) The following verbal description based on a physical interpretation of Fick's law, the drift equation, and the Einstein relationship will help to explain how the biopotential arises and how it differs from other voltage-producing processes. It will also help to explain biopotential electrodes used in medical instrumentation.

Single-Cell Membrane Potential

The way in which the diffusion and drift processes give rise to a membrane potential is illustrated in Figure 2.4. Here we see the hypothetical case of

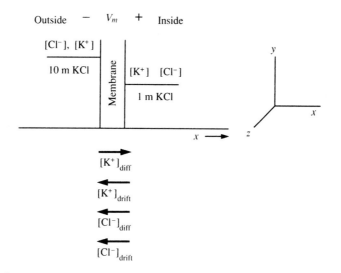

FIGURE 2.4
Ionic currents due to drift and diffusion forces.

a 10-molar potassium chloride (KCl) solution outside a membrane and a 1-molar solution inside.

The x-y plane is shown. The y-z plane is perpendicular to the paper. The membrane separating the two KCl solutions is in the y-z plane. A high concentration of ions of $[K^+]$ and $[Cl^-]$ appears on the outside of the cell, while a low concentration appears on the inside. This means that the slope of the ionic concentrations is negative, since in both cases the concentration decreases as x increases. According to Fick's law, the negative chlorine ions $[Cl^-]$ flow from outside to inside, causing a diffusion current flowing to the left, as shown by the arrow in the figure; the arrow points in the direction of conventional positive-charge current flow. Likewise, the positive potassium ions $[K^+]$ diffuse from outside to inside, causing a conventional diffusion current flowing to the right, shown by the arrow pointing right in the figure. These positive ions collect on the inside of the membrane, thereby causing a voltage that is positive on the right and negative on the left. This voltage has a positive slope; it increases as x increases. In accordance with the drift equation, this voltage produces drift currents. The positive voltage repels the positive $[K^+]$ ions, causing a drift current indicated by the arrow pointing left, labeled $[K^+]_{drift}$. This voltage also attracts negative $[Cl^-]$ ions, moving them to the right across the membrane, producing a conventional current to the left, as indicated by the arrow pointing left, labeled $[Cl^-]_{drift}$. V_m, in this case, is assumed positive in the direction indicated in the figure. If V_m were predominantly determined by the negative ions in the electrolyte, it would be a negative number.

At equilibrium, which is the condition of a cell membrane at rest, the total current across the membrane must be zero. Otherwise the regions, no matter how large, would eventually fill, since ions are matter. Therefore, the total current is zero. That is,

$$J_{K(drift)} + J_{K(diff)} + J_{Cl(drift)} + J_{Cl(diff)} = 0$$

This condition leads to Goldman's equation, stated here as

$$V_m = -\frac{kT}{q} \ln\left(\frac{P_K[K^+]_i + P_{Cl}[Cl^-]_o}{P_K[K^+]_o + P_{Cl}[Cl^-]_i}\right)$$

where the subscript i indicates inside the cell, o designates outside, and

$$
\begin{aligned}
k &= \text{Boltzmann's constant} \\
T &= \text{absolute temperature (K)} \\
q &= \text{the charge on a proton} \\
P_K &= \text{the permeability of potassium} \\
P_{Cl} &= \text{the permeability of chlorine} \\
[K^+] &= \text{the concentration of potassium ions} \\
[Cl^-] &= \text{the concentration of chlorine ions}
\end{aligned}
$$

Permeability is a measure of the ease with which ions pass through the cell membrane.

Resting Potential in a Cell

In a similar argument, we can extend the preceding equation for three ions as follows:

$$V_m = -\frac{kT}{q} \ln\left(\frac{P_K[K^+]_i + P_{Na}[Na^+]_i + P_{Cl}[Cl^-]_o}{P_K[K^+]_o + P_{Na}[Na^+]_o + P_{Cl}[Cl^-]_i}\right) \tag{2.4}$$

Goldman's equation specifies the cell membrane voltage for actual concentrations of potassium, chlorine, and sodium. It shows that membrane potential depends strongly on temperature. Since the permeabilities of different cell types vary, the corresponding membrane potentials vary as well. This relationship is the basis for understanding many aspects of transducer behavior, including surface electrodes, discussed in Chapter 4. It also explains the behavior of chemical electrodes used in clinical instrumentation.

In a living cell, when the approximations $P_{Na} \approx 0$ and $P_{Cl} \approx 0$ hold, Goldman's equation reduces to a simple form as

$$V_m = -\frac{kT}{q} \ln\left(\frac{[K^+]_i}{[K^+]_o}\right) \qquad (2.5)$$

This is called the *Nernst equation*, and it is often valid as an approximation to the Goldman equation. A direct derivation of the Nernst equation from the basic laws governing biopotentials is given as Exercise 12.

EXAMPLE 2.1 Suppose a frog skeletal muscle has the following ion concentrations and permeabilities of the membrane:

Ion	Inside (mmol/liter)	Outside (mmol/liter)	Permeability (cm/s)
Na^+	11	146	1.9×10^{-8}
K^+	150	4.35	2.1×10^{-6}
Cl^-	5	125	3.9×10^{-6}

Compute the membrane voltage from inside to outside the cell at 37 °C (310 K).

SOLUTION Boltzmann's constant $k = 1.38 \times 10^{-23}$ J/K
An electronic charge $q = 1.602 \times 10^{-19}$ C
The temperature $T = 310$ K

Then

$$V_m = -0.0267 \ln\left(\frac{2.1(10^{-6})(150) + 3.9(10^{-6})(125) + 1.9(10^{-8})(11)}{2.1(10^{-6})(4.35) + 1.9(10^{-8})(146) + 3.9(10^{-6})(5)}\right)$$

$$= -86.5 \text{ mV}$$

Considering potassium, $[K^+]$ in this equation yields

$$V_m = -0.0267 \ln\left(\frac{[K^+]_i}{[K^+]_o}\right)$$

$$= -0.0267 \ln\left(\frac{150}{4.35}\right) = -94.5 \text{ mV}$$

These two results verify the idea that the resting potential in a cell is caused primarily by potassium flow. We see that if potassium is considered alone, the result is −94.5 mV, whereas if we also take into account Cl and Na, the result is −86.5 mV. The accuracy is improved by 9.2% when all ions are accounted for. Under certain circumstances, the approximation given by the Nernst equation is better than this.

Action Potential and Muscle Contraction

Living cells are encased in a high-resistance membrane, which, at rest, has a potential caused by the flow of sodium and chlorine ions into the cell and potassium ions out of it. The resting potential, V_m, as computed by the Goldman equation (Equation 2.4) normally has values between −50 mV and −100 mV. If the potential is raised across the membrane by about 20%, then a stimulus threshold is exceeded and the cell membrane resistance changes, causing a change in the membrane potential. This new membrane potential, called the action potential, is shown in Figure 2.5. As long as the action potential exists, the cell is said to be *depolarized*. In a tissue, the depolarization disturbance of one cell is propagated to the next until the entire tissue depolarizes. In muscle, where cells are situated in an orderly ar-

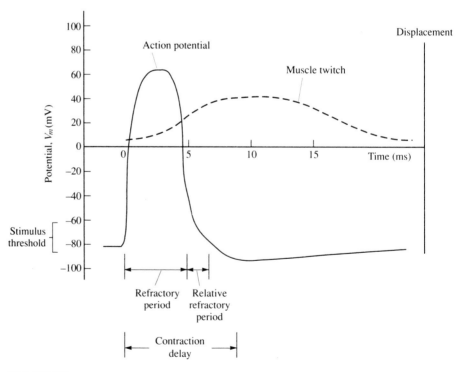

FIGURE 2.5
The relationship between the action potential and muscle contraction.

rangement, the tissue contracts and becomes shorter in length after some delay following a depolarization. A typical delay of 10 ms between the action potential depolarization and the subsequent muscle twitch is indicated in the figure. A stimulus voltage generally does not affect a cell while it is changing its polarization. The *refractory period* is the time duration of cell nonresponse to further stimuli. During the *relative refractory period*, a higher stimulus is required to reinitiate an action potential and the subsequent contraction of muscle.

2.2 BIOPOTENTIALS IN THE HEART

The electrical activity of the heart is integral to the operation of several types of medical instruments, including the electrocardiograph, the pacemaker, and the defibrillator. Very small electrical disturbances can cause this vital organ to cease pumping blood necessary to sustain life.

The heart consists of two major smooth muscles, the atrium and the ventricle, which form a syncytium, or fusion of cells, that conducts depolarization from one cell to an adjacent cell. Because of ionic leakage in the smooth muscle membrane, the tissue of the heart depolarizes spontaneously from its resting state, and effectively oscillates, or beats. The sinoatrial (SA) node beats at a rate of from 70 to 80 beats per minute (bpm) at rest; the atrioventricular (AV) node beats at 40 to 60 bpm, and the bundle branch oscillates at 15 to 40 bpm.

The SA node normally determines the heart rate, since it beats at the fastest rate and causes stimulation of the other tissue before it reaches its self-pacing threshold. Thus, the SA node can be considered the heart's pacemaker. The path of the depolarization of cells in a heart is illustrated in Figure 2.6.

The depolarization of the SA node spreads throughout the atrium and reaches the AV node in about 40 ms. Because of the low conduction velocity of the AV node tissue, it requires about 110 ms for the depolarization to reach the bundle branches pointed out in the figure, called the *Purkinje system*. The ventricles then contract, the right ventricle forcing blood into the lungs, the left ventricle pushing blood into the aorta and subsequently through the circulation system. The contraction period of the heart is called *systole*.

The action potentials in the ventricle hold for 200 to 250 ms. This relatively long time allows the ventricular contraction to empty blood into the arteries. The heart then repolarizes during a rest period, called *diastole*. Then the cycle repeats.

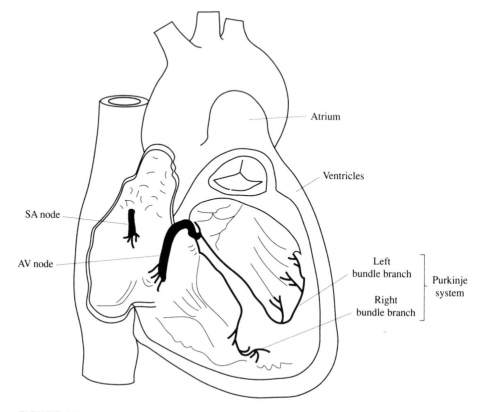

FIGURE 2.6
The depolarization path through the heart.

2.3 THE ELECTROCARDIOGRAM

During *diastole*, while the heart is at rest, all of the cells are polarized so that the potential inside each cell is negative with respect to the outside. Normally, depolarization occurs first at the SA node, making the outside of the tissue negative with respect to the inside of the cells, and also making it negative with respect to the tissue not yet depolarized. This imbalance results in an ionic current, *I*, causing the left arm (LA) to measure positive with respect to the right arm (RA), as illustrated in Figure 2.7(a). The resulting voltage is called the *P-wave*.

After about 90 ms, the atrium is completely depolarized, and the ionic current measured by lead *I* reduces to zero. The depolarization then passes through the atrioventricular node, causing a delay of about 110 ms. The

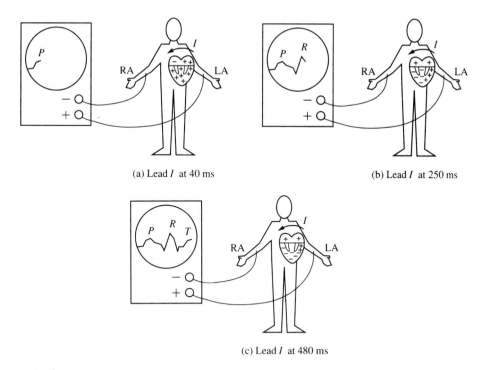

(a) Lead *I* at 40 ms

(b) Lead *I* at 250 ms

(c) Lead *I* at 480 ms

FIGURE 2.7
Ionic currents as the source of an electrocardiogram.

depolarization then passes into the right ventricular muscle, depolarizing it and making it negative relative to the still-polarized left ventricular muscle, as illustrated in Figure 2.7(b). Again, the direction of *I* causes a plus-to-minus voltage from LA to RA called the *R-wave.*

The complete waveform in Figure 2.8 is called an *electrocardiogram* (ECG), with labels *P, Q, R, S,* and *T* indicating its distinctive features. The *P*-wave arises from depolarization of the atrium. The *QRS* complex arises from depolarization of the ventricles. The magnitude of the *R*-wave within this complex is approximately 1 mV. The *T*-wave (Figure 2.7c) arises from repolarization of the ventricle muscle. During the *T*-wave, partial repolarization of the cardiac muscle causes ionic currents, and a corresponding ECG potential, as previously described for the *R*-wave. The *U*-wave that sometimes follows the *T*-wave is a second-order effect of uncertain origin and is of little diagnostic significance. The intervals, segments, and complexes of the ECG are defined in Figure 2.8. Typical durations are as follows:

Feature	Duration (ms)
QRS complex	70 to 110
R-R interval	600 to 1000
P-R interval	150 to 200
S-T interval	320

The *QRS* duration, *P-R* interval, and *S-T* interval depend on the depolarization rate of the heart and are relatively constant for an individual, regard-

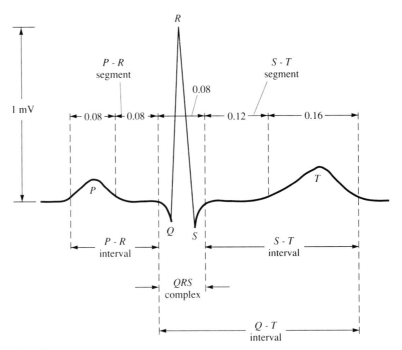

Intervals:
P - R   Beginning of *P*-wave to beginning of *QRS* complex.
S - T   End of *S*-wave to end of *T*-wave.
Q - T   Beginning of *Q*-wave to end of *T*-wave.

Segments:
P - R   End of *P*-wave to beginning of *Q*-wave.
S - T   End of *S*-wave to beginning of *T*-wave.

Complex:
QRS   Beginning of *Q*-wave to end of *S*-wave.

Durations:
Average durations shown on drawing, in seconds.

FIGURE 2.8
ECG definitions. (Courtesy Hewlett-Packard Company)

less of his or her exercise level. The ranges above reflect individual differences in a normal population.

2.4 ELECTRICAL SHOCK

An understanding of electrical shock is important to everyone working with and around electrical equipment. Patients and hospital equipment users are especially susceptible to shock because they must make physical contact with the hardware. The physiological effects of shock range from discomfort to injury to death, if the heart or respiratory system is affected. An *electrical shock* is an unwanted or unnecessary physiological response to current. Electrical shock may cause an unwanted cellular depolarization and its associated muscular contraction, or it may cause cell vaporization and tissue injury. A cell is depolarized when the membrane potential is changed by approximately 20%. The question is, how much current is required to create this threshold?

To conveniently estimate the stimulus current in a cell, a spherical model (Figure 2.9a) may be used. The cell membrane is modeled as a dielectric with dielectric constant ϵ,

$$\epsilon = \epsilon_0 \epsilon_r$$

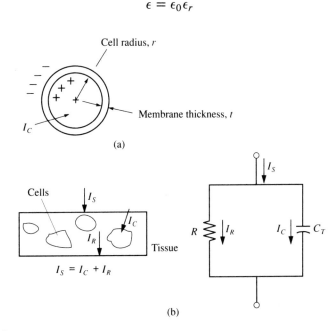

(a)

(b)

FIGURE 2.9
A cell model illustrating high-frequency effects on cell membrane current.

The capacitance of the sphere enclosed by the membrane is given by

$$C = \epsilon \frac{\text{Area}}{t} = \epsilon_0 \epsilon_r \frac{4\pi r^2}{t} \tag{2.7}$$

where $\epsilon_0 = 8.85 \times 10^{-12}$ F/m, ϵ_r is the relative dielectric constant, t is the membrane thickness, and r is the radius. The stimulus current I_C entering the cell to initiate the action potential is given by

$$I_C = \frac{V_{mt}}{Z} \approx V_{mt}(j2\pi fC) \tag{2.8}$$

where V_{mt} is the threshold potential required to depolarize the cell. This approximation holds for frequencies, f, sufficiently high for the current I_S to be considered steady state, and allows us to calculate the high-frequency effects.

EXAMPLE 2.2   A cell membrane has a thickness t of 0.1 μm and a radius r of 10 μm. Assuming a relative dielectric constant ϵ_r of 2, compute the cell capacity C.

SOLUTION

$$C = 2(8.85 \times 10^{-12})4(10 \times 10^{-6})^2\pi/(0.1 \times 10^{-6})$$

$$= 0.222 \text{ pF}$$

A model of tissue may be regarded as a set of cells in an interstitial fluid. The fluid is a conducting electrolyte, as shown in Figure 2.9(b), where I_S is the total stimulus current into the tissue, I_R is the component through the interstitial fluid, and I_C is the sum of all currents entering the cells in the tissue.

EXAMPLE 2.3   A tissue 1 cm^2 in area contains 450×10^6 cells with characteristics as described in Example 2.2. The conductance of the interstitial fluid is 1 siemens (mho) per square centimeter ($\mho$/cm^2). Make an equivalent circuit for this tissue.

SOLUTION   The total capacitance, C_T, is the sum of the capacitances of each cell from Example 2.2. These capacitances are added because the reference is taken as the inside of the cell. Thus,

$$C_T = (450 \times 10^6)(0.22 \times 10^{-12})$$

$$= 100 \text{ } \mu\text{F/cm}^2$$

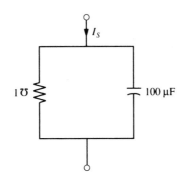

FIGURE 2.10
An equivalent circuit of tissue passing high-frequency current.

and the equivalent circuit is as illustrated in Figure 2.10. Notice that if the area doubles, the conductance also doubles.

From this tissue model, we can also estimate the current levels necessary to produce an electrically induced muscle contraction. From Figure 2.10, the stimulus threshold may be estimated at 20 mV. We can then use Equation (2.8) to estimate the stimulus current.

EXAMPLE 2.4 If the stimulus for an action potential in the individual cells of the tissue in Example 2.3 is 20 mV, compute the stimulus current necessary to depolarize all of the cells simultaneously at a frequency of 60 Hz. The syncytium of these cells may, for example, represent a muscle.

SOLUTION

$$I_S = (20/Z_T)(10^{-3})$$

and, from Figure 2.10, the tissue impedance Z_T is

$$Z_T = 1/[1 + j2\pi(60)(10^{-4})]$$

Therefore,

$$|I_S| = |(20 \times 10^{-3})[1 + j2\pi(60)(10^{-4})]| = 20 \text{ mA}$$

In this case a 20-mA current would cause an involuntary contraction of the muscle. This is consistent with let-go current given in the safety tips in Box 1, which lists the effects of arm-to-arm currents, applied as shown in Figure 2.11. These are 60-Hz currents entering one hand and traveling through

 University of Ulster LIBRARY

Box 1

SAFETY TIPS

Electrical currents passing through surface electrodes from one arm to the other have serious physiological consequences. At 60 Hz, such currents above 5 mA are considered dangerous. Specific physiological effects are listed in the following table:

Type of current	Current range (mA)	Physiological effect
Threshold	1–5	Tingling sensation
Pain	5–8	Intense or painful sensation
Let-go	8–20	Threshold of involuntary muscle contraction
Paralysis	>20	Respiratory paralysis and pain
Fibrillation	80–1000	Ventricular and heart fibrillation
Defibrillation	1000–10,000	Sustained myocardial contraction and possible tissue burns

---

the vital organs of heart, respiration control center, and brain. Similar effects would occur if the current passed from the right or left arm to a foot, from the hand to the head, and from the head to a foot. In each case, currents could pass through the vital organs of respiration and the heart. Such currents, however, traveling from the bicep brachii to a hand or between

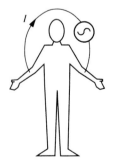

FIGURE 2.11
Current passed from arm to arm, described in Box 1.

two abdominal points, for example, would not cause the life-threatening effects of respiratory paralysis or heart failure, provided that the currents did not pass through these vital organs.

In general, the physiological effects of current on the body for several seconds range from a tingling sensation at 1 to 5 mA applied to the surface, to tissue injury due to burns when more than 1 A is applied. A surface current above 5 mA is considered dangerous because it may cause pain or injury (see Box 1). Let-go current (8 to 20 mA) causes involuntary muscle contractions. It may, for example, prevent a person receiving such a current from releasing himself or herself from the source of shock. At 20 mA, widespread muscle contraction in the respiratory system and interference with respiratory control signals from the brain could prevent breathing, and would lead to death if sustained. Above 80 mA, currents reach parts of the heart and cause ectopic beats to occur. If this happens at several sites on the heart simultaneously, the heart may begin to fibrillate. The SA node then loses control of the pacing so that the heart continues to flutter without pumping blood. The fluttering will continue until therapeutic action is taken to reverse it. One method of reversing it, called defibrillation, requires the application of a current exceeding 1 A across the thorax. This causes simultaneous contraction of all of the heart muscle. When the current is removed, the SA node is able to regain control and pace the heart normally. (Defibrillation is covered in greater detail in Chapter 8.)

In summary, it is clear that currents above 5 mA should be considered hazardous. Currents above 20 mA passing through a vital organ can be fatal. The electrical effects listed in the safety tip box are called *macroshocks* because they are distributed over large areas. The thresholds listed are for current durations greater than 1 s. If the shock duration is reduced to 0.1 s, the fibrillation threshold increases ten times. This fact is used to design circuit interrupters to prevent injuries due to shock.

High-Frequency Effects

Although most electrical currents that might contact a patient are of low frequency (around 60 Hz), the effects of high frequencies cannot be ignored. Since electrosurgical scalpels operate at frequencies in the order of 500 kHz, the question arises as to whether a muscle contraction or heart fibrillation might be stimulated by a scalpel.

As frequency is increased in a conductor, the current tends to flow near the surface. This is called the *skin effect*. Compared with the effects of currents flowing within the human body, the skin effect does not seem important. On the other hand, the 500-kHz current generated by an electrosurgical unit (ESU) flows strongly in the core of the body.

We can look to the model of tissue in Figure 2.9 for one of the more important reasons why currents cause less muscle contraction at ESU frequencies, and so are less dangerous. The let-go current as a function of frequency is plotted in Figure 2.12, indicating that it increases at high frequency. Example 2.5 interprets the data in Figure 2.12 by showing that the current needed to create the threshold for the action potential on the cells increases according to the computed value in the figure.

EXAMPLE 2.5   Extend the calculation in Example 2.4 and compute I_S as a function of frequency.

SOLUTION

$$I_S = 0.020 \; (1 + j \, 2\pi f \times 10^{-4})$$

$$= 0.020 + j \, 1.26 \times 10^{-5} \; \text{f}$$

A calculation of I_S versus frequency is plotted as computed data in Figure 2.12. For example, a frequency of 500 kHz produces $I_S = 6.3$ A. The

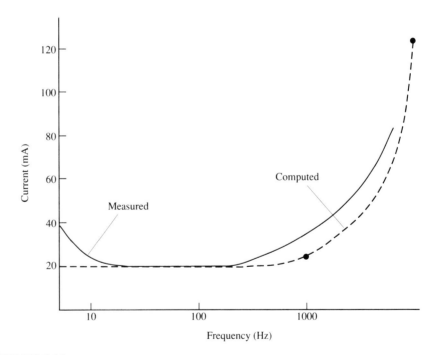

FIGURE 2.12
An example let-go current measured from arm to arm as a function of frequency compared with Example 2.5 calculations.

conclusion from this calculation is that at 500 kHz it is necessary to drive 6.3 A into the tissue in order to reach the threshold for an action potential. Such high currents cause the cells to vaporize rather than depolarize. Therefore, the muscle would not contract at these current levels, and electric shock manifested as muscle contractions or heart fibrillations would not occur. Thus, we would not expect an ESU to produce shock in patients from currents intended for surgical cutting. Any shock hazard would come from stray currents at low frequency. ESUs are designed to eliminate such low-frequency currents.

Microshock and Macroshock

The electrical shock situations we have just described are called macroshock. A much subtler electrical shock situation (one that may sometimes be more dangerous because it is difficult to detect) is *microshock*. The two situations differ as indicated in the following definitions:

> *Macroshock.* A physiological response to a current applied to the surface of the *body* that produces unwanted or unnecessary stimulation, muscle contractions, or tissue injury.
>
> *Microshock.* A physiological response to a current applied to the surface of the *heart* that results in unwanted stimulation, muscle contractions, or tissue injury.

Microshock is most often caused when currents in excess of 10 μA flow through an insulated catheter to the heart, as illustrated in Figure 2.13. The catheter may be an insulated, conductive-fluid–filled tube, or a solid-wire pacemaker cable as illustrated in Figure 2.13(a). The microshock results be-

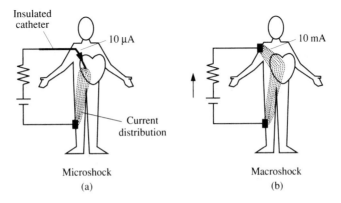

FIGURE 2.13
The current density accompanying microshock versus that accompanying macroshock.

cause the current density at the heart can become high in the situation depicted there, in which the catheter is touching the heart. To produce macroshock, much larger current is required, because the current distributes itself throughout the body, as shown in Figure 2.13(b). Obviously, the current density at the heart is much lower in this case, and more current is required to cause a shock. This accounts for the thousand-to-one ratio of macroshock current to microshock current levels.

REFERENCES

Bahill, A. T. *Bioengineering: Biomedical, Medical and Clinical Engineering*. Englewood Cliffs, NJ: Prentice-Hall, 1981.

Carr, J. J., and Brown, J. M. "The Heart and Circulatory System." Chapter 2 in *Introduction to Biomedical Equipment Technology*. New York: John Wiley & Sons, 1981.

Clark, J. W. "The Origin of Biopotentials." Chapter 4 in *Medical Instrumentation, Applications and Design*, edited by J. G. Webster. Boston: Houghton Mifflin, 1978.

Dalziel, C. F. "Electrical Shock." In *Advances in Biomedical Engineering*, Vol. 3, edited by J. H. V. Brown and J. F. Dickson. New York: Academic Press, 1973.

Guyton, A. C. "The Heart." Part III of *Textbook of Medical Physiology*. 3rd ed. Philadelphia: W. B. Saunders, 1966.

Sze, S. M. *Physics of Semiconductors*. 2nd ed. New York: John Wiley & Sons, 1981.

EXERCISES

1. Show that the units $[C]$ in moles per liter, x in meters, J in amperes per meter squared, and D in liter amperes per mole meter $[(\text{liter} \cdot A)/(\text{mol} \cdot m)]$ are a consistent set of units.

2. In Figure 2.4 the charge on the ions is negative. In what direction does the corresponding diffusion current, taken in a conventional sense, flow?

3. Show that the units given for Equation (2.2) form a consistent set.

4. In Figure 2.4, the concentration of potassium outside the cell is lower than inside the cell. No other ions are present.
   (a) What is the direction of the diffusion current?
   (b) What is the direction of the drift current?
   (c) What is the polarity of the membrane potential relative to the direction defined in the figure?

5. In Figure 2.4 there is a lower concentration of chlorine outside the cell than inside. No other ions are present. The positive terminal of a voltmeter is connected by means of a microelectrode inside the cell; the negative terminal is placed in the interstitial fluid.

(a) What is the polarity of the voltage on the voltmeter?

(b) What is the direction of the diffusion current?

(c) What is the direction of the drift current?

6. A red blood cell has the following ionic concentrations: inside, $[Na^+] = 19$, $[K^+] = 136$, and $[Cl^-] = 78$ mmol/liter; outside, $[Na^+] = 155$, $[K^+] = 5$, $[Cl^-] = 112$ mmol/liter. The permeability for $[Na^+]$ is 2×10^{-8}, $[K^+]$ is 2×10^{-6}, and $[Cl^-]$ is 3.9×10^{-6} cm/s. Compute the membrane voltage measured from inside to outside the cell at a temperature of 37 °C.

7. In Exercise 6, suppose that only the potassium ion contributes significantly to the membrane potential, and compute the potential based on that assumption. Compute the percentage of error introduced and evaluate the validity of the Nernst equation based on this calculation.

8. In Figure 2.8 determine by graphical measurement the difference between the *P-R* interval and the *P-R* segment. Then find the difference between the *S-T* interval and the *S-T* segment.

9. If a threshold detector is to be used to isolate the *R*-wave in the ECG given in Figure 2.8, to what minimum value must it be set?

10. A surface current is presented through a 1-cm^2 area of the skin having a resistance of 50 kΩ. The current above 5 mA at 60 Hz is considered dangerous. What voltage applied from one arm to the other would be considered dangerous?

11. A person in a bathtub touches the metal surface of a room heater. The wet surfaces reduce the person's skin resistance to 1000 Ω. What is the maximum voltage above ground allowed on the metal of the heater before a macroshock hazard is present?

*12. Suppose that in a particular living cell, the membrane potential is caused entirely by the action of the potassium ion, which has a concentration $[K^+]_i$ inside and $[K^+]_o$ outside. Under this assumption, use Equations (2.1), (2.2), and (2.3) to derive the Nernst equation (Equation 2.5) directly.

*Exercise is considered more difficult than average.

3

Hospital Equipment Safety and Organization, and a Logical Approach to Troubleshooting

A hospital is more than simply a building in which health care is delivered. It is a high-tech center that must be superbly organized in order to operate effectively. A typical modern community hospital contains more than 3000 pieces of medical equipment used by hundreds of physicians, health care workers, other staff, and even the patients themselves, in order to help cure disease and save lives. In order to avoid electrical shock, burns, excessive radiation, toxic exposure, fire, explosion, and other hazards, many of the devices must be handled with extreme care. Serious accidents can be kept to a minimum if hospital personnel are properly trained to exercise caution, and if regulations and procedures are strictly adhered to.

Our objective in this chapter is to alert health care professionals to existing hazards and to describe the various means available to provide protection against them.

3.1 ELECTRICAL HAZARDS OF MEDICAL INSTRUMENTS

One of the main hazards connected with the use of medical equipment is electrical shock. The physiological effects of electrical current on the body were described in the preceding chapter, where we defined macroshock as the undesirable effects of a current greater than 5 mA at 60 cycles applied to the surface of the body. These effects range from discomfort and pain to tissue injury, heart fibrillation, and death if a vital body part, such as the heart or respiratory center, is affected. A macroshock to a limb of a technician repairing equipment may also cause secondary injury, such as cuts on the hand as the person pulls away from the equipment. Or worse, a fall could result, if the technician were on a ladder while being jolted by

TABLE 3.1
Skin Resistance at 60 Hz

Condition	Skin resistance per square centimeter of electrode
Dry skin	93 kΩ
Electrode gel on skin	10.8 kΩ
Penetrated skin	200 Ω

an electrical current. We also defined microshock as the undesirable effects of a current greater than 10 μA applied directly to the heart. Microshock can cause a heart fibrillation and can result in a patient's death. It is, however, a hazard only to patients who are in a critical-care situation, because the current must be applied directly to the heart.

Shock is defined in terms of current because the voltages that produce the current are highly variable. The variance in voltage is caused by wide variation in skin resistance among individuals and among differing clinical situations. For example, the skin resistance at 60 cycles may vary from 93 kΩ down to 200 Ω, depending on the condition, as indicated in Table 3.1. (See Spach, 1966.)

EXAMPLE 3.1 Using the skin resistance values given in Table 3.1, compute the voltage levels that would deliver a macroshock current of 5 mA, I_S, between two surface electrodes for the cases of dry skin, electrode-gel-treated skin, and penetrated skin. Let the electrode area be the typical value of 15.5 cm^2.

SOLUTION The voltage source drives two skin electrodes and must overcome a skin resistance R_s and viscera resistance R_v of 200 Ω.

$$V_T = (2R_s + R_v)I_S \qquad (3.1)$$

Applying Equation (3.1) to the cases cited requires that the skin resistances of Table 3.1 be divided by 15.5 to account for the larger electrode surface area. The resulting voltages are as follows:

Situation	Dangerous voltage (V)
Dry skin	61.0
Electrode gel on skin	7.96
Penetrated skin	1.0

These results indicate dangerous voltage levels for 15.5-cm^2 electrodes. If the skin is penetrated with a needle, or if there is a wound, even a 1-volt source is dangerous in the case illustrated.

All electrical and electronic devices in the hospital are sources of potentially harmful current. Most of this equipment is energized by the building wiring. Therefore, an understanding of the shock hazards begins with a discussion of this wiring.

The electrical power bus consists of three wires as shown in Figure 3.1: a *hot wire* H at 110 or 220 V, 60 cycle, usually color-coded black; a *neutral wire* N, usually color-coded white, connected to ground through a pipe embedded in the earth; and a *ground wire* G, usually color-coded green. The neutral wire carries the return current from the equipment loads, and normally carries the same current as the hot lead. The G-wire is connected to the external parts of the equipment to bleed away any leakage that may occur and to prevent the external parts from acquiring a high voltage in case of a short or fault in the circuit. It normally carries very small current, though in fault situations it may cause large currents.

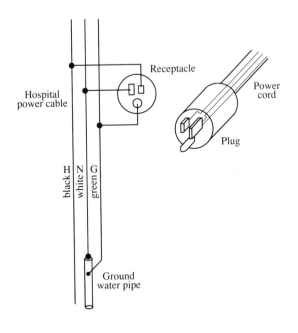

FIGURE 3.1
A power bus.

Macroshock Hazards

Macroshock occurs more often with two-wire systems than with three-wire systems. (See Figures 3.2a and b.) With two-wire equipment it is always dangerous to get between the hot H and neutral N wires. Touching H and N wires simultaneously with two limbs can direct currents through vital organs of circulation and respiration. Because N wires are internally grounded, touching H and G wires can produce macroshock. In some commercial equipment, such as inexpensive a.c./d.c. radios, which are often brought to the hospital by patients, the power-cord plug may be reversed so that the hot lead becomes attached to the chassis. In this case, a macroshock hazard exists when the chassis and ground are touched simultaneously.

Figure 3.3 illustrates additional hazardous situations that result from faults that may occur in the equipment. In part (a), the H lead shorts to the patient lead P. Thus a macroshock results if the patient touches ground or the chassis. In part (b), the hot wire H and neutral N are reversed because the two-wire plug has been reversed. A grounded patient is therefore shocked upon touching the chassis. In part (c) the H wire is shorted to the chassis, causing the shock configuration shown as the patient touches either neutral or ground and the chassis. In part (d) the neutral wire accidentally shorts to the equipment case leading to a shock situation of H to chassis or H to ground. If the H line faults to N, no shock occurs unless the patient touches H or N and ground.

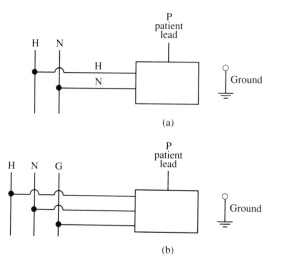

FIGURE 3.2
Power bus connections to (a) two-wire and (b) three-wire equipment.

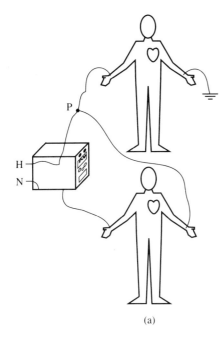
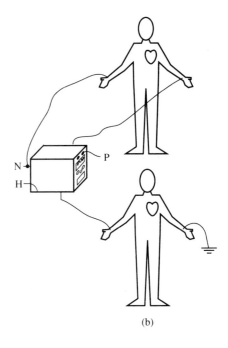

(a)

(b)

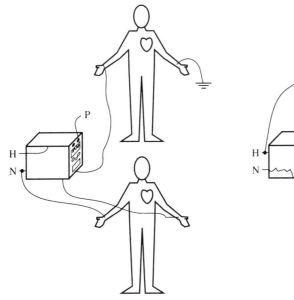
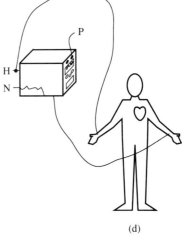

(c)

(d)

FIGURE 3.3
Macroshock situations other than touching H and N, or H and G wires for two-wire units.

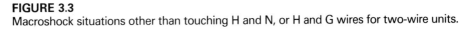

The primary defense against the hazards of a two-wire plug is to add a third ground wire, as shown in Figure 3.2(b). This wire is usually connected to the chassis of the equipment and ensures that it will not rise to a high voltage. Another method is to double-insulate the chassis — that is, to place a layer of insulation between the circuit-board chassis and the equipment case exposed to the user. To prevent a hot chassis on this type of equipment, two-prong plugs have prongs of different sizes so they cannot be reversed.

The addition of a ground wire protects against the hazard of high voltage on the chassis. Assuming the equipment is not faulty, the only macroshock danger occurs when a person gets between the hot lead and ground, neutral, or chassis. Of course, when the third wire faults (is broken) the haz-

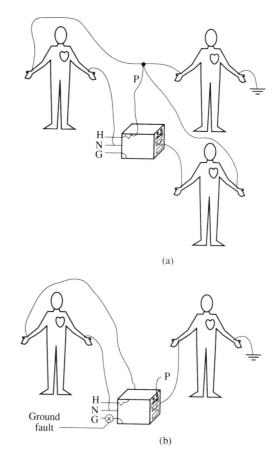

FIGURE 3.4
Macroshock situations other than touching H and N, or H and G for three-wire units.

ards of the two-wire equipment are once again present, except for plug reversal, which is prevented by the shape of the three-prong plug. Other macroshock hazard faults would occur if the hot lead were to short to the patient lead, as illustrated in Figure 3.4(a), or, in the double-fault case, if the hot lead were to short to the chassis with the ground lead open, as illustrated in Figure 3.4(b).

Microshock Hazards

Microshock occurs when a current applied to the heart causes depolarizations to originate from sites other than the sinoatrial (SA) node of the heart. The resulting fibrillations can impair circulation and can ultimately be fatal.

Microshock is apt to occur if the heart receives currents above 10 μA. The conditions leading to such a situation include all of those that induce macroshock, as discussed previously. Additional conditions (Figure 3.5) include the leakage of current and slight elevations of the chassis voltage resulting from high power-line current.

Leakage current is caused by inductive, capacitive, or resistive coupling of electronic circuit currents to the chassis or the patient lead on equipment. Inductive coupling may exist in the power supply transformer, or between the windings of equipment motors and the chassis or leads. Likewise, circuit wires and the metal of the equipment could form a capacitive coupling. Resistive coupling of current from the circuit arises from dirt, oil, or fluids that may get into the equipment and cause a conductive pathway.

EXAMPLE 3.2   In Figure 3.5(b), suppose the electronic circuit has a strong capacitive coupling of 1000 pF between the power line and the patient lead. The catheter resistance is 10 kΩ and the skin resistance is 10 kΩ. Compute the leakage current that passes through the patient's heart. Assume a viscera resistance of 200 Ω.

SOLUTION   The equivalent circuit for the case in question allows calculation of the leakage current magnitude I_L. Here,

$$|I_L| = \left| \frac{120 \angle 0°}{20,200 - \dfrac{j}{2\pi(60)(1000 \times 10^{-12})}} \right| = 45.2 \ \mu A$$

This leakage current exceeds the minimum safe value and could cause a fibrillation of the heart.

Figures 3.5(a) and 3.5(c) illustrate the microshock hazard that occurs when a person gets between two pieces of equipment. The chassis voltages

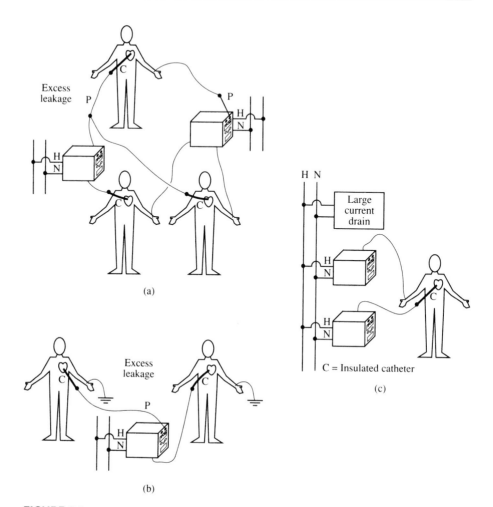

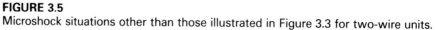

FIGURE 3.5
Microshock situations other than those illustrated in Figure 3.3 for two-wire units.

between the two pieces of two-wire equipment could be considerable because of power-line currents in the different power buses that cause leakage current and elevate chassis voltage. This effect is virtually eliminated by the third wire in three-wire equipment.

EXAMPLE 3.3   In Figure 3.5(b) the N wire is connected to the chassis of the equipment. The 120-V instrument draws 500 W. Compute the voltage of the chassis with respect to ground. The power-cord resistance is 0.25 Ω.

SOLUTION   The neutral N wire current is

$$I_N = \frac{500}{120} = 4.17 \text{ A}$$

The voltage drop across the neutral to ground is then $0.25(4.17) = 1.04$ V.

The preceding example shows that the chassis may be elevated 1.04 V above ground. In a catheterized patient, this voltage could easily drive more than 10 μA through the patient's heart. Furthermore, leakage currents from the patient leads need to be considered. Protection against the effects of leakage current is achieved by periodically inspecting equipment and measuring the leakage current. Figure 3.5(c) illustrates the case in which elevated chassis voltage could be caused by large currents existing in the power bus. For example, a ventilation fan may draw over 10 A. Equipment that operates safely with the fan turned off could acquire an elevated voltage when the fan was turned on. To guard against this, a third wire is added to ground the chassis of the equipment, as illustrated in Figure 3.6(a). Even with the third wire, the leakage hazard still exists. For this reason, periodic inspection of leakage currents in medical equipment is a necessity.

Two subtle faults can occur that introduce microshock faults into three-wire equipment. First, the ground wire or neutral wire may break. Since the power cord is vulnerable to metal fatigue from being moved around and to abuse, breakage in the cord is not rare. Therefore, periodic inspection of the power cord is a necessity. Figure 3.6(a) illustrates microshock hazards due to a broken ground wire. Elevated voltages may exist between the chassis and ground or between the two pieces of equipment that are sufficient to cause a microshock in a catheterized patient.

Second, as Figure 3.6(b) illustrates, a microshock hazard may result from a fault in equipment not used in patient care. For example, suppose an air conditioning unit opens in the neutral and uses the ground lead to supply the large current needed to drive it. This is the case of a neutral fault that occurs while the ground wire remains intact. This fault would pour a large current into the ground lead. Two medical equipment units attached to this ground could have elevated voltage between their chassis. In this case, the medical equipment would have tested normal, and the elevated voltage constituting a microshock situation would be due to equipment outside the medical area. To protect against this situation, the medical circuits may be isolated from such large-current equipment. As a last defense, however, the user may shunt the two pieces of equipment with a ground wire connected exclusively between the units attached to a catheterized patient.

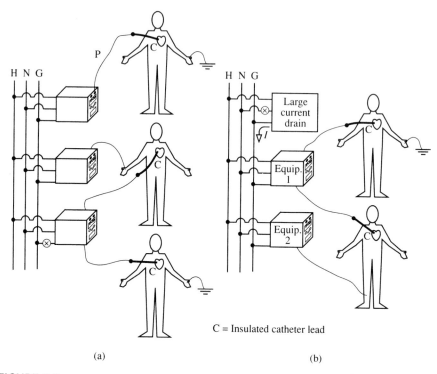

(a)   (b)

FIGURE 3.6
Microshock situations other than those illustrated in Figure 3.4 for three-wire units.

3.2 DEVICES TO PROTECT AGAINST ELECTRICAL HAZARDS

Several devices are available to protect patients and health care workers from hazardous electrical currents. These range from devices to protect against high-voltage macroshock hazards to procedures that minimize the probability that a microshock will occur.

Ground Fault Interrupter

A ground fault interrupter (GFI) protects against a shock that occurs if a person touches the hot lead with one hand and the ground with the other. The GFI opens the power lead if the hot lead current differs by more than approximately 2 mA from the neutral lead current for a duration of longer than 0.2 s. The GFI shown in Figure 3.7 consists of a magnetic coil on which the hot lead and the neutral lead are wound with the same number of turns, but in opposite directions. When the system is normal, I_N is equal to I_H, and the magnet flux, ϕ, in the coil due to these currents cancels. Un-

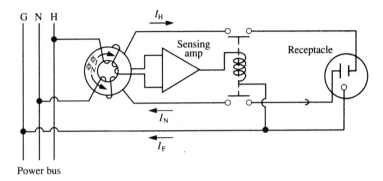

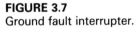

FIGURE 3.7
Ground fault interrupter.

der this condition, the sensing coil does not have a voltage induced in it. However, when the hot lead faults, or is touched by a person, the fault current I_F is shunted to ground. Then we have

$$I_N = I_H - I_F$$

and I_H is not equal to I_N. Under this fault condition the corresponding fluxes in the coil are unequal, and a net flux exists in the coil. This induces a voltage into the sensing amplifier. If the current I_F exceeds 2 mA for 0.2 s, the relay opens the line and prevents a macroshock from injuring the person, as well as preventing further damage to the equipment. The GFI can be conveniently mounted in the power receptacle. It is required in wet areas.

Isolation Transformer

The isolation transformer provides a second means of protecting against an H-lead to G-lead macroshock. It also prevents sparks when the H lead touches ground, a particularly important protection in an explosive or flammable environment, such as when flammable anesthetics or excessive oxygen is present. Figure 3.8(a) clearly shows that a fault such as a short circuit from either secondary lead of the transformers to ground will carry no current. Therefore, a secondary lead to ground spark, or shock, is prevented.

However, when the isolation transformer is in use, and equipment is plugged into the secondary, the stray capacitance and input impedance of the hardware tend to make a conductive path to ground. This reduces the isolation by completing the circuit from either secondary lead to ground and then to the other secondary lead. If a fault should now occur on the secondary, a hazardous current could flow.

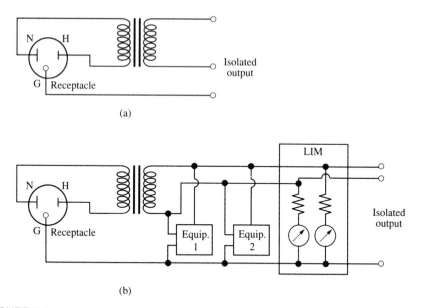

(a)

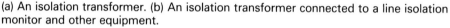

(b)

FIGURE 3.8
(a) An isolation transformer. (b) An isolation transformer connected to a line isolation monitor and other equipment.

Line Isolation Monitor

A line isolation monitor (LIM) puts a relatively large impedance from either secondary lead through an ammeter to ground of the isolation transformer. If there is a conductive path through the equipment shown in Figure 3.8(b), the meter in the LIM will read a current. The meter on the LIM is calibrated to read what current would flow through a short-circuit fault if it should occur from either secondary to ground. This number will vary according to the leakage in the equipment attached to the secondary and any faults that may exist between the secondary leads and ground. An alarm in the LIM is usually set off when it is calculated that a short-circuit fault between a secondary lead and ground would draw 2 to 5 mA of current. This alarm merely indicates that the backup system has failed and the equipment is no longer isolated. It does not mean that the dangerous currents are already flowing. Therefore, if the equipment is critically needed, the LIM alarm may, sometimes, justifiably be overridden.

Receptacle Tester

The LIM and GFI are permanently attached to the power lines in order to warn of potential hazards or to open the circuit when hazardous current flows. Other types of equipment are available for inspecting equipment and circuits for hazardous conditions. For example, the receptacle tester may be inserted in the power receptacle to check for defects in the wiring, such as polarity reversals, shorts, or opens. Light-emitting diodes (LEDs) in series with a directional diode and a limiting resistor R are used to give a coded indication of a receptacle fault. If the receptacle is normal, the LEDs in Figure 3.9 will all be OFF when H is negative. However, when H is positive, LEDs 1 and 3 go ON, blinking at 60 times a second. The observer will perceive both LEDs 1 and 3 as being ON steadily in this case, since the time response of the eye will cause the blinks to merge. Also, 2 will be perceived as OFF. An H to G short will turn all LEDs OFF, as will an open H lead. The light responses for several fault states possible in the figure are as follows:

Possible wiring defect	LED state		
	1	2	3
Normal	ON	OFF	ON
H to G short	OFF	OFF	OFF
H, N reversed	OFF	ON	ON

Determination of the other LED states corresponding to receptacle faults is given as Exercise 13.

The receptacle also needs to be tested for the grasping tension it exerts on the plug, and the device for this is the *receptacle contact tester*, which consists of a plug blade attached to a spring scale. As the plug is retracted from the receptacle, the scale is read to ensure that the tension it is required to overcome exceeds approximately 8 oz.

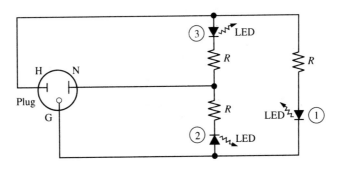

FIGURE 3.9
A power receptacle tester.

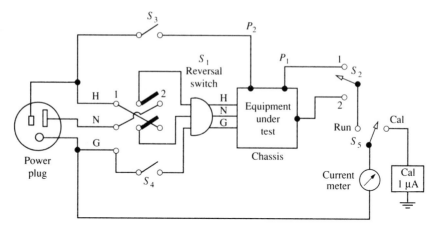

FIGURE 3.10
Block diagram of a generic safety analyzer.

Electrical Safety Analyzer Equipment

The equipment discussed in the preceding section is mostly used as protection against macroshock. The safety analyzer, as illustrated by the block diagram in Figure 3.10, is primarily used to test medical equipment for leakage currents that can cause microshock to patients. The safety analyzer is calibrated by placing switch S_5 in the calibrate position while adjusting the meter for 1 μA. The equipment under test (EUT) is plugged into the safety analyzer. To measure the chassis to ground leakage on the EUT, S_4 is opened while S_1 is in position 1, S_2 is in position 2, and S_3 is opened. The ground leakage is then also measured with the hot and neutral leads reversed by means of switch S_1. Switch S_2 may then be moved to position 1 to measure the leakage current in the patient lead P_1. The leakage current between patient leads when the hot lead is applied to one of the P-leads is measured when S_3 is closed.

3.3 AN EQUIPMENT SAFETY PROGRAM

The clinical engineering department in a hospital should take responsibility for establishing an equipment safety program. Such a program should conform to safety regulations established by government agencies and professional organizations. The program is necessary to ensure the safety of patients and health care workers in the hospital. Specific regulations must be met in order to secure accreditation and license to operate.

The instrumentation described in the preceding sections is used to make safety tests and to ensure safety in the hospital. Here we present a sample program in order to discuss the issues involved. A specific safety program would need to be geared to a particular clinical situation and would of course differ from that described here.

Hospital Regulations

The many instruments, medicines, and procedures used to deliver health care in a hospital for the benefit of patients may also present hazards. In order to protect patients and health care workers, hospital regulations have been developed to cope with hazards of electricity, radiation, magnetism, toxics, infectious agents, pressure, flame, heat, explosion, and energy interruptions.

Legally enforceable regulations are issued by these U.S. government agencies: (1) Occupational Safety and Health Administration (OSHA), founded in 1971; and through the Federal Drug Administration (FDA) by the Medical Device Amendments of 1976 to the Food, Drug and Cosmetic Act. Both of these mechanisms arose as a result of the increased environmental awareness during the 1970s. In addition, local building codes for fire, electrical, and structural safety are enforced in hospitals.

Furthermore, voluntary regulations are issued by civic and professional groups for the protection of the public and the professions. Although such regulations are not always legally enforceable, they are effective because failure to comply may result in a withdrawal of third-party funding and insurance, a damaged reputation, a loss of professional staff, and a loss of clients. In some cases, voluntary regulations are the only rules in evidence, because the cost of rigid enforcement cannot be justified in terms of the risk involved. This, coupled with the fact that voluntary regulations do work, makes voluntary compliance all the more important. Furthermore, when these regulations are adopted as local building codes, they acquire the force of law.

Several agencies that issue regulations for health care facilities are:

- National Fire Protection Association (NFPA)
- Joint Commission on Accreditation of Healthcare Organizations (JCAHO)
- Underwriters' Laboratories (UL)
- Association for the Advancement of Medical Instrumentation (AAMI)

Apart from the economic incentives for following the "voluntary" regulations, compliance leads to better-run hospitals and reduces the risk of their being accused of neglect in a lawsuit.

It is beyond the scope of this chapter to state the essential regulations that apply to health care facilities. Indeed, these regulations fill volumes and are stated with inclusive precision for specific cases. Comprehensive documents are listed as end-of-chapter references. (See AAMI, 1985, and NFPA, 1984.)

Inspections of Equipment

The frequency of electrical safety inspections generally depends upon the degree of vulnerability of the equipment user and patient to hazards associated with the equipment. In general care areas, tests are done every year. In wet areas, where the patient's skin resistance is likely to be low, tests are done every six months. In critical areas, where the skin might be penetrated in surgery by a catheter or a needle or injury, tests are also done every six months.

Equipment testing begins with concern for the integrity of the power system. A receptacle tester, as discussed in the previous section, is used to test for power-line opens, shorts, or wiring errors. In order to prevent excessive leakage current and shock hazards, medical instrumentation either has a power cord with a three-prong plug or is double-insulated. Double-insulated equipment has its hot and neutral power leads connected to electronics insulated from the chassis and the chassis insulated from the external case of the equipment. With these provisions, the power-cord leakage should test less than 100 μA. Existing equipment in the hospital may have a power-cord leakage as high as 500 μA. These cases need to be documented to ensure safe use of such equipment.

Specifications on hospital equipment to be used in patient areas typically take into account that a 5-mA current applied through the surface of the body is dangerous and that currents in excess of 10 μA applied to a catheterized heart can be dangerous. Leakage currents are measured with the safety analyzer (Figure 3.11). A typical set of leakage current values that meet specifications of equipment safe to use in patient areas is given in Table 3.2. The leakage of the individual patient lead, the leakage of all leads together, and the chassis leakage are measured with the a.c. line power normally connected to the equipment. The driven patient leads are connected to the power line in order to determine how much current the 120 V would drive through them. Equipment used outside the patient's vicinity may exhibit as much as 500 μA leakage current.

TABLE 3.2
Leakage Current Values for Equipment
Used with Patient

Description	Leakage current (μA)
Individual patient lead	10
Driven patient lead	20
Current between patient leads	50
All patient leads connected together	100
Chassis leakage to ground	100

The leakage current specifications on hospital equipment are a function of the current frequency due to the high-frequency effects, as discussed in Chapter 2. The leakage current specifications follow the equation

$$I = I_{lk} f \qquad (3.2)$$

where I is the leakage current allowed at a frequency f, given in kilohertz. I_{lk} is the leakage current for frequencies below 1 kHz.

Leakage currents in equipment may be measured with a safety analyzer such as is illustrated in Figure 3.11.

Emergency Power Systems

The reliability of power companies in the United States is so high that we almost take the availability of 60-cycle ($\sim$) power for granted. However, power is occasionally interrupted by severe weather such as high winds, lightning, snow, and ice. In less-developed countries, power outages are common, sometimes lasting for several hours during the business day. Uninterrupted power, however, is necessary for many modern medical instruments, among them artificial blood circulators, ventilators, operating room equipment, intensive care units, external pacemakers, kidney dialysis machines, and artificial hearts. Injury to patients relying on any of these devices would obviously occur if the power were to fail for an extended period.

To protect against such interruptions, hospitals use two independent sources of power. An in-house *emergency power source* may consist of an internal combustion engine driving an electrical generator. The time it takes for the emergency source to switch on when an outage occurs is typically

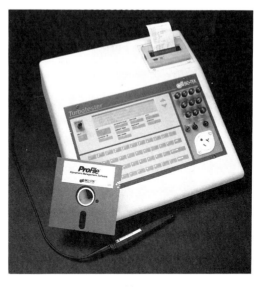

(a)

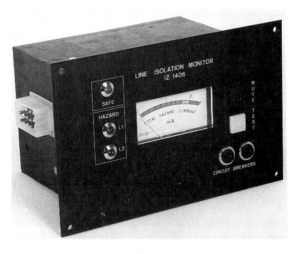

(b)

FIGURE 3.11
(a) An electrical safety analyzer to test equipment. (Courtesy of Bio-Tek Instruments, Inc.)
(b) A line isolation monitor. (Courtesy of Bender, Inc.)

less than 10 seconds. The reliability of the emergency power system should be ensured by exercising the emergency generator for 30 minutes every 30 days and by inspecting batteries on the engine every seven days. Other causes of power interruption, such as ground fault interrupters, should not turn off critical equipment but should have automatic reset systems with alarms to warn of hazards or else have backup systems.

Oxygen Safety

A widely used gas in the hospital, oxygen must be handled carefully, because it supports flame and fire, is stored at high pressure, and can be toxic when misused.

In order to prevent fire and explosion with oxygen, the ambient temperature where the gas is used or stored should be kept below 130 °F. As a rule of thumb, one can ordinarily just keep skin contact with a surface at that temperature. A second precaution is to keep any flammable substance out of the oxygen system, including flammable gases. Oil must be kept off the oxygen system valves, because it is highly combustible in the presence of oxygen. As a safety precaution, if the valves become frozen from high-pressure gas release, for example, a flame torch must not be used to thaw them; wet rags would provide a safe alternative. Many materials normally resistant to flame will burn in an oxygen-rich atmosphere. Examples include human tissue, body oils, silicon rubber, oil-based cosmetics, polyvinyl chloride, alcohols, acetone, asbestos-containing paint, glass epoxy compounds, tent canopies, and suction tubing. Since some of these materials are invariably present in the hospital—for example, in oxygen tents, on respirators, and near anesthesia machines—it is essential to eliminate sources of ignition in the oxygen-enriched atmosphere. Common sources of ignition that must be kept away from oxygen are open flame, static electricity, burning tobacco, electric radiant heaters, electric shavers, electric bed controls, hair dryers, remote TV controls, and telephones. Hearing aids, external pacemakers, and other equipment worn by patients can also be sources of ignition. Of course, any other potential sources of ignition should likewise be eliminated.

Safety in the Operating Room

The operating room (OR) is carefully designed and maintained to protect the patient from hazards including fire, explosion, mechanical injury, toxic overdose, anoxia, and infection. Many of these hazards arise from anesthesia and surgery.

Protection against infection is achieved by sterilization. Surgeons and surgical assistants scrub their hands and arms, wear sterile gloves, gowns, caps, masks, and foot coverings. The operating room has a *sterile region* where the patient, instruments for surgery, and anesthesia machine are located. The periphery of the operating room is usually a nonsterile area where equipment and technicians who do not come in contact with the patient are located. Personnel confined to this region also wear gowns, caps, masks, and foot coverings, but do not need to scrub.

Instruments may be sterilized in the OR with either steam, ethylene oxide gas, or a liquid, glutamic aldehyde. Steam sterilization may be done under pressure to produce superheated steam temperatures up to 144 °C. After treatment for approximately 15 minutes, the instruments are dried at high temperatures. The resulting temperature stress, which may be damaging to the instruments, may be avoided by sterilizing at low temperatures with ethylene oxide (ETO) gas. Although the temperature in this treatment may be reduced below 60 °C, exposure time is increased to several hours. Careful ventilation of the ETO from the instrument is then necessary since the gas is hazardous. A gas sterilizer is illustrated in Figure 3.12.

Anesthetics and anesthesia delivery equipment also present safety hazards. An example block diagram of an anesthesia machine appears in Figure 3.13. The anesthetic, in this case nitrous oxide (N_2O), is mixed with oxygen and fluorocarbons and then delivered to the patient on the inspiration cycle. Exhalation passes through a one-way valve, through a CO_2 absorber, and is delivered again to the patient. The anesthetic is constantly monitored and adjusted for the correct mixture. A portion of the anesthetic is exhausted and usually delivered to the outside through vent ducts.

The most commonly used anesthetic is nitrous oxide, used in combination with fluorocarbons such as halothane, enflurane, or methoxyflurane. These are nonflammable but should not be vented into the OR, since they may have deleterious effects on OR personnel. Although flammable

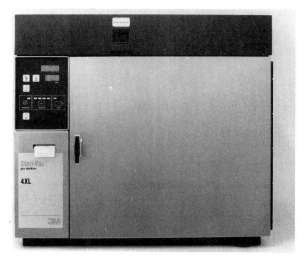

FIGURE 3.12
A gas sterilizer. (Courtesy of 3M Corporation)

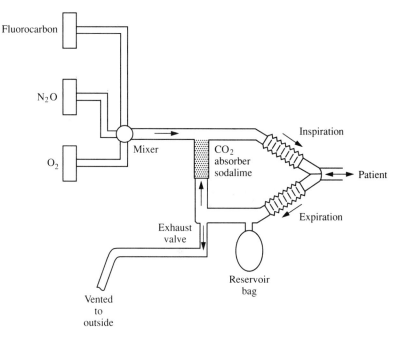

FIGURE 3.13
An anesthesia machine.

anesthetics such as ether and cyclopropane are no longer in common use, operating rooms are still designed to avoid fire hazards from these anesthetics. Any oxygen-enriched atmosphere, especially at elevated pressures, justifies continued caution.

Hazards of Gases

Before the 1970s gases were exhausted into the OR. Now waste gases are drawn through an exhaust ventilator to the outside.

The OR is specifically designed to provide protection against fire from flammable gas, toxic effects of anesthesia that may escape inadvertently into the atmosphere, and the dangers of electrical spark ignition and shock. To monitor operating room personnel for exposure to toxic material, a dosimetry indicator, such as that illustrated in Figure 3.14, may be used.

The ventilating system of the OR usually produces a positive pressure to sweep contaminated air out through doors, openings, and exhaust vents. It also regulates the temperature and humidity.

To reduce the probability of flame due to sparks, the humidity should be kept above 50%; in nonflammable areas it may be allowed to drop to 30%. Since oxygen, and most flammable anesthetics, are heavier than air, they tend to sink to the floor. Exhaust vents in the OR are therefore

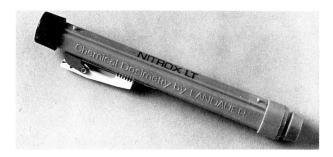

FIGURE 3.14
A pocket chemical dosimetry device. (Courtesy of R. S. Landauer, Jr. & Co.)

mounted within three inches of the floor, which helps to keep dangerous gas from reaching the faces of people working there. The air inlet is near the OR ceiling, and ventilation should exceed eight air changes per hour. In general, the ventilating system should keep the toxic and flammable gases in the OR below five feet.

To keep explosive gas out of contact with electrical outlets in the OR, since sparks may be created when power cords are plugged in or pulled out, outlets are placed five feet above the floor. Furthermore, all switches and wires are enclosed in screens to prevent ignition due to sparks. Hot spots, such as fixed lighting, are located more than eight feet above the floor. To guard against sparks that could cause a fire from static charges induced by shoes, clothing, and equipment, a conductive floor with a resistance of less than 1 megohm should be installed in an OR qualified for flammable anesthetics. This high-resistance conductive path bleeds off any buildup of static charge.

The resistance of the floor is specified to be on average greater than 25 kΩ, measured with an electrode 2.5 inches in diameter, and at no point should it be less than 10 kΩ. The lower limit on the resistance offers protection against macroshock to OR personnel by limiting shock current should they come in contact with a high voltage.

An isolation transformer is used to maintain an open circuit between the ground and the return path of currents in the electrical equipment. This reduces the probability that a spark will be created by faults in the equipment. It also reduces the possibility that operating room personnel who wear conductive clothing will receive shocks.

Because of the gas hazards in the OR, personnel must be careful to avoid bringing in any objects that might be sources of ignition or static charges.

All portable equipment in the OR should be labeled for "flammable" or "nonflammable" use. Electrosurgical units or lasers are not to be used with flammable anesthetics, because they cut with a spark; neither are appliances such as portable drills. Portable x-ray machines require special approval for use with flammable anesthetics. Equipment with hot spots is either permanently mounted above the five-foot level in the OR, or mounted on portable devices that keep it above that level.

Any foot treadle switch should be explosion-proof unless nonflammable anesthetics are being used, and it should be splash-proof. Flexible power cords may sometimes be used in the OR when the extension receptacles are permanently attached to equipment.

To further prevent static sparks, all accessory devices should be either conductive or antistatic, if the use of conductive materials is impractical. For example, antistatic sheets should be used, as should conductive footwear with a resistance of less than 500 kΩ to prevent sparks. Sparks from hot wires coming into contact with ground may be avoided by use of an isolation transformer, isolating the OR power currents.

Before 1950, the anesthetics in use, primarily chloroform and diethyl ether, were flammable. It was then that the previously mentioned techniques to protect against fire in the OR were developed. With the introduction of nonflammable anesthesia, the requirement to use these techniques was sometimes relaxed. However, in cases where an oxygen-rich environment exists, such as in pressure chambers, at other than atmospheric pressure, the fire hazard returns, and fire safety precautions should be taken. Other common flammable substances found in the hospital are aldehydes, ketones, esters, benzene, toluene, and oils. Other flammable gases include cyclopropane, ethyl chloride, and ethylene. Therefore, precautions against fire hazards are always prudent. Halothane is used in the OR to reduce the flammability of anesthetics. The common nonflammable anesthetic nitrous oxide is toxic. Clinical personnel should not breathe air containing more than 5 parts per million (ppm), and the temperature of exposed surfaces in its presence should be below 130 °F. Ethylene oxide, another toxic gas used for sterilizing procedures in the OR, had an exposure limit of less than 50 ppm in 1982, but this was changed to 2 ppm in 1987.

Pressure Chambers

High-pressure facilities, called hyperbaric chambers, are used in medical procedures to facilitate oxygen transfer in the blood. The partial pressure of oxygen in the blood, $^PO_2$, is greatly increased when the patient is placed in a hyperbaric chamber. For example, in a 100% oxygen atmosphere, $^PO_2$ increases from 650 mmHg to 2000 mmHg as the pressure increases from 1 to 3 atmospheres (atm). This allows the use of blood with less hemoglobin when large quantities of blood are required.

Under conditions of 100% oxygen at 3 atm, the danger of fire is acute. Thus, a hyperbaric chamber should have a noncombustible floor and be equipped with fire extinguishers and fire detectors. Flameproof clothing and conductive footwear are required, as are individual breathing supplies for occupants. One is cautioned not to introduce cotton, wool, synthetic fabrics, flammable hairspray, or skin oil into the environment. X-ray and electrosurgical equipment are not allowed in these chambers. In general, the chamber must be rated safe for 100% oxygen at 3 atm of pressure.

3.4 PREVENTIVE MAINTENANCE

Preventive maintenance is done on medical equipment to make sure that it is safe and in proper working order. The inspections necessary to ensure that safety specifications are met are a part of the preventive maintenance procedure. Furthermore, equipment should be inspected to ensure that it is calibrated accurately. Physicians use the output data from medical equipment to make diagnoses and to prescribe treatment of disease, so inaccurate data from the equipment can clearly lead to serious mistakes. Preventive maintenance can protect a patient by reducing the likelihood of these mistakes.

Preventive maintenance procedures are recommended by the manufacturers of equipment and are usually given in the equipment service manual. Every biomedical equipment shop should have a program of regular preventive maintenance that goes beyond the basic safety checks described in the previous section.

The frequency of preventive maintenance depends on how vital the instrumentation is and on the frequency of observed failures. Preventive maintenance of equipment used to maintain vital functions such as patient blood circulation or breathing should be more frequent than that of equipment that does not come in contact with the patient. Also, if a particular kind of equipment is observed to fail frequently, it should be scheduled for more frequent inspections.

In spite of all precautions taken, however, equipment will fail. In fact, certain parts of equipment are *wearing parts*, and, like automobile tires, must be changed periodically. X-ray tubes, chemical electrodes, and air filters are examples of wearing parts in medical equipment. In any case, when the equipment becomes inoperative, it is necessary to do troubleshooting and repair.

3.5 A LOGICAL APPROACH TO TROUBLESHOOTING

Troubleshooting is done either by analysis based on circuit theory or by recall of previous cases, sometimes called the case-study approach. These are two different logical processes that can be used to fix broken equipment.

The case-study approach would be used if a piece of equipment were known to have a chronic, or repetitive, problem. In this case one would naturally check to see if it had reoccurred before looking for other problems. This is an example of the approach often used by physicians in diagnosing disease. Equipment repair records are used to systematically store such information. The records form a database that can be accessed with the shop computer as an aid to troubleshooting.

The other basic method of troubleshooting uses logical analysis of given evidence. In this procedure data relating to the problem is gathered and used to isolate the cause analytically. Because circuit theory is basic to the design of medical equipment, it could, in principle, be used to deduce every problem with the hardware. However, that process may be more complicated than is necessary. A systematic approach to troubleshooting uses both methods, analysis and recall.

A flow diagram outlining logical steps to troubleshooting is presented in Figure 3.15. In troubleshooting you would follow the steps indicated until the problem is identified. At whatever step this happens, you would skip down to step 25, fix the equipment, and assess the need for future preventive maintenance.

Step one in the diagram implies that in troubleshooting, all available resources should be used. This begins with assessing the environment. Is there an emergency or a hazard involved? It is important also to interview the person who reported the problem, and to use diplomacy and tact so that issues of personal blame do not arise. Others who have been involved with the equipment may also be interviewed.

Equipment is organized at various levels, the most complex being the system level. A *system* consists of units. Each unit might be a different type of equipment such as an electrocardiograph or a pressure monitor. Each *unit* consists of modules that perform particular functions within the equipment. One module may consist of a transducer, and another the signal processing section of the unit. The *modules* consist of circuit boards and discrete elements, and circuit boards themselves consist of discrete elements. The troubleshooting process is the effort to find the discrete element or elements that have failed. The logical process described here is to start at the system level and work down to the discrete element.

Logical Steps in Troubleshooting

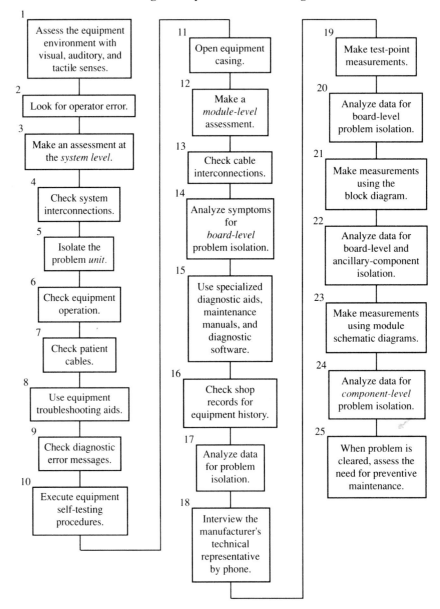

FIGURE 3.15
A general troubleshooting flowchart.

At the system level, interconnecting cables, which are vulnerable to breakage, loosening, and corrosion, should be checked early in the troubleshooting process. It is then necessary to isolate the subsystem unit that may be causing the problem.

At the unit level, patient cables and other cables attached to the equipment should be checked. At this point you may want to refer to the equipment service manual for equipment troubleshooting aids. Many medical instruments display error messages that aid in troubleshooting. Sometimes these appear automatically; other times self-testing procedures must be externally executed. At this point (step 11 in the figure) it will be necessary to open the equipment casing, if the trouble has not been located. After a visual and tactile assessment, it is good policy again to check the cables. One good test of a cable is to invert it in its connector, if possible. If the symptoms of the problem change, the cable is probably bad.

Troubleshooting at the *circuit-board* level is facilitated if the equipment block diagram provided in the service manual is used as a guide. Troubleshooting flowcharts are often provided to expedite the process. Data for problem analysis may be gathered from designated test points. The equipment's maintenance history may give some clue. Further information may be obtained by telephoning the manufacturer's representative, who should have a broad perspective on the kinds of problems that the equipment may be susceptible to. As indicated in step 22, this data can be used to isolate the problem either to a particular board or to an ancillary component that is often too large or that gets too hot to be attached to a board because of heat sink requirements.

If a particular circuit board has been found to be the source of the problem, it may be replaced by a board known to be good. Before a board swap is made, however, a visual inspection should be performed to look for any evidence of short circuits or overheating. Checks should be made for power supply over-voltage, which could damage a new board. Antistatic spray should be used to prevent damage due to static charge buildup. Circuit boards are expensive, and all precautions should be taken not to damage them during troubleshooting procedures.

If a board swap does not correct the problem or change the symptoms, the old board should be put back, and the analysis process should be continued.

When a circuit board has been found to be faulty, component-level troubleshooting should be done. This involves detailed signal tracing, voltage and resistance measurements, and use of the equipment schematic showing interconnections between the individual components. This task is sometimes highly specialized. Before it is undertaken, a decision has to be made either to fix the board in house or to send it back to the manufacturer. This depends on the complexity of the board, how it is manufactured, and the cost of one option versus the other. Since shipping circuit boards is easily done, and the manufacturer may have specialists who can fix the board most economically, this option should always be considered.

When the source of the problem is discovered, the repair procedure will involve systematic disassembling and reassembling of the equipment. To disassemble the equipment, number each part as you remove it. Then to reassemble, replace the parts in the reverse order, in order to be sure you are putting all the parts back together correctly.

Equipment repair requires manual dexterity and an ability to solder parts. After the troubleshooting and repair procedures have been completed, the need for future preventive maintenance of the equipment should be assessed.

REFERENCES

Association for the Advancement of Medical Instrumentation (AAMI). *Essential Standards for Biomedical Equipment Safety and Performance.* Arlington, VA: AAMI, 1985.

Carr, J., Brown, J. M. *Introduction to Biomedical Equipment Technology.* New York: John Wiley & Sons, 1981.

Feinberg, B. N. "Electrical Performance and Safety Testing of Electromedical Equipment." Chapter 16 in *Applied Clinical Engineering.* Englewood Cliffs, NJ: Prentice-Hall, 1986.

Freeman, J. J., *et al.* "Safety Program." In *Clinical Engineering*, edited by J. G. Webster and A. M. Cook. Englewood Cliffs, NJ: Prentice-Hall, 1979.

Leeming, M. N., and Perron, E. *Electrical Safety Program Guide.* Shelburne, VT: Bio-tek Instruments, Inc., 1974.

Olson, W. H. "Electrical Safety." Chapter 13 in *Medical Instrumentation*, edited by J. G. Webster. Boston: Houghton Mifflin, 1978.

National Fire Protection Association (NFPA). *NFPA 99 Health Care Facilities.* Quincy, MA: NFPA, 1984.

Seippel, R. G. *Transducer Interfacing.* Englewood Cliffs, NJ: Prentice-Hall, 1988.

Spach, M. S., *et al.* "Skin-Electrode Impedance and Its Effect on Recording Cardiac Potentials." *Circulation* 34 (Oct. 1966): 649–656.

UL554 Laboratories. *Standard for Safety; Medical and Dental Equipment.* Chicago: Underwriters' Laboratories, 1974.

EXERCISES

1. A cell membrane has a thickness t of 0.09 μm and a radius r of 8 μm. The relative dielectric constant is 3. If the cell may be considered a spherical capacitor, compute its capacitance.

2. A certain type of tissue has a 15-mV threshold for the action potential. Its impedance follows the $Z_T = 1/(1 + j6.28 \times 10^{-4} f)$. Compute the stimulus current at 60 Hz and 600 Hz. How does this explain why an electrosurgical unit does not cause an electrical shock under normal use?

3. An individual has a skin resistance of 100 kΩ on the hand holding a 1-cm^2 electrode. The same electrode on the forearm creates a resistance of 50 kΩ. When electrode gel is added to the electrode, the resistance goes down to 5 kΩ; and when the skin is penetrated by the electrode, the resistance falls to 50 Ω. If a stimulus current of 5 mA is considered dangerous, what voltage level is considered dangerous in each case?

4. The cross-sectional area of a torso is approximately 600 cm^2. What is the current density through the heart when 15 mA is applied across the limbs—the arm and the leg? How does this calculation explain why microcurrents applied to the heart can cause fibrillations?

5. The worst-case microshock situation resulting from stray capacitance leakage from 120-V, 60-cycle ($\sim$) power-line voltage is assumed to be a direct contact of the equipment chassis to a pacemaker lead wire embedded in cardiac muscle. If the heart resistance and skin resistance may be considered negligible, compute the maximum allowed stray capacity, C_{max}, which keeps the leakage current through the heart below 10 μA.

6. Calculate the value of resistance connected from the hot lead on a 120-V, 60-$\sim$ power line to ground but not connected directly to the neutral, which will normally cause a GFI to trip the circuit open.

7. In Figure 3.6(b), the large current drain is caused by a ventilation fan run by a 120-V, 60-$\sim$ source. The neutral and ground wires are connected normally in the fan housing. However, a fault occurs, opening the neutral causing the line current to flow in the ground lead. The fan presents a 3000-W load. The resistance of the ground lead between equipment units 1 and 2 is 0.3 Ω. Compute the voltage difference between the grounded chassis of equipment units 1 and 2.

8. In Figure 3.6(b), a 5000-Ω catheter is connected from the equipment unit 1 chassis to a patient's heart. The body resistance is 300 Ω and the skin resistance is 20 kΩ. Assume that the ground current computed in Exercise 7 is flowing. Compute the microcurrent that goes into the patient's heart. Assess the danger level of these currents.

9. An LIM places 1 MΩ from the 120-V, 60-∿ hot lead to ground and 1 MΩ on the neutral lead to ground. The current measured in the 1-MΩ resistor is 0.05 mA. What is the value of fault current that would flow if the hot lead were then shorted to ground?

10. What value of stray capacitance to ground could cause a 2-mA fault current in an isolation transformer if it appears from neutral to ground? A fault is considered to be a short to ground. Assume a 120-V power line.

11. A power cord is wrapped around a patient's leg so that it contacts 2 cm^2 of his skin. A *cordohmeter*, a device for measuring insulation resistance, applies 200 V to the inner conductor of the power cord and measures 5 μA to a 1-cm^2 electrode placed on the outer insulation of the cord. How much leakage current flows into the patient from a 120-V power line?

12. List the switch positions in the block diagram of a safety analyzer (Figure 3.10) necessary to measure the following quantities on a piece of equipment under test (EUT).

	Switch positions				
	S_1	S_2	S_3	S_4	S_5
Chassis leakage with ground fault					
Patient lead leakage normal equipment					
Driven lead-to-lead leakage					
Chassis leakage, hot to neutral reversed					

13. A receptacle tester has the circuit shown in Figure 3.9. Indicate which LEDs are ON or OFF for fault conditions indicated in the table.

	LED		
	1	2	3
Hot open			
Neutral open			
No possible wiring			
Ground open			
Hot and ground reversed			
Hot and neutral reversed			
Hot open and neutral hot			

4 Medical Instrument Transducers and Component-Level Troubleshooting

Transducers in medical instrumentation are very important, because they come in direct contact with the patient. In the vast majority of cases, the function of the transducer is to convert a physiological parameter—an extremely weak potential, a pressure, a fluid flow rate, a temperature, a chemical concentration, a tissue displacement—into a voltage. This voltage must be large enough to be accurately processed by electronic equipment.

To perform this task, the transducer must be strategically placed into an electronic circuit such as a Wheatstone bridge (described later in this chapter) or into a differential amplifier (described in the next chapter). Transducer principles are illuminated by simple and direct electronic circuit analysis of these circuits. This analysis leads to an understanding of transducers and associated equipment schematics, both to facilitate the design of new configurations and to troubleshoot existing equipment.

A transducer of medical equipment often poses problems for users and maintenance personnel. Because it comes into contact with the patient, safety issues are raised. It is often subject to physical wear and abuse. Its performance is often affected by patient motion and tension. Noise and interference factors arise, because the physiological parameters being measured are often very small. Accuracy and calibration become critical, because the data being measured may be used to diagnose disease and prescribe treatment.

4.1 ELECTRODE TRANSDUCERS

An electrode transducer couples the voltage on the surface of the body to an electronic instrument. The surface potentials on the body range from 1 microvolt (μV) on the skull to 1 millivolt (mV) across the arms to 0.1 V on exposed viscera. The electrodes are either *invasive*, and penetrate the skin, as in the case of a needle electrode, or *noninvasive* surface electrodes, which do not penetrate the skin. The type most frequently used in the clinical environment is the surface electrode.

The Surface Electrode

The surface electrode may consist of a metal plate coated with an electrolyte solution. Sometimes, however, it may consist of a metal plate separated from the surface of the body by an insulator, thereby forming a capacitive coupling. Two types of metal surface electrodes, both requiring an electrolyte gel applied to the skin, are shown in Figure 4.1. The suction-cup electrode (a) can be readily moved about and is held in place against the skin by suction. The metal surface electrode (b) is attached to a limb using the elastic strap. Adhesive electrodes are formed by filling the hole in a donut-shaped adhesive tape with electrode gel backed by metal attached to the electrode-lead cable. Several common means of attaching the electrodes are illustrated in Figure 4.2.

To understand the principle of operation of the metal-electrolyte surface electrode, consider Figure 4.3. A metal-to-electrode potential is formed by electrons that leave the electrolyte and enter the metal, leaving behind a distribution of charge that varies as a function of position, as shown in the figure. This charge distribution is similar to that of a capacitor, being positive over one surface and negative over another. Therefore, the equivalent electrical circuit for this junction contains a capacitor, C_d. This charge distribution also causes an electric potential called the *half-cell po-*

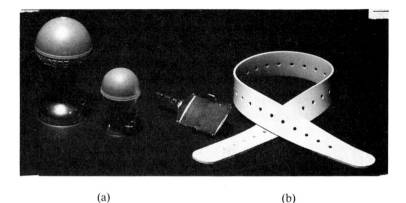

(a)   (b)

FIGURE 4.1
(a) Suction-cup electrodes. (b) Metal-plate surface electrode attached with an elastic strap. (Courtesy Bowen and Company, Inc.)

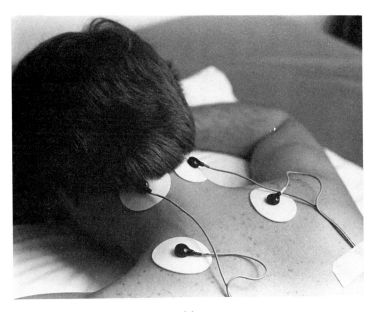

(a)

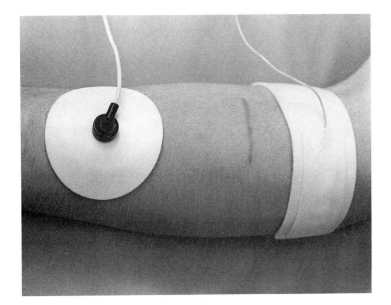

(b)

FIGURE 4.2
(a) Adhesive surface electrodes for measuring electromyographs. (b) A surface electrode with a large return pad. (c) (next page) Multiple-site attachment of adhesive surface electrodes. (Courtesy of Consolidated Medical Corporation)

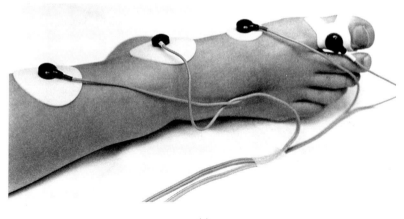

(c)

FIGURE 4.2 (continued)

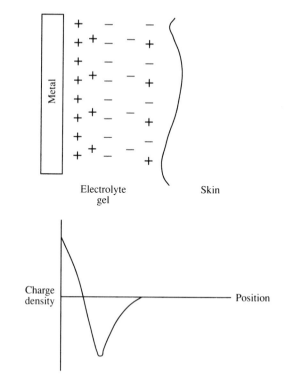

FIGURE 4.3
Surface electrode charge distribution.

tential, E_{hc}. A leakage resistance, R_d, exists across the equivalent capacitance. A series resistance in the equivalent circuit, R_s, represents the electrolyte fluid in charge equilibrium. The arrangement of these equivalent circuit elements is given in Figure 4.4.

The electrode impedance for this equivalent circuit is given by rules for combining impedances, as

$$Z = R_s + \frac{\dfrac{R_d}{j2\pi f C_d}}{R_d + \dfrac{1}{j\pi f C_d}}$$

Rearranging these terms gives

$$Z = R_s + \frac{R_d}{1 + j2\pi f C_d R_d} \qquad (4.1)$$

This impedance formula gives a precise description of the electrical behavior of a surface electrode. It is especially important to note that the impedance is a function of frequency.

To facilitate calculation of this equation for specific R_s, R_d, and C_d as a function of frequency f, a hand-held calculator program is provided in Appendix A, Program A-1. The flow diagram appears in Figure 4.5.

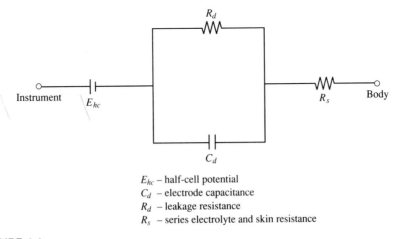

E_{hc} – half-cell potential
C_d – electrode capacitance
R_d – leakage resistance
R_s – series electrolyte and skin resistance

FIGURE 4.4
Surface electrode equivalent circuit.

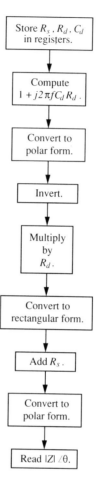

FIGURE 4.5
Flow diagram for calculation of Equation (4.1) using Program A-1 in Appendix A.

Half-Cell Potential and Equivalent Circuit Elements

The half-cell potential, E_{hc}, is measured with reference to a hydrogen-jet electrode placed in an electrolyte near the metal under test. The plus-to-minus voltage drop from the metal under test to the reference electrode is measured with a high-input impedance voltmeter. The measured values of E_{hc} for several metals are given in Table 4.1.

Pairs of these metals can be immersed in an electrolyte to produce a potential source, as in an ordinary battery. On surface electrodes, they produce an unwanted polarization potential.

TABLE 4.1
Half-Cell Potentials, E_{hc},
Measured at 25 °C

Metal	E_{hc} (V)
Aluminum	−1.7
Hydrogen	0.00
Copper	+0.34
Silver	+0.80

EXAMPLE 4.1   Aluminum and silver are immersed in an electrolyte and separated by a large distance. Calculate the potential drop from the aluminum to the silver, E_0.

SOLUTION   Figure 4.6 shows the orientation of the half-cell potentials. Applying Kirchhoff's voltage law to Figure 4.6 yields

$$E_0 = -E_{hc1} + E_{hc2}$$

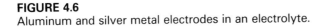

FIGURE 4.6
Aluminum and silver metal electrodes in an electrolyte.

The values of the half-cell potentials taken from Table 4.1 yield the aluminum-to-silver voltage drop:

$$E_0 = -0.80 - 1.7 = -2.5 \text{ V}$$

In actual practice, the measured voltage E_0 would differ from this value because of impurities in the metal and the electrolytes, as well as variations from standard conditions of pressure and temperature. The polarization potential is also sensitive to patient motion, which disturbs the metal-to-electrolyte interface. As long as the patient remains still, the polarization potential represents a d.c. component that can be isolated from the a.c. component of the biopotential under measurement, such as an ECG.

The other equivalent circuit elements R_d and C_d are shown in Figure 4.4. Measured data shows that the other equivalent circuit elements in the figure, in particular the electrode capacitance C_d and the electrode resistance R_d, are not constant. Rather, they are inversely proportional to the square root of the frequency. For example, for a stainless steel electrode in a 0.9% NaCl solution, Geddes and Baker data can be approximated by the formulas

$$R_d = \frac{7269}{\sqrt{f}(0.157)} \qquad \text{(in } \Omega/\text{cm}^2)$$

and

(4.2)

$$C_d = \frac{25.2}{0.157\sqrt{f}} \qquad \text{(in } \mu\text{F/cm}^2)$$

for frequencies f within approximately 50% of 60 Hz. The values of R_d and C_d are also a function of current but remain nearly constant for current densities of less than 1 mA/cm^2.

An approximation to the values of the components in the equivalent circuit of an electrode as given in Figure 4.4 can be made by matching the measured magnitude of the impedance versus frequency to calculated values. The measured impedance is obtained by attaching electrodes to two body sites and measuring the ratio of the voltage to current as a function of frequency. Example data might be as in Figure 4.7, where half the measured magnitude is shown. This, then, represents the impedance of one electrode as a function of frequency.

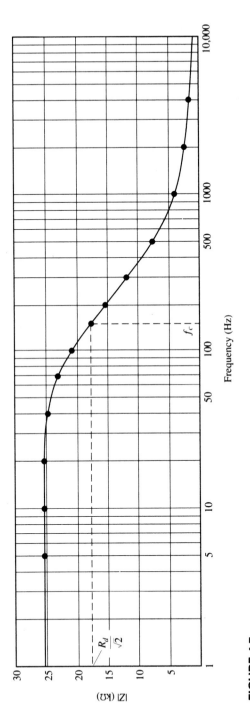

FIGURE 4.7
Magnitude of the impedance of a surface electrode.

EXAMPLE 4.2   The magnitude of the impedance of a single metal surface electrode immersed in an electrolyte is given in Figure 4.7. The half-cell potential is measured as -0.583 V. From this graphical data, compute the equivalent circuit elements as defined in Figure 4.4: R_d, C_d, and R_s. Let this approximation neglect the fact that R_d and C_d are functions of frequency as given in Equation (4.2).

SOLUTION   The data in Figure 4.7 shows that the impedance, $|Z|$, is relatively constant both at low frequency and at high frequency. Therefore, the first step is to analyze the low-frequency asymptote of the equivalent circuit in Figure 4.4. At frequencies approaching zero, we have

$$R_d \ll \frac{1}{j\omega C_d}$$

Also, since R_d is in parallel with it, we can neglect the capacitive reactance. Thus, for a low frequency, we have the formula

$$|Z_0| = R_d + R_s \qquad (4.3)$$

where $|Z_0|$ is the impedance when $f = 0$.
   From Figure 4.7, we see that $|Z|$ at low frequencies is such that

$$R_d + R_s = 25.4 \text{ k}\Omega$$

On the other hand, at high frequencies we have

$$\frac{1}{j\omega C_d} \ll R_d$$

That is, the capacitor effectively shorts out R_d, so that for high frequency,

$$|Z_H| = R_s \qquad (4.4)$$

where $|Z_H|$ is the impedance on the high-frequency asymptote. From Figure 4.7, $|Z|$ at high frequency is such that $R_s = 400\ \Omega$. Substituting this for R_s in Equation (4.3) gives

$$R_d = 25.4 \text{ k}\Omega - 0.4 \text{ k}\Omega = 25 \text{ k}\Omega$$

Thus we have determined the resistance elements of the equivalent circuit.
   Next, the approximation is made that $R_s \ll R_d$ as justified by the calculated values, and the equivalent circuit form is as shown in Figure 4.8. The

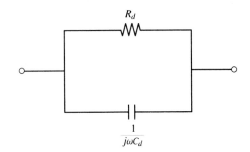

FIGURE 4.8
The critical-frequency approximation.

approximate equivalent circuit is at the critical frequency, f_c. This approximation is valid when

$$R_d = \frac{1}{2\pi f_c C_d}$$

Solving for C_d gives

$$C_d = \frac{1}{2\pi f_c R_d} \qquad (4.5)$$

To find f_c from the data in Figure 4.7, note that in Equation (4.1), when we neglect R_s and set $f = f_c$, we have approximately

$$|Z| = \frac{R_d}{\sqrt{2}}$$

Thus f_c is found graphically by locating a line at

$$\frac{R_d}{\sqrt{2}}$$

and noting the intersection at f_c on the graph, as indicated in Figure 4.7. There f_c is found to be 159 Hz. Computing C_d from Equation (4.5) then yields

$$C_d = 4 \times 10^{-8} \text{ F}$$

EXAMPLE 4.3   An Ag-AgCl electrode has an equivalent circuit as follows (referring to Figure 4.4): $E_{hc} = -0.349$ V, $R_d = 25$ kΩ, $R_s = 410$ Ω, and $C_d = 4 \times 10^{-8}$ F. Compute the magnitude of the impedance as a function of frequency.

SOLUTION   The use of Equation (4.1) at $f = 159$ Hz yields

$$Z = 410 + \frac{25{,}000}{1 + j2\pi(159)(4)(10^{-8})(25{,}000)}$$

$$= 17.97 \; \angle -44° \quad \text{(in kΩ)}$$

The other values, plotted in Figure 4.7, can be calculated with the computer Program A-1 in Appendix A.

4.2 THERMAL TRANSDUCERS

Thermistors, a form of thermal transducers, result from the property of some materials that they change resistance as a function of temperature. Conductors, such as copper, tend to have a *positive temperature coefficient*: their resistance increases as their temperature increases. This is caused by the fact that at higher temperatures, the atoms of the material vibrate more and have more collisions with the electrons passing through. Certain semiconductors, on the other hand, have a *negative temperature coefficient*, because at higher temperature more electrons are freed from their bonds to atoms. These free electrons are then available for conduction, causing the resistance of the material to decrease as temperature increases. Various encapsulations of thermistors are illustrated in Figure 4.9.

The resistance of a semiconductor material, R_t, is given by the relation

$$R_t = R_{t0} \exp\left[\beta\left(\frac{1}{T} - \frac{1}{T_0}\right)\right] \tag{4.6}$$

where T is the absolute temperature in degrees Kelvin, K,
   T_0 is the reference temperature in K units,
   R_{t0} is the resistance of the thermistor at T_0, and
   β is the material constant, typically 3000–5000 K.

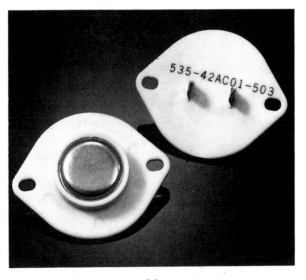

(a)

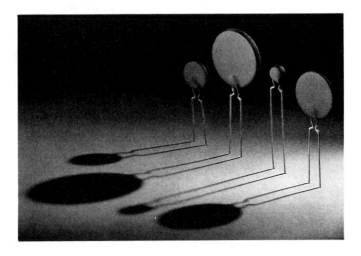

(b)

FIGURE 4.9
(a) A thermistor with a stainless steel top to keep it free of contaminants. (b) Resistive thermistors in ceramic cases. (c) (next page) Glass-encapsulated silicon-based resistive thermistors. (d) Chip thermistors for surface bonding, or epoxy bonding. (Courtesy of Fenwal Electronics)

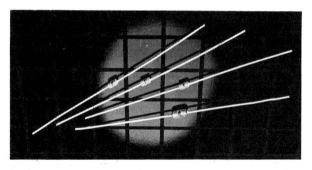

(c)

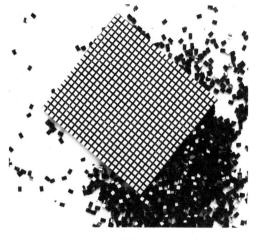

(d)

FIGURE 4.9 (continued)

Equation (4.6) shows that as temperature T increases, R_t decreases. It also shows that the resistance R_t is nonlinear. However, since temperatures vary only slightly inside the human body, the thermistor may be approximately linear over a sufficient temperature range to be usable as an approximately linear device in many applications.

EXAMPLE 4.4 A thermistor has a resistance of 10 Ω at 98 °F (37.6 °C), or 310 K. The material constant $\beta = 4000$ K. Make a plot of R_t versus temperature in the range from 300 to 320 K.

SOLUTION

$$R_t = 10 \exp\left[4000\left(\frac{1}{T} - \frac{1}{310}\right)\right]$$

For $T = 302$ K, $R_t = 14.08$ Ω, according to this equation.

Calculations of R_t for several values of β are plotted in Figure 4.10 as a function of the absolute temperature T.

Variations of the material constant β affect the linearity. β can be changed in a semiconductor by process variations such as altering the doping level. Also, a resistor that is constant as a function of temperature may be used to improve linearity. The linearizing resistor is placed in parallel with the thermistor. The value of the resistor that produces an inflection

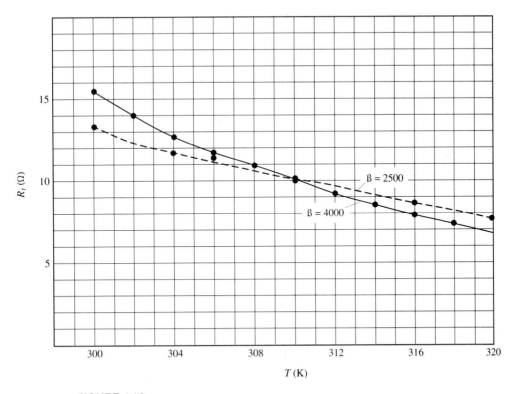

FIGURE 4.10
A plot of thermistor resistance versus temperature for Example 4.4.

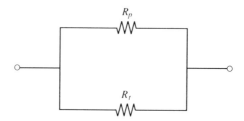

FIGURE 4.11
R_p linearizes R_t.

point at the reference temperature, T_0, for the parallel combination is given by

$$R_p = R_{t0} \frac{\beta - 2T_0}{\beta + 2T_0} \tag{4.7}$$

where R_{t0} is the thermistor resistance at the reference temperature. The linearizing circuit is shown in Figure 4.11.

EXAMPLE 4.5   Compute the values of R_p needed in parallel with the thermistor in Example 4.4 for several values of β, in order to linearize it.

SOLUTION

$$R_p = 10 \frac{\beta - 2(310)}{\beta + 2(310)}$$

Calculation of R_p for various β gives the following:

β (K)	R_p (Ω)
2500	6.03
3000	6.57
3500	6.99
4000	7.32

EXAMPLE 4.6   For the case $\beta = 4000$, plot the parallel combination of R_p and R_t versus temperature. Which is more linear, the parallel combination R_{tp}, or R_t versus T?

SOLUTION   The parallel combination

$$R_{tp} = \frac{R_p R_t}{R_p + R_t} \tag{4.8}$$

For $\beta = 4000$, $R_p = 7.32$ in the previous example. At $T = 306$ K, $R_t = 11.84$ Ω, and then

$$R_{tp} = \frac{(7.32)(11.84)}{7.32 + 11.84} = 4.52$$

The plot of R_t and R_{tp} on the same scale in Figure 4.12 shows that R_t with a β of 4000 is approximately linear over a range of 4 K, whereas the parallel combination R_{tp} is linear over more than 20 K.

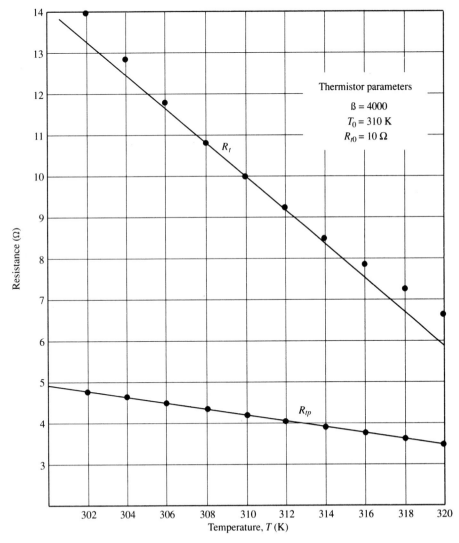

FIGURE 4.12
A thermistor R_t compared with the linearized version, R_{tp}.

R_{tp} is clearly more linear. However, this advantage must be traded off with the fact that R_{tp} is also less sensitive to temperature changes, as is apparent in Figure 4.12.

A thermistor may also be linearized by digital techniques. Digital techniques are sometimes preferable, because other circuit nonlinearities can be compensated for in the same process. The resistance-versus-temperature characteristic for several types of thermistor is shown in Figure 4.13. The

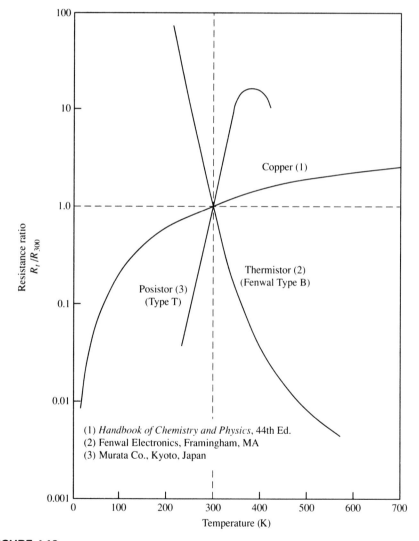

FIGURE 4.13
The resistance-versus-temperature curves for an example thermistor, a posistor, and copper. (From Geddes and Baker, *Principles of Applied Medical Instrumentation*, 2nd ed. New York: John Wiley & Sons. ©1975. p. 17. Used by permission.)

copper wire and the posistor have a positive temperature coefficient, and the thermistor has a negative temperature coefficient, as shown in the figure. A *positive temperature coefficient* means that the resistance increases as the temperature increases. A *negative temperature coefficient* means that the resistance of the thermistor decreases as temperature increases.

4.3 THE WHEATSTONE BRIDGE

Two properties of the Wheatstone bridge that make it useful in thermistor applications are that (1) the output voltage can be made to vary around a well-defined null resulting when the bridge is balanced; and (2) the output voltage is a linear function of small resistance changes in the bridge. The bridge circuit consists of an applied source V_a and four impedances Z_1, Z_2, Z_3, Z_x, as shown in Figure 4.14.

The definition for balance is that $V_{OUT} = 0$ for all values of V_a. By application of the voltage division principle, the output voltage is calculated in Figure 4.14. The branch plus-to-minus voltage drop from node B to node D is

$$V_{BD} = \frac{Z_1}{Z_x + Z_1} V_a \qquad (4.9)$$

Similarly, the branch voltage V_{CD} is

$$V_{CD} = \frac{Z_2}{Z_2 + Z_3} V_a \qquad (4.10)$$

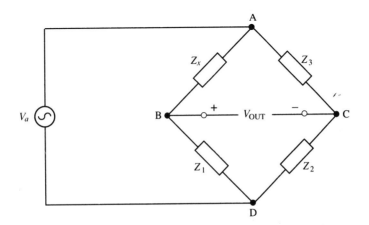

FIGURE 4.14
A Wheatstone bridge with phasor impedances.

The plus-to-minus voltage drop $V_{OUT} = V_{BC}$, and

$$V_{BC} = V_{BD} - V_{CD} = V_{OUT} \qquad \text{(4.11)}$$

Inserting (4.11) into (4.9) and (4.10) yields

$$V_{OUT} = \left[\frac{Z_1}{Z_x + Z_1} - \frac{Z_2}{Z_2 + Z_3} \right] V_a \qquad \text{(4.12)}$$

To achieve the balanced condition, we set $V_{OUT} = 0$ in Equation (4.12), yielding

$$\frac{Z_1}{Z_x + Z_1} = \frac{Z_2}{Z_2 + Z_3}$$

Algebraic manipulation of this equation gives

$$Z_1 Z_2 + Z_1 Z_3 = Z_2 Z_x + Z_2 Z_1$$

Then,

$$Z_x = \frac{Z_3 Z_1}{Z_2} \qquad \text{(4.13)}$$

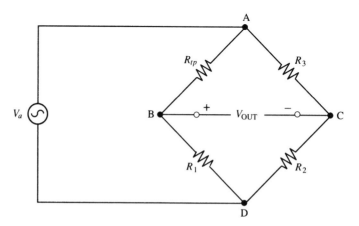

FIGURE 4.15
A linearized thermistor, R_{tp}, in a Wheatstone bridge.

Equation (4.13), then, is the condition for balance of a Wheatstone bridge. If this condition is met, the output voltage will be a null, or zero. This will also be true if the voltage generator has an internal impedance, since when $V_{OUT} = 0$, V_a drops out of Equation (4.12).

A thermistor is often chosen so that its resistance balances the bridge at a reference temperature but causes the bridge to become unbalanced when the temperature changes from the reference value and the condition in Equation (4.13) is no longer satisfied.

Since a thermistor is resistive, the Wheatstone bridge employing it uses resistors such that $R_{tp} = Z_x$, $R_1 = Z_1$, $R_2 = Z_2$, and $R_3 = Z_3$. The output voltage for such a bridge is obtained by analyzing the circuit in Figure 4.15.

EXAMPLE 4.7   The thermistor linearized as indicated in Example 4.5 is placed in the Wheatstone bridge of Figure 4.15 in place of R_{tp}. The material constant $\beta = 4000$ K. The reference resistance $R_{t0} = 10 \ \Omega$ at $T_0 = 310$ K. Make a plot of the output voltage V_{OUT} versus temperature T for $V_a = 10$ V and

$$300 \text{ K} < T < 320 \text{ K}$$

The resistor values are $R_1 = 4 \ \Omega$, $R_2 = 1 \ k\Omega$, and $R_3 = 1 \ k\Omega$.

SOLUTION   The branch resistance from node B to node C in Figure 4.15 is infinite. Then, by voltage division, the output voltage V_{OUT} is given by

$$V_{OUT} = \left[\frac{R_1}{R_1 + R_{tp}} - \frac{R_2}{R_2 + R_3} \right] V_a \qquad (4.14)$$

To plot V_{OUT} versus T_1, it is necessary to use Equations (4.8), (4.7), and (4.6). For example, for $T = 306$ K, Equation (4.6) yields

$$R_t = 11.84 \ \Omega$$

This into Equation (4.7) yields

$$R_p = 7.32 \ \Omega$$

Both of these values into Equation (4.8) yield

$$R_{tp} = 4.52 \ \Omega$$

These three values into Equation (4.14) then yield

$$V_{\text{OUT}} = -0.31 \text{ V}$$

To complete the graph, it is convenient to use a programmable calculator. A flow diagram is given in Figure 4.16 for Program A-2, given in Appendix A.

A plot of V_{OUT} versus T resulting from these calculations is given in Figure 4.17.

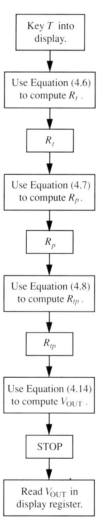

FIGURE 4.16
Flow diagram for Example 4.7 for the calculation using Program A-2 in Appendix A.

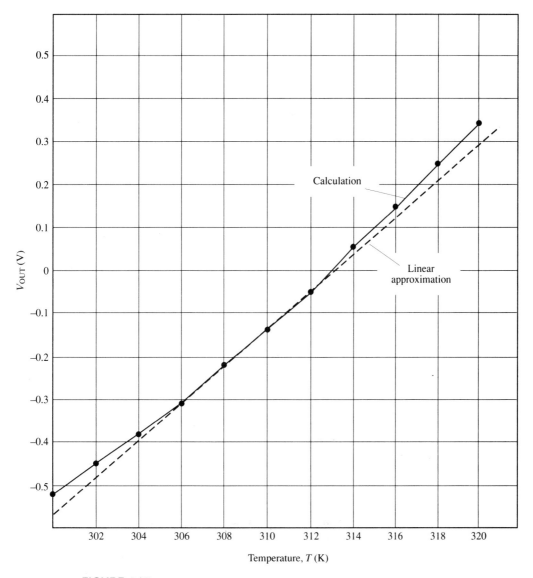

FIGURE 4.17
The output voltage due to a linearized thermistor as a function of temperature, as computed in Example 4.7.

Sensitivity of a Wheatstone Bridge

Several kinds of transducers, including the thermistor analyzed above and the strain gauge that will be analyzed, operate on the principle that the measured parameter causes a small change in the resistance of the device. In a thermistor, for example, a small change in temperature causes a corresponding change in thermistor resistance. A Wheatstone bridge is commonly used to measure the change in an output voltage, ΔV_{OUT}, due to the change in output resistance of the transducer, ΔR_x. The sensitivity of the bridge, S_R, is defined by Equation (4.15) as the change in output voltage per unit resistance change:

$$S_R = \frac{\Delta V_{\text{OUT}}}{\Delta R_x} \tag{4.15}$$

To compute the bridge sensitivity, a typical bridge circuit is analyzed in Figure 4.18.

When $\Delta R_x = 0$, $V_{\text{OUT}} = 0$. For other values of ΔR_x, $V_{\text{OUT}} = \Delta V_{\text{OUT}}$, the change from zero, and

$$\Delta V_{\text{OUT}} = \left[\frac{R_x - \Delta R_x}{R_x + \Delta R_x + R_x - \Delta R_x} - \frac{R_x}{R_x + R_x} \right] V_a$$

Grouping terms,

$$\Delta V_{\text{OUT}} = \left[\frac{R_x}{2R_x} - \frac{\Delta R_x}{2R_x} - \frac{R_x}{2R_x} \right] V_a$$

or

$$\Delta V_{\text{OUT}} = \frac{-\Delta R_x}{2R_x} V_a$$

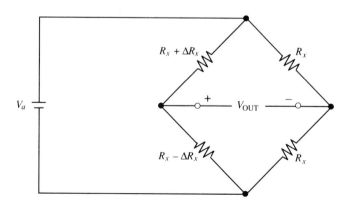

FIGURE 4.18
Two strain gauges in a Wheatstone bridge.

The sensitivity by Equation (4.15) is then

$$S_R = \frac{-V_a}{2R_x} \quad \text{(in V/Ω)} \tag{4.16}$$

It is clear from this result that the sensitivity is proportional to the excitation voltage, V_a, on the bridge circuit, and is affected by R_x.

It can also be shown that if the transducer causes a variation in only one resistor arm of the bridge, the sensitivity is reduced by half. (See Exercise 13.)

EXAMPLE 4.8 A transducer is represented by Figure 4.18(a). $R_x = 1$ kΩ, and the excitation voltage on the Wheatstone bridge is 20 V. Calculate the sensitivity in volts per ohm.

SOLUTION Using Equation (4.16), we have

$$S_R = \frac{-20}{2(10^3)} = -0.01 \quad \text{(in V/Ω)}$$

4.4 STRAIN GAUGES

A *strain gauge* is a device that measures changes in the length of an object. In the strain gauges considered here, the length change causes a change in resistance in the gauge. For example, Weston strain gauges, such as shown in Figure 4.19, are wrapped around an arm or leg to measure changes in their diameter, which in turn may be used to measure blood volume. A volume-measuring instrument of this type is called a *plethysmograph*. A finger-mounted strain gauge for measuring small changes in blood volume flowing through the finger is shown in Figure 4.20.

Strain, S, is defined as the fractional change in the length of an object in the direction of the applied force, as given in Equation (4.17), where l is the length,

$$S = \frac{\Delta l}{l} \tag{4.17}$$

The *gauge factor G* is defined as the percentage, or fractional, change in resistance divided by the percentage, or fractional, change in length. This

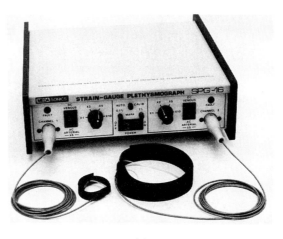

(a)

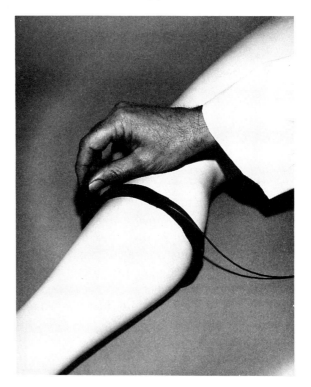

(b)

FIGURE 4.19
(a) A strain gauge plethysmograph. (b) Strain gauges for attachment to a limb. (Courtesy Meda Sonics Inc.)

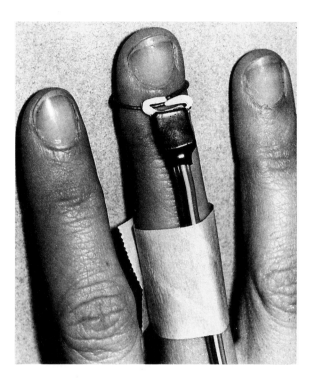

FIGURE 4.20
A finger-mounted strain gauge for measuring small volume changes. (Courtesy of D. E. Hokanson, Inc.)

is expressed mathematically in the following equation, where R is the resistance:

$$G = \frac{\dfrac{\Delta R}{R}}{S} \tag{4.18}$$

Therefore, combining these two equations, we have

$$\frac{\Delta R}{R} = \frac{G \Delta l}{l} \tag{4.19}$$

where l is the resting length of the strain gauge wire, R is the resting resistance of the strain gauge wire, Δl is the change in wire length, and ΔR is the corresponding change in gauge resistance. In Table 4.2, the gauge factor and strain are listed for several representative materials used in strain

TABLE 4.2
Gauge Factors and Young's Modulus

Material	Gauge factor, G	Young's modulus (lb/in.^{2})
Constantan	2.1	$24 \times 10^{+6}$
Nickel	-12 to -20	$30 \times 10^{+6}$
Silicon	~ 120	$27 \times 10^{+6}$

gauges. Another property of strain gauge materials that is relevant to medical application is the measure of the strain induced by an applied force. The typical strain gauge element consists of a wire (or metal cylinder) of length l, as shown in Figure 4.21, where f is the applied force stretching the bar of cross-sectional area A. Stress is defined as the pressure applied to a body. The stress, or pressure, required to double the length of a bar is called Young's modulus, M. That is, when $\Delta l = l$,

$$\frac{f}{A} = M \qquad (\text{in N/m}^2)$$

Here $l =$ the rest length of the bar, and $l + \Delta l$ is the length of the bar under stress, M. For other values of stress,

$$\Delta l = \frac{fl}{AM} \qquad (4.20)$$

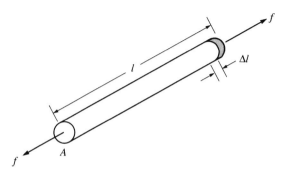

FIGURE 4.21
A bar under tensile force.

EXAMPLE 4.9 A constantan wire strain gauge has a rest length of 1 in. What is the change in length when an applied force of 2 lb is applied? The diameter of the wire is 5 mils (5×10^{-3} in.).

SOLUTION

$$\Delta l = \frac{2 \text{ lb}}{\pi \left(\dfrac{5(10^{-3})}{2} \right)^2 \text{in.}^2} \left(\frac{1 \text{ in.}}{24(10^6) \dfrac{\text{lb}}{\text{in.}^2}} \right)$$

$$\Delta l = \frac{2}{\pi 25(6)} = 4.24 \, (10^{-3}) \qquad (\text{in inches})$$

Combining Equation (4.17) with (4.20) gives

$$S = \frac{f}{AM}$$

Combining this with Equation (4.19) gives

$$\frac{\Delta R}{R} = \frac{Gf}{MA} \qquad\qquad (4.21)$$

where G = the gauge factor,
M = Young's modulus,
f = the force applied to the strain gauge, and
A = the cross-sectional area of the gauge wire.

Inspection of Table 4.2 and Equation (4.20) shows that Young's modulus, M, does not change much among the materials listed. However, the gauge factor changes radically. Clearly, silicon is much more sensitive to pressure than constantan. But silicon is also very sensitive to temperature change, whereas constantan is less so. Therefore, to take advantage of the pressure sensitivity of silicon, it is often necessary to design circuitry to compensate for changes in temperature that affect silicon.

EXAMPLE 4.10 A wire as shown in Figure 4.21 has a rest length of 1 in., a diameter of 5 mils, and in both cases a resting resistance of 1 kΩ. Compute the change in resistance for (a) constantan and (b) silicon. One pound tensile force is applied.

SOLUTION   For part (a) from Equation (4.21) we calculate

$$\Delta R = \frac{1000(2.1)(1)(4)}{24(10^6)(\pi)(5 \times 10^{-3})^2}$$

Thus $R = 4.46 \ \Omega$ for constantan. Likewise, for part (b)

$$\Delta R = \frac{1000(120)(1)(4)}{27(10^6)(\pi)(5 \times 10^{-3})^2}$$

So $R = 226.35 \ \Omega$ for silicon.

The silicon has a resistance change approximately 50 times larger for the same change in applied force. However, it is much more sensitive to temperature changes.

The Strain Gauge in a Wheatstone Bridge

The strain gauge producing the resistance $\Delta R_x + R_x$ in Figure 4.22 produces an output voltage V_{OUT}:

$$V_{\text{OUT}} = \left[\frac{R_1}{R_1 + R_x + \Delta R_x} - \frac{R_2}{R_2 + R_3} \right] V_a \qquad \textbf{(4.22)}$$

where, from Equation (4.19),

$$\Delta R_x = \frac{G \Delta l}{l} R_x \qquad \textbf{(4.23)}$$

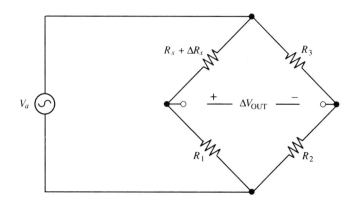

FIGURE 4.22
A strain gauge in one arm of a Wheatstone bridge.

EXAMPLE 4.11 A strain gauge has a gauge factor, G, of 4, the rest length is 0.9 in., and the rest resistance is 2 kΩ. It is placed in the Wheatstone bridge of Figure 4.22. Plot the output voltage V_{OUT} as a function of the elongation length Δl. $R_1 = 1$ kΩ, $R_2 = 2$ kΩ, $R_3 = 3$ kΩ, and $V_a = 10$ V.

SOLUTION A calculator program of Equation (4.22) and (4.23) follows the flow diagram in Figure 4.23. The program is listed in Appendix A, Program A-3. A sample calculation when $\Delta l = 0.04$ in. is from Equation (4.22):

$$\Delta R_x = \frac{4(0.04)(2000)}{0.9} = 355.55$$

Putting this into Equation (4.22) yields

$$V_{OUT} = \left[\frac{1000}{1000 + 2000 + 355.5} - \frac{2000}{2000 + 3000} \right] 10$$

$$= -1.019 \text{ V}$$

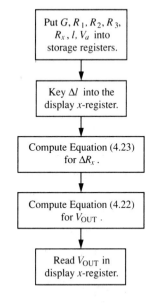

FIGURE 4.23
Flow diagram for Example 4.11 (Appendix A, Program A-3).

A plot of V_{OUT} resulting from several values of Δl is given in Figure 4.24. The plot shows that the output voltage of the Wheatstone bridge is a linear function of strain when Δl is small.

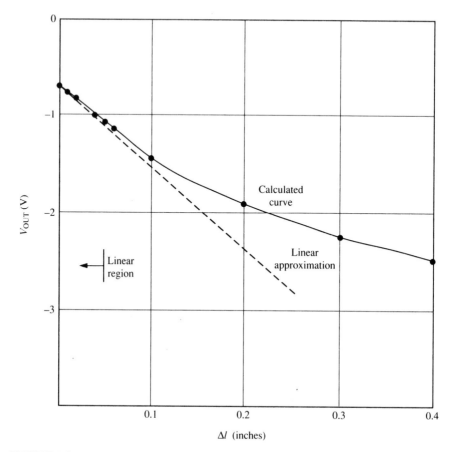

FIGURE 4.24
Output voltage due to the elongation of a strain gauge.

Sensitivity of a Strain Gauge

The sensitivity of a strain gauge, S_g, with respect to the output voltage change it causes in an electrical circuit, is defined as the ratio of the output voltage, ΔV_{OUT}, in Figure 4.22 to the change in length of the strain gauge, Δl, in Figure 4.21. That is,

$$S_g = \frac{\Delta V_{OUT}}{\Delta l} \tag{4.24}$$

EXAMPLE 4.12   Compute the strain gauge sensitivity, S_g, for the linear portion of the strain gauge of Example 4.11. Use the graphical data of Figure 4.24.

SOLUTION Inspection of the data of Figure 4.24 shows that the strain gauge is nearly linear for elongations less than approximately 0.05 in. The strain gauge sensitivity taken from Figure 4.24 for small displacements is

$$S_g = \frac{-0.67 + 0.76}{0 - 0.01} = -9.0 \text{ V/in.}$$

Inspection of Figure 4.24 shows that the strain gauge becomes nonlinear for elongations greater than 0.05 in.

In medical applications, strain gauges fall into one of two categories: bonded or unbonded. The *bonded* strain gauge is attached along its entire length with a cement, or bonding compound, to the body, or surface that elongates. The *unbonded* strain gauge is connected at the end points or at several points along the body or surface that elongates or contracts under stress.

A pressure transducer using a strain gauge as an element is illustrated in Figure 4.25. A fluid such as blood from a catheter enters the dome and displaces the diaphragm. This in turn stretches the gauge wires attached to the case on one end, and a shaft from the diaphragm at the other end. An example value of the sensitivity of such a pressure transducer is 375 μV/mmHg. This is based on a sensitivity of 50 μV/mmHg when attached to a Wheatstone bridge excited by 7.5 V. Applied pressures typically range from −50 to 300 mmHg. The effect of this transducer in a Wheatstone bridge is illustrated in Exercise 13. Disposable pressure transducers are constructed similarly and are calibrated with laser-trimmed resistors molded into the structure in the form of a Wheatstone bridge.

4.5 THE DIFFERENTIAL CAPACITIVE TRANSDUCER

A differential capacitor can be used to produce an appreciable imbalance in a bridge circuit for an extremely small physical displacement of the central plate of the differential capacitor. A schematic for a differential capacitor appears in Figure 4.26.

The differential capacitor consists of two capacitors, C_1 and C_2, placed back to back and sharing a common plate. The motion of this common plate due to a displacement of a body to which it is attached causes a decrease in one capacitor and an increase in the other according to the capacitance formulas,

$$C_1 = \epsilon \frac{A}{d - x} \tag{4.25}$$

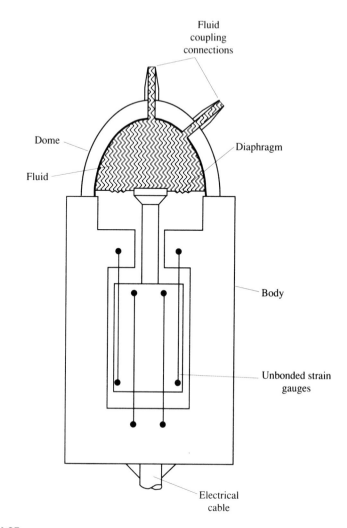

FIGURE 4.25
Resistive strain gauge pressure transducer.

and

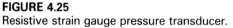

$$C_2 = \epsilon \, \frac{A}{d + x} \qquad\qquad (4.26)$$

where A is the capacitor area and ϵ is the dielectric constant. Here C_1 is increased by a positive x displacement, while C_2 is simultaneously decreased

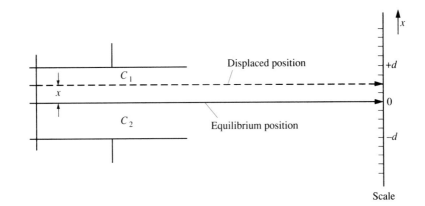

FIGURE 4.26
Differential capacitor transducer.

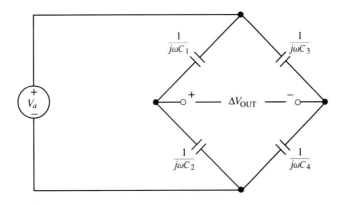

FIGURE 4.27
Differential capacitor in a bridge circuit.

by the same positive x displacement in Figure 4.26. To translate the displacement x into a voltage output for a Wheatstone bridge, consider Figure 4.27. The voltage output V_{OUT} is

$$V_{\text{OUT}} = \left[\frac{\dfrac{1}{j\omega C_2}}{\dfrac{1}{j\omega C_1} + \dfrac{1}{j\omega C_2}} - \frac{\dfrac{1}{j\omega C_4}}{\dfrac{1}{j\omega C_3} + \dfrac{1}{j\omega C_4}} \right] V_a$$

Multiplying the top and bottom of these two terms by $C_1 C_2$ and $C_3 C_4$, respectively, and canceling $j\omega$ gives

$$V_{OUT} = \left[\frac{C_1}{C_1 + C_2} - \frac{C_3}{C_3 + C_4} \right] V_a \tag{4.27}$$

Putting Equations (4.25) and (4.26) into Equation (4.27) then gives

$$V_{OUT} = \left[\frac{\dfrac{1}{d-x}}{\dfrac{1}{d+x} + \dfrac{1}{d-x}} - \frac{C_3}{C_3 + C_4} \right] V_a$$

and, by simplifying algebra, this becomes

$$V_{OUT} = \left[\frac{1}{1 + \dfrac{d-x}{d+x}} - \frac{C_3}{C_4 + C_3} \right] V_a$$

or

$$V_{OUT} = \left[\frac{d+x}{2d} - \frac{C_3}{C_4 + C_3} \right] V_a \tag{4.28}$$

It is clear from this equation that the output voltage is proportional to the displacement, x, plus a constant term. The sensitivity of the differential transducer S_x is defined as the change in output voltage, ΔV_{OUT}, divided by the change in displacement. That is, from Equation (4.28) we have

$$S_x = \frac{d V_{OUT}}{dx} = \frac{V_a}{2d} \quad \text{(in V/m)} \tag{4.29}$$

EXAMPLE 4.13   A differential capacitor consists of three metal plates, each with an area of 2 cm^2 in air. Compute the equilibrium capacity for an equilibrium displacement, d, of 1 mm. Also compute the sensitivity for a 10-V a.c. bridge bias, V_a.

SOLUTION

$$C_{\text{equi}} = \frac{\epsilon A}{d}$$

$$= \frac{8.8(10^{-12}) \text{ F/m}}{10^{-3} \text{ m}} (2 \times 10^{-2})^2 \text{ m}^2$$

$$= 1.76 \ (10^{-12}) \text{ F}$$

The sensitivity is

$$S_x = \frac{10}{2(10^{-3})} = 5000 \text{ V/m}$$

In conclusion, it is clear that the differential capacitor is perfectly linear and is very sensitive to displacements.

A differential capacitor can be used in a pressure transducer to measure pressure, P. An example is illustrated in Figure 4.28. The movable diaphragm changes position such that the displacement x is proportional to pressure. From Equation (4.29), the sensitivity, $S_P = dV_{\text{OUT}}/dP$, becomes

$$S_P = \frac{k_c V_a}{2d} \tag{4.30}$$

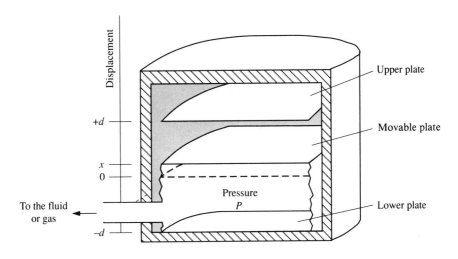

FIGURE 4.28
Capacitive pressure transducer.

S_P has units of volts per millimeter of mercury (V/mmHg), and k_c is a proportionality constant.

4.6 INDUCTIVE TRANSDUCERS

The motion in a diaphragm due to displacement or pressure can also be transformed into a voltage by changing an inductance. A widely used form of this is the linear variable differential transformer (LVDT) illustrated in Figure 4.29. Changes in the applied pressure move the transformer core or ferrous material such that the top inductor increases by ΔL, the change in the inductance, when the bottom inductor decreases by the same amount. Analysis of the equivalent-circuit Wheatstone bridge (Figure 4.30) yields

$$V_{\text{OUT}} = \left[\frac{j\omega(L - \Delta L)}{j\omega(L + \Delta L) + j\omega(L - \Delta L)} - \frac{R}{R + R} \right] V_a$$

which directly reduces to

$$V_{\text{OUT}} = \frac{-\Delta L}{2L} \, V_a$$

In the LVDT, the pressure, P, is proportional to the change in the inductance. The proportionality constant is defined as k_1. The formula is

$$V_{\text{OUT}} = \frac{k_1 P V_a}{2L} \tag{4.31}$$

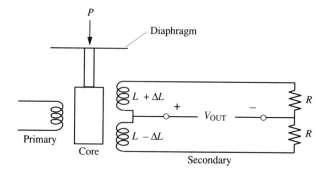

FIGURE 4.29
Schematic of linear variable differential transformer.

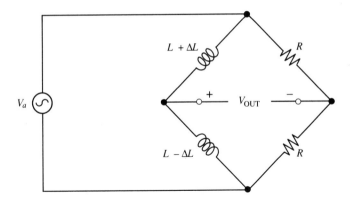

FIGURE 4.30
LVDT equivalent circuit.

The sensitivity of the transducer $S_1 = dV_{OUT}/dP$. Therefore,

$$S_1 = \frac{k_1 V_a}{2L}$$

Commercially available pressure transducers for measuring blood pressure, using the LVDT principle, are capable of measuring pressures from -100 to 400 mmHg. With $V_a = 5$ V, the sensitivity $S_1 = 200$ μV/mmHg is a representative value. The applied voltages may range from 5 to 20 V at frequencies from 1.5 to 15 kHz.

4.7 TROUBLESHOOTING AT THE COMPONENT LEVEL

In the hierarchy of troubleshooting levels described in Section 3.5 of the previous chapter, starting with the system level and working down, troubleshooting of transducers is done at the component level. Since they are the point of contact between the patient and the instrument, transducers are often vulnerable to damage. Troubleshooting techniques apt to be effective with them are visual inspection, interview of the operator, and voltage or resistance measurement. Since transducers are often moved about and have delicate parts, they are subject to wear and abuse.

While troubleshooting a surface electrode, an inspector should check its attachment to the skin to make sure the electrode gel is adequate and has not dried out. The adhesive connection should be secure. Excessive hair under the electrode, or a scarred or bony surface, can cause a poor signal connection. Visual inspection of cable connections for frays, breaks, or corrosion may reveal a problem.

Problems in thermistors can arise from poor thermal conductivity between the body tissue monitored and the thermistor. A secure mechanical connection free of air gaps is essential. The thermistor is usually placed in one branch of a Wheatstone bridge. A voltage check of the bridge output and resistance measurements on its components could reveal thermistor-related faults. Nonlinearity of the thermistor, for example, could be caused by a failure in a linearizing resistor attached across the thermistor.

The sensitivity of the thermistor can also be affected by faults in the bridge branch components. Another possible cause of poor sensitivity is a drop in the excitation voltage of the bridge. Because the transducer cable is vulnerable to wear, this could cause loss of thermistor sensitivity. To isolate the problem you could use circuit analysis, voltage or resistance checks. The final proof that a component is faulty is that changing the part either changes the symptoms of the problem or causes it to disappear.

Troubles in a strain gauge are also affected by mechanical contact with the patient. Elimination of these problems is usually the responsibility of the equipment operator. Problems with the balancing bridge and the excitation voltage are similar to those affecting thermistors.

The operation of pressure transducers often depends on having the pressure being measured transmitted through a fluid column. Any air bubbles in the line seriously degrade both the transducer sensitivity and its frequency response. (See Chapter 11, Figure 11.27.)

Bubbles often can be seen visually, and flushed. This must be done when the transducer is removed from the patient, so as to remove any hazard of transferring bubbles into the bloodstream.

In summary, troubleshooting transducers is a component-level task. It is usually done at the beginning of a signal tracing procedure. Because of the visibility of the transducer-body interface, visual inspection is often an effective troubleshooting method.

REFERENCES

Cobbold, R. S. C. *Transducers for Biomedical Measurements.* New York: John Wiley & Sons, 1974.

Geddes, L. A., and Baker, L. E. *Principles of Applied Biomedical Instrumentation.* New York: John Wiley & Sons, 1968.

Neuman, M. R. "Biopotential Electrodes." In *Medical Instrumentation, Application and Design*, edited by J. G. Webster. Boston: Houghton Mifflin, 1978.

Peura, R. A., and Webster, J. G. "Basic Transducers and Principles." Chapter 2 in *Medical Instrumentation, Application and Design*, edited by J. G. Webster. Boston: Houghton Mifflin, 1978.

Seippel, R. G. *Transducer Interfacing.* Englewood Cliffs, NJ: Prentice-Hall, 1988.

EXERCISES

1. A thermistor has a resistance of 25 Ω at body temperature, 37 °C. The material constant is 3500 K. This thermistor is linearized with a resistor R_p given by Equation (4.7) and is placed in the position R_{tp} in the given Wheatstone bridge (Figure 4.31).

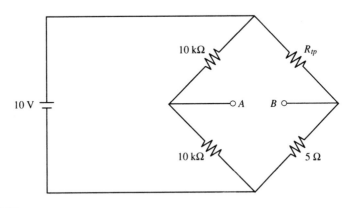

FIGURE 4.31

(a) Compute R_{tp} for $T = 35$ °C and $T = 39$ °C.
(b) Compute V_{AB} at the temperatures given in part (a).
(c) Assuming the thermistor is linear between these temperatures, compute the sensitivity in units of V/°C.

2. In the Figure 4.32 bridge circuit, find the Thevenin equivalent at the output terminals *A-B*. Draw the Thevenin equivalent circuit and label the unknown values. If a 5-kΩ resistor is attached to terminals *A* and *B*, compute the current flowing through I_{AB}.

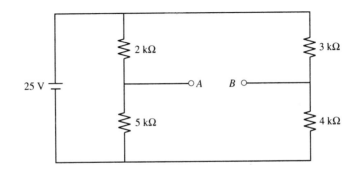

FIGURE 4.32

3. The half-cell potential of silver is 0.799 V, and the half-cell potential of gold is 1.68 V. If silver and gold are placed in an active electrolyte, what is the electrode offset voltage, V_{OS}, as indicated in Figure 4.33?

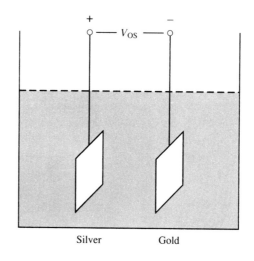

FIGURE 4.33

4. In the circuit of Figure 4.34, a measurement shows that the magnitude of the impedance $|Z|$ is given by $|Z| = 7.0 \text{ k}\Omega$ at a frequency of 200 Hz. Compute the capacitance, C_d.

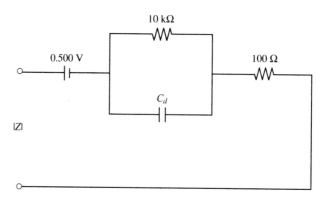

FIGURE 4.34

5. In the circuit of Figure 4.35, the capacitor, C, is adjusted until $V_{AB} = 0$, a balance. Compute the value of C.

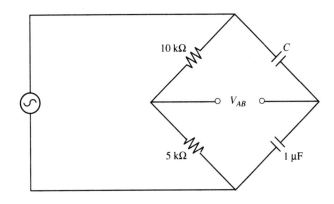

FIGURE 4.35

6. The circuit of Figure 4.36 represents the equivalent circuit of a metal surface electrode against skin treated with an electrolyte gel. A measurement of the magnitude of the impedance Z is given by $|Z| = 7.07$ kΩ, at a frequency of 400 Hz.

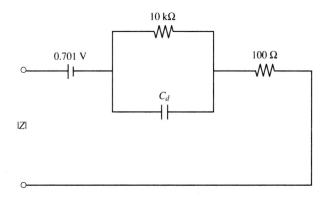

FIGURE 4.36

(a) Compute the capacitance C_d.
(b) Give the value of the half-cell potential.
(c) Compute the magnitude of the skin impedance, Z, at a frequency of $f =$ 200 Hz. Assume C_d remains constant as a function of frequency.

7. In the circuit of Figure 4.37, find V_{AB} when $V_1 = 30$ V and $V_2 = 20$ V.

8. Compute the formula for the thermistor graphed in Figure 4.38 in the form temperature $T = mR_T + b$; that is, find the slope m and the intercept b.

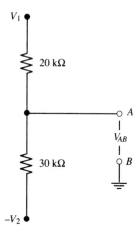

FIGURE 4.37

9. The thermistor of Figure 4.38 is used in the Wheatstone bridge (Figure 4.39) to measure the temperature. Find the temperature of the thermistor when the voltage V_{AB} in the bridge containing the thermistor is adjusted to a null.

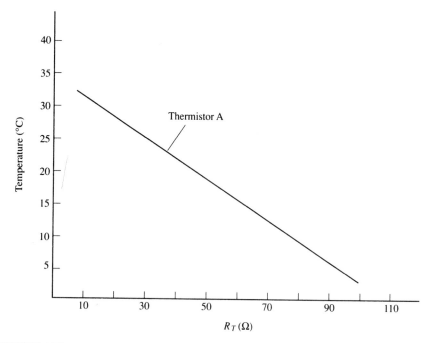

FIGURE 4.38

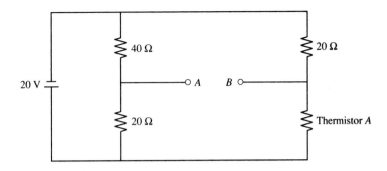

FIGURE 4.39

10. Compute the value of the loop currents I_1 and I_2 in the network of Figure 4.40.

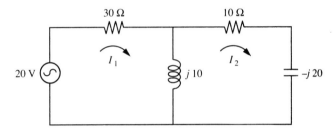

FIGURE 4.40

11. A thermistor has the characteristic $R_T = 300\ T + 5000\ \Omega$. Two such thermistors are arranged in a bridge in Figure 4.41.
    (a) Compute V_{AB} when $T = 15\ °C$.
    (b) Compute V_{AB} when $T = 18\ °C$.
    (c) Assuming the output voltage is a linear function of temperature, compute the bridge sensitivity, S, in units of V/°C.

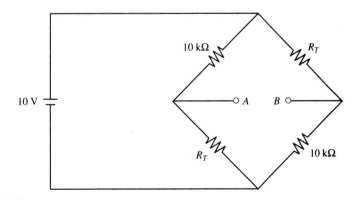

FIGURE 4.41

12. A strain gauge has a gauge factor $G = 5$, which measures the ratio of the percentage change in resistance to percent change in length. The rest length is 1.2 in., the rest resistance R_x is 3 kΩ, and it is placed as indicated in Figure 4.42.

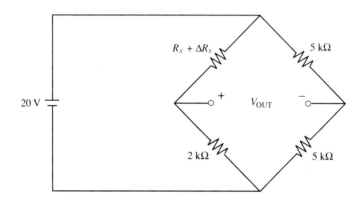

FIGURE 4.42

(a) Find the output voltage V_{OUT} when the strain gauge is at rest and not elongated.

(b) Find the output voltage when the strain gauge is lengthened by 0.04 in.

(c) From parts (a) and (b), calculate the strain gauge sensitivity S in units of V/in.

*13. In Figure 4.22, show that the sensitivity, S_R, of the strain gauge that causes ΔR_x is given by

$$S_R = \frac{-V_a R_1}{(R_1 + R_x)^2} \quad (\text{in V}/\Omega)$$

14. A thermistor changes resistance from 100 Ω at 10 °C to 101 Ω at 12 °C. The thermistor is placed in Figure 4.22 as $R_x + \Delta R_x$, and $R_1 = 100$ Ω, $R_2 = 1$ kΩ, and $R_3 = 2$ kΩ. Compute the sensitivity in volts per degree Celsius, S_t. Let $V_a = 10$ V.

5

Biopotential Amplifiers

One of the most fundamental and widely used tools of measurement is the balance scale. More than 5,000 years ago, balance scales were used to compare the weights of objects, such as grain or precious metals, with standard weights. In Chapter 4, we considered the Wheatstone bridge as a balanced circuit capable of making sensitive difference measurements on transducer outputs. When electronic components, such as field effect transistors (FETs) and other transistors, are used, the Wheatstone bridge can be made into what is called a *differential amplifier*.

A differential amplifier, often abbreviated *diff amp*, is an electronic amplifier in which the output voltage is proportional to the difference between two input voltages. Diff amps are particularly useful for measuring biopotentials, since many biopotentials of clinical and medical diagnostic significance consist of the difference in voltage on two body sites. The ECG, for example, is measured as the difference in surface potential between two limbs. The electroencephalogram (EEG) is the difference in surface potential on two skull sites. Likewise, the electromyogram (EMG) records the difference between two potentials measured on a muscle. The diff amp is ideal for measuring these difference potentials and is thus often used in medical instrumentation.

Diff amps are widely used because of the advances in semiconductor chip fabrication techniques as well. In 1970, the number of active elements that could be fabricated on a chip was about one thousand. By 1987 this number had increased to over one million. This increase in efficiency has led to a reduction in the cost of the diff amp, from about $350 in the 1950s, when vacuum tubes were used, to about 35 cents in 1987. Along with the

1000-to-1 reduction in cost has come an equally dramatic reduction in size, as illustrated in Figure 5.1. Here, a semiconductor chip diff amp is compared with a vacuum-tube model of the 1950s. Furthermore, integrated-circuit diff amps have such low power-drain requirements that it is feasible to have battery-powered medical instruments, such as pacemakers. These advantages of low cost, low power drain, and small size have stimulated the use of diff amps in medical equipment, and have indeed contributed significantly to the increase in the number of electronic medical instruments in use today.

The symbol for the diff amp is given in Figure 5.2(b), and the mathematical definition of the diff amp is

$$V_{\text{OUT}} = A_d(V_2 - V_1) \qquad (5.1)$$

where V_1 and V_2 are input voltage drops measured to ground, V_{OUT} is the output voltage, referenced to ground, and A_d is the differential voltage gain.

A particularly convenient property of the diff amp is that it tends to eliminate *common-mode voltage* interference. Common-mode voltages are

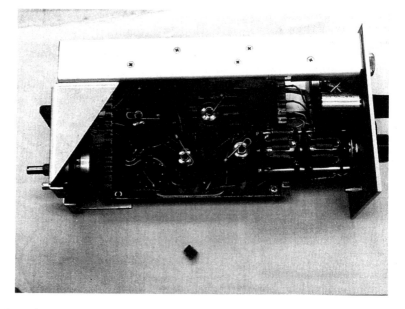

FIGURE 5.1
(Above) A 1950s diff amp made of vacuum tubes. (Below) An integrated-circuit chip as a diff amp.

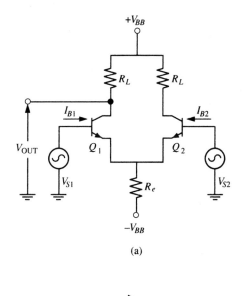

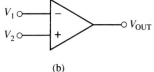

(a)

(b)

FIGURE 5.2
(a) A transistor circuit diff amp. (b) The circuit symbol for a diff amp.

those that have the same value on all diff amp input terminals. This means that if V_1 and V_2 are common-mode voltages, then $V_1 = V_2$, and the output V_{OUT} due to them is zero, by Equation (5.1). That is, the output voltage due to common-mode interference tends toward zero in a diff amp. How this fact helps reduce interference in biopotential amplifiers is explained in Section 5.3.

5.1 A TRANSISTOR DIFFERENTIAL AMPLIFIER

A diff amp is usually fabricated as an integrated circuit on a chip. However, to illustrate the concept and increase your understanding of the diff amp, let us consider the transistor diff amp circuit given in Figure 5.2(a). This amplifier is a balanced circuit with the transistors Q_1 and Q_2, and the collector resistors R_L being identical. It uses two power supplies with voltages V_{BB} and $-V_{BB}$, respectively. The output voltage is measured as the plus-to-minus voltage drop from one of the collectors to ground. The fact that V_{OUT} is measured to ground is an advantage, since it then can be used as an input to successive amplifier stages for further processing.

The transistors are assumed to have a small emitter resistance, r_e, such that $\beta r_e \ll r_b$, and it can be neglected in Figure 5.3(a). An a.c. equivalent circuit representation for the transistors, using lowercase "r" for resistance, is given in this figure, as modified from Figure 1.28 in Chapter 1. Here, the a.c. collector resistance, r_c, is assumed to be much greater than R_L and can be neglected in the equivalent circuit. r_b is the base resistance, and I_B is the value of an ideal current source. Here $\beta_{ac} \approx \beta_{dc}$ and is written as β.

The a.c. equivalent circuit for the differential amplifier is formed by replacing the bias supply with a short circuit, and by replacing the transis-

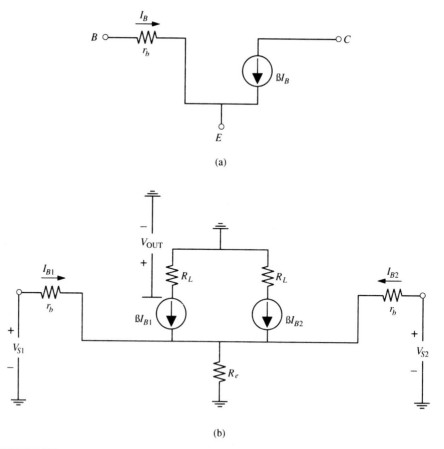

(a)

(b)

FIGURE 5.3
(a) An approximate equivalent circuit of a transistor. (b) The small-signal equivalent circuit of a diff amp.

tors Q_1 and Q_2 with their a.c. equivalent circuit, as given in Figure 5.3(a). Figure 5.3(b) is used to compute the a.c. component of the output voltage, V_{OUT}, considered as a phasor. The d.c. component could then be found by analyzing Figure 5.2 with $V_{S1} = V_{S2} = 0$, as is done in Exercise 6.

In order to determine the output voltage V_{OUT} of the differential amplifier as a function of the difference between the two input signal voltages V_{S1} and V_{S2}, we apply Kirchhoff's voltage law (KVL) to three loops in Figure 5.3, where resistors R_L and R_e are external to the transistor equivalent circuit. First note that the current going through R_e is

$$I_{B1} + \beta I_{B1} + \beta I_{B2} + I_{B2}$$

Then we may write the loop equation involving V_{S2} as

$$V_{S2} = I_{B2} r_b + (I_{B1} + \beta I_{B1} + \beta I_{B2} + I_{B2}) R_e$$

Rewriting this gives

$$V_{S2} = I_{B2} r_b + (\beta + 1)(I_{B1} + I_{B2}) R_e \qquad (5.2)$$

Likewise, the loop equation involving V_{S1} yields

$$V_{S1} = I_{B1} r_b + (\beta + 1)(I_{B1} + I_{B2}) R_e \qquad (5.3)$$

Then, across the load resistor,

$$V_{OUT} = -I_{B1} \beta R_L \qquad (5.4)$$

Equations (5.2), (5.3), and (5.4) are three equations containing the three unknowns, the base currents I_{B1}, I_{B2}, and V_{OUT}, and can be solved for any of these variables in terms of the known parameters of the amplifier. The most interesting and relevant result from these equations for increasing our understanding of the diff amp is that

$$V_{OUT} = \frac{-\beta R_L}{2 r_b} (V_{S1} - V_{S2}) \qquad (5.5)$$

The derivation of this equation, given in Box 1 for further information, results when two assumptions are taken: first, $\beta \gg 1$; and second, $r_b \ll \beta R_e$.

The conclusion drawn from Equation (5.5) is that the circuit in Figure 5.2 fulfills the definition of a diff amp. The output voltage V_{OUT} is proportional to the difference of two input voltages, V_{S1} and V_{S2}. From Equation (5.1) we then conclude that the differential gain of this diff amp is

$$A_d = + \frac{\beta R_L}{2r_b} \qquad (5.6)$$

EXAMPLE 5.1   The diff amp in Figure 5.2 has $R_L = 500 \ \Omega$, $R_e = 1000 \ \Omega$, $V_{BB} = 10$ V, $\beta = 60$ for each transistor, and $r_b = 1000 \ \Omega$. Determine whether the assumptions necessary to obtain a differential amplifier characteristic are valid.

SOLUTION   The two assumptions to be tested are $\beta \gg 1$ and $\beta R_e \gg r_b$. $\beta = 60$ satisfies the first assumption and $\beta R_e = 60(1000) = 60,000$ is much greater than $r_b = 1000 \ \Omega$. Therefore, both assumptions are satisfied and the circuit will behave like a diff amp.

EXAMPLE 5.2   In the previous example, determine the differential amplifier gain, A_d.

SOLUTION   Application of Equation (5.6) gives

$$A_d = + \frac{60(500)}{2(1000)} = +15$$

Inverting and Noninverting Amplifiers

The differential amplifier can be connected in either the inverting or noninverting mode. The *inverting mode* is achieved by shorting the source V_{S2} to ground, thereby making $V_{S2} = 0$ in Equation (5.5). In this case, illustrated in Figure 5.4, the approximate gain becomes (from Equation 5.5)

$$V_{OUT} = - \frac{\beta R_L}{2r_b} V_{S1}$$

The minus sign here indicates that the output voltage is 180° out of phase with the input. That is, the output voltage is inverted in phase, hence the name inverting mode.

The differential amplifier symbol in Figure 5.4(b) is shown connected in the inverting mode. The two node voltages on the symbol are measured as plus-to-minus voltage drops to ground. For the connection shown, the approximate gain, A_I, is

$$A_I = - \frac{\beta R_L}{2r_b} \qquad (5.7)$$

Box 1

FOR FURTHER INFORMATION

In order to show that Equation (5.5) describes the diff amp in Figure 5.3, assume first that $\beta \gg 1$.

Then Equation (5.4) is put into Equation (5.3), yielding

$$V_{S1} = \frac{-V_{OUT} r_b}{\beta R_L} + \beta R_e \frac{-V_{OUT}}{\beta R_L} + I_{B2} R_e \beta$$

This equation is then solved for I_{B2}, yielding

$$I_{B2} = \frac{V_{S1}}{\beta R_e} + \left(\frac{r_b}{\beta R_L} + \frac{R_e}{R_L} \right) \frac{V_{OUT}}{\beta R_e} \qquad (5.4.1)$$

Since we want the output voltage as a function of the difference of the input voltages, Equation (5.3) is subtracted from Equation (5.2), yielding

$$V_{S2} - V_{S1} = r_b(I_{B2} - I_{B1}) \qquad (5.4.2)$$

Equations (5.4) and (5.4.1) are now put into Equation (5.4.2), yielding

$$V_{S2} - V_{S1} = r_b \frac{V_{S1} + \left(\dfrac{r_b}{\beta R_L} + \dfrac{R_e}{R_L} \right) V_{OUT}}{\beta R_e} + r_b \frac{V_{OUT}}{\beta R_L}$$

Then, multiplying through,

$$V_{S2} - V_{S1} = r_b \left[\frac{V_{S1}}{\beta R_e} + \left(\frac{r_b}{\beta^2 R_L R_e} + \frac{1}{\beta R_L} \right) V_{OUT} \right] + \frac{r_b V_{OUT}}{\beta R_L}$$

and rearranging the terms gives

$$V_{S2} - V_{S1} - \frac{r_b}{\beta R_e} V_{S1} = \left(\frac{r_b}{\beta R_e} \frac{1}{\beta R_L} + \frac{1}{\beta R_L} \right) V_{OUT} r_b + \frac{r_b V_{OUT}}{\beta R_L} \qquad (5.4.3)$$

One more simple and practical assumption simplifies this equation and makes the amplifier more useful. That is, let r_b be much less than βR_e ($r_b \ll \beta R_e$). This can be done with a high current gain, β, transistor. With this assumption, Equation (5.4.3) becomes

$$V_{OUT} = \frac{\beta R_L}{2 r_b} (V_{S2} - V_{S1}) \qquad (5.5)$$

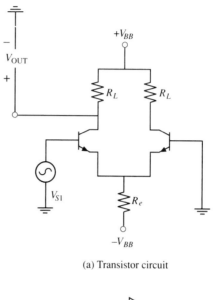

(a) Transistor circuit

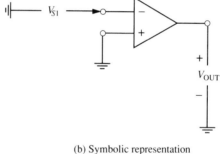

(b) Symbolic representation

FIGURE 5.4
A diff amp in an inverter connection.

Here the gain is negative. On the other hand, if the source number 1 is shorted to ground, the output V_{OUT} becomes

$$V_{OUT} = \frac{\beta R_L}{2r_b} V_{S2}$$

by Equation (5.5), in which $V_{S1} = 0$. In this case the symbolic representation in Figure 5.5(a) has a gain A_{NI}, with

$$A_{NI} = +\frac{\beta R_L}{2r_b} \tag{5.8}$$

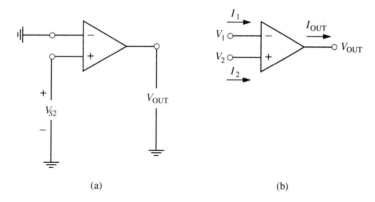

(a)   (b)

FIGURE 5.5
(a) A diff amp in a noninverting connection. (b) The symbol for a diff amp in which all voltages are measured with reference to a common ground as plus-to-minus voltage drops.

Here the positive gain means that the output voltage is in phase with the input voltage, and the amplifier operates in its *noninverting* mode. In both Equations (5.7) and (5.8) the assumptions made were that $\beta \gg 1$ and $r_b \ll \beta R_e$.

5.2 OPERATIONAL AMPLIFIER ANALYSIS

Differential amplifiers can be produced on integrated circuit chips at very low cost. These chips often have a metal-oxide-semiconductor (MOS) construction, in which the metal of the input gate is separated from the semiconductor by glass (SiO_2), an insulator. This makes it possible to produce very high input impedances in amplifiers made from these chips. Furthermore, the gain can be made very high, all at low cost when the power requirements are low and the frequency range is within that used in biopotential amplifiers. It therefore becomes economical and practical to define an ideal differential amplifier as a component for circuit analysis. This is in addition to the other circuit components, resistors, R, capacitors, C, and inductors, L. All of these circuit components are defined in an ideal sense. The reason these ideal definitions are practical is that it is possible to economically design devices that actually approach this ideal performance. Of course, actual R, L, and C components and actual diff amps are not exactly ideal. However, circuit analysis based on these ideal assumptions is greatly simplified, and in most cases, the calculations are accurate enough for purposes of design and troubleshooting.

An *ideal differential amplifier* is defined as one for which (1) the driving point impedance of each input is infinite, (2) the gain is infinite ($A_d \rightarrow \infty$), and (3) the output voltage is given in Figure 5.5(b) by

$$V_{OUT} = A_d(V_2 - V_1) \qquad (5.9)$$

Since the output voltage is a physical quantity, and must remain finite, we have

$$V_2 - V_1 = \frac{V_{OUT}}{A_d} = \frac{V_{OUT}}{\infty} \rightarrow 0$$

The immediate implications of these ideal assumptions is that $V_2 \approx V_1$. Also, because the input impedance is infinite at both ports, $I_1 \approx 0$ and $I_2 \approx 0$, and because Equation (5.9) is assumed to hold true, the output voltage V_{OUT} remains constant regardless of what load is attached to the output port. This is exactly the property of an ideal voltage source such as you would study in electrical circuit theory. And such sources have a zero output impedance. Therefore we can conclude that the ideal diff amp has zero output impedance.

In order to analyze an RLC circuit containing *ideal* differential amplifiers, only two additional rules other than those for RLC circuits are needed. These are relative to Figure 5.5(b):

$$Rule\ \#1 \qquad V_1 \approx V_2$$

$$(5.10)$$

$$Rule\ \#2 \qquad I_1 \approx 0,\ I_2 \approx 0$$

These rules, in addition to Kirchhoff's laws for voltage and current (KVL and KCL), plus Ohm's law for R, L, and C elements, are all that we need to analyze any network containing these ideal components.

Amplifiers that use ideal differential amplifier chips as components, along with other R, L, and C components, are called *operational amplifiers*, or op amps. The term "operational" is used because these circuits perform mathematical operations on the input voltage. Such operations may include multiplication or integration. In Figure 5.6, a simple operational amplifier is analyzed by application of Rules #1 and #2. In Figure 5.6, Z_i and Z_f

are complex impedances. Since V_2 is grounded, $V_2 = 0$, and by the Rule #1, $V_1 = 0$ also. Applying KCL to node 1 yields

$$I_{IN} = I_F + I_1$$

and by Rule #2, $I_1 = 0$, so

$$I_{IN} = I_F$$

Then, applying Ohm's law to the input branch,

$$\frac{V_S - V_1}{Z_i} = I_{IN} = \frac{V_S}{Z_i} \tag{5.11}$$

because $V_1 = 0$. Then Ohm's law is applied to the feedback branch as

$$\frac{V_1 - V_{OUT}}{Z_f} = I_F = -\frac{V_{OUT}}{Z_f}$$

Combining this with Equation (5.11) gives us

$$\frac{V_S}{Z_i} = -\frac{V_{OUT}}{Z_f}$$

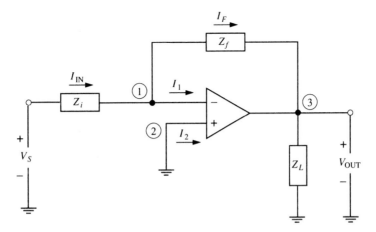

FIGURE 5.6
An op amp loaded with impedance Z_L.

The voltage gain A of the circuit is then $A = V_{OUT}/V_S$, or

$$A = -\frac{Z_f}{Z_i} \tag{5.12}$$

The gain, A, is a complex number, and therefore has both a magnitude and a phase. Furthermore, since circuit impedances are often a function of frequency, the operational amplifier gain is as well.

The input impedance of this amplifier, Z_{IN}, is defined as

$$Z_{IN} = \frac{V_S}{I_{IN}} \tag{5.13}$$

From Equation (5.11) we have

$$\frac{I_{IN} Z_i}{I_{IN}} = Z_{IN} = Z_i \tag{5.14}$$

In general, the input impedance is a complex number called a *phasor*. Furthermore, Equation (5.12) shows that the output voltage is the same value regardless of the value of the load impedance, Z_L. This means that the output impedance is zero, since the amplifier behaves like an ideal voltage source. Therefore,

$$Z_{OUT} = 0 \tag{5.15}$$

EXAMPLE 5.3   The operational amplifier in Figure 5.6 consists of only resistors and the ideal diff amp chip. $Z_i = 100\ \Omega$, $Z_f = 5000\ \Omega$, and $Z_L = 50\ \Omega$. Compute the amplifier gain A, the input impedance Z_{IN}, and the output impedance Z_{OUT} of this amplifier.

SOLUTION   Application of Equation (5.12) yields a gain $A = -5000/100 = -50$, and Equation (5.14) shows that $Z_{IN} = 100\ \Omega$. Also, $Z_{OUT} = 0$.

Equations (5.12) and (5.14) are widely applicable, and worth memorizing, along with the corresponding circuit configuration. Of course, slight changes in the circuit that are often present make these formulas irrelevant, so it is important to develop skill in directly using Kirchhoff's laws, Ohm's law, and the rules for diff amps. These laws and rules always work if properly applied.

EXAMPLE 5.4 Compute the output voltage in the circuit of Figure 5.7.

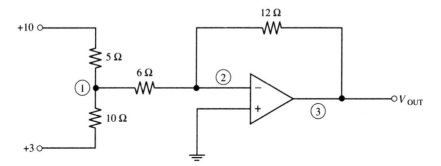

FIGURE 5.7

SOLUTION Write KCL at node 1 as

$$\frac{V_1 - 10}{5} + \frac{V_1 - 3}{10} + \frac{V_1 - 0}{6} = 0$$

Solving for V_1 gives $V_1 = 4.928$. Then write KCL at node 2 where $V_2 = 0$ by Rule #1:

$$\frac{0 - 4.928}{6} + 0 - \frac{V_{OUT}}{12} = 0$$

$$V_{OUT} = -9.856 \text{ V}$$

In this case the basic circuit laws are more convenient to use than a specific gain formula for the circuit.

Operational Amplifier Voltage and Current Sources

The ideal differential amplifier can be wired as either a voltage source or a current source, as long as it is not driven out of its linear range. The voltage source is shown in Figure 5.6 as described previously. The Thevenin equivalent of this circuit is given in Figure 5.8. The Thevenin impedance equals the Z_{OUT}, in this case zero. The Thevenin voltage source, V_{OC}, is then

$$V_{OC} = -\frac{Z_f}{Z_i} V_{IN}$$

The current source is configured in Figure 5.9(a). Applying the voltage rule for diff amps, Equation (5.10), makes node 1 voltage equal to node 2 voltage. Therefore $V_{IN} = V_2$. The current through the resistor, I_R, is then

$$I_R = \frac{V_2}{R} = \frac{V_{IN}}{R}$$

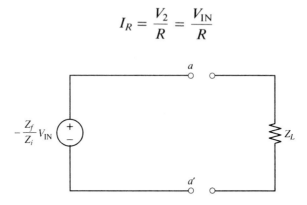

FIGURE 5.8
Op amp Thevenin equivalent voltage source driving a load Z_L.

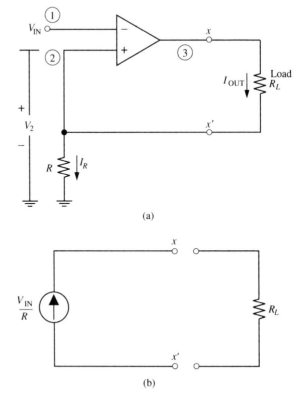

(a)

(b)

FIGURE 5.9
(a) A constant current source. (b) A current source representation.

Also, by the current rule for ideal diff amps (Equations 5.10), $I_{OUT} = I_R$. Therefore, we have

$$I_{OUT} = \frac{V_{IN}}{R} \tag{5.16}$$

Notice that the output current, I_{OUT}, taken as the current through the load, R_L, by Equation (5.16) does not depend upon the value of R_L. Thus, since the current is independent of the load resistance, R_L, we conclude that (1) the circuit in Figure 5.9(a) to the left of terminals x-x' is a current source; and (2) the output impedance approaches infinity for currents within the linear range of the diff amp. The Norton equivalent of the operational amplifier current sources is shown in Figure 5.9(b).

Operational Amplifiers in Tandem

Because the op amp of Figure 5.6 acts like an ideal voltage source, it is particularly easy to string several stages of amplification in tandem as multistage amplifiers. The successive stages do not distort the voltages in previous stages, because the output impedance of each stage is zero. This is illustrated by Example 5.5.

EXAMPLE 5.5 Two operational amplifiers connected in tandem are arranged as shown in Figure 5.10. For the given input node voltage, compute the output voltage. Then find the gain of stage 1, A_1, stage 2, A_2, and finally the total gain, A_T. The differential amplifiers are ideal.

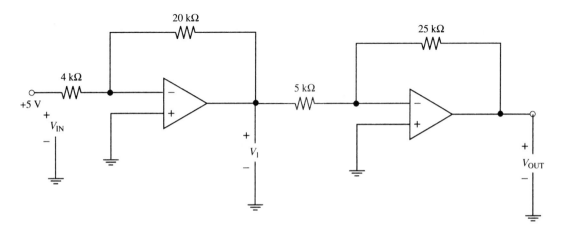

FIGURE 5.10
Op amps connected in tandem.

SOLUTION

$$\frac{5-0}{4000} = \frac{0-V_1}{20,000}$$

and, therefore, $V_1 = -25$ V. Then from KCL we have

$$\frac{-25-0}{5000} = \frac{0-V_{\text{OUT}}}{25,000}$$

The gain of stage 1 is $A_1 = -5$. The gain of stage 2 is $A_2 = -5$. The gain of the multiple stages is $A_T = V_{\text{OUT}}/V_{\text{IN}}$, where $V_{\text{IN}} = 5$ V here. Therefore, the gain of the entire amplifier $A_T = 125/5 = +25$.

The conclusion we may draw from a similar general analysis of these tandem amplifiers is that the total gain is the product of the individual stages: $A_T = A_1 A_2$. This results from the fact that the output impedance of the ideal amplifier is zero. Of course, if the amplifier were operated outside its linear range, the ideal assumptions would no longer be valid, and the conclusion drawn above would not hold.

EXAMPLE 5.6   Find the output node voltage V_{OUT} in Figure 5.11 resulting from the input node voltages indicated, using KVL, KCL, and/or the rules for ideal differential amplifiers.

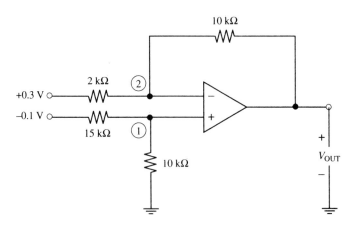

FIGURE 5.11

SOLUTION   The current rule (Equations 5.10) for diff amps leads to

$$V_1 = \frac{-10,000}{15,000 + 10,000}(0.1) = -0.04 \text{ V}$$

Since the current entering the positive lead is zero, and the current through the 15-kΩ resistor equals that through the 10-kΩ resistor, they therefore form a voltage divider.

Then, since $V_2 = V_1$, by the voltage rule for diff amps (Equations 5.10) we have $V_2 = -0.04$ V. Then, applying KCL to node 2, we have

$$\frac{0.3 - (-0.04)}{2000} = \frac{-0.04 - V_{OUT}}{10,000}$$

$$V_{OUT} = -1.74 \text{ V}$$

EXAMPLE 5.7 Determine whether the circuit in Figure 5.12 could be called a "summer." That is, for the node voltage inputs given, compute the output voltages V_{OUT}.

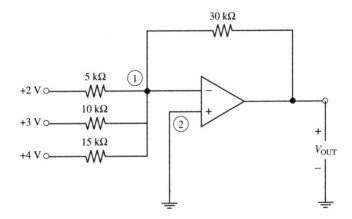

FIGURE 5.12

SOLUTION Since node 1 voltage equals node 2 voltage, we have, from the application of KCL to node 1,

$$\frac{V_1 - 2}{5000} + \frac{V_1 - 3}{10,000} + \frac{V_1 - 4}{15,000} = \frac{V_{OUT} - V_1}{30,000}$$

where $V_1 = 0$. Solving for V_{OUT} gives $V_{OUT} = -29$ V. Since -29 V is not the sum of $2 + 3 + 4$, this circuit is not a "summer." However, if all resistors were the same value, it would be a "summer" in the sense that the output would equal the inverse of the sum of the input voltages.

High-Input-Impedance Amplifiers with Controlled Gain

As a rule, the higher the input impedance of a signal processing amplifier, the better. The basic reason for this is that when the input impedance of an amplifier is high, it will draw very little current from previous transducers or amplifiers. This means it will not disturb the voltages and the currents of those devices, and is in a sense "invisible'" to them. Specifically, in the case of medical instrumentation, the biopotential is most often measured through a high impedance. Skin surface electrodes for noninvasive bio-potential measurement are in series with skin resistances of about 100 kΩ. Furthermore, needle and microelectrodes usually have high impedances because of their narrow dimensions, often several megohms (MΩ). The input impedance of practical amplifiers, on the other hand, as in Figure 5.6, is lower than this. In order to avoid the distorting effects of amplifier loading on the body potential source, it is often necessary to use a high-input-impedance buffer.

The simplest buffer using op amps is shown in Figure 5.13. In this circuit the input impedance ideally would be infinite, and its output impedance would be zero. By the voltage rule for diff amps, V_1 at node 1 in Figure 5.13 equals V_{IN} and is tied directly to V_{OUT}. Thus we have for the buffer

$$V_{OUT} = V_{IN}$$

This buffer amplifier therefore has a gain of one. This amplifier preserves the high input impedance of the ideal diff amp while reducing its gain to the more practical value of one.

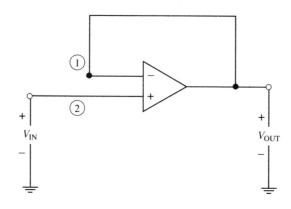

FIGURE 5.13
A buffer circuit.

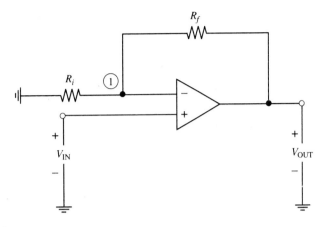

FIGURE 5.14
A noninverting amplifier.

An amplifier that gives more control over the gain while preserving the high input impedance is shown in Figure 5.14. The gain is computed by finding the ratio $A = V_{\text{OUT}}/V_{\text{IN}}$. The rule for ideal diff amps gives the node 1 voltage $V_1 = V_{\text{IN}}$. Application of KVL at node 1 gives

$$\frac{V_{\text{IN}} - 0}{R_i} + \frac{V_{\text{IN}} - V_{\text{OUT}}}{R_f} = 0$$

Solving this for the ratio $V_{\text{OUT}}/V_{\text{IN}}$,

$$\frac{V_{\text{OUT}}}{V_{\text{IN}}} = \left(\frac{R_f}{R_i} + 1\right) = A \tag{5.17}$$

The gain of this amplifier may therefore be controlled by R_f and R_i, as with the op amp in Figure 5.6. However, here the input impedance ideally approaches infinity. This is often considered an improvement over the amplifier in Figure 5.6, which has an input impedance of R_i.

EXAMPLE 5.8   In Figure 5.14, $R_f = 25\ \Omega$ and $R_i = 5\ \Omega$. The input voltage is 3 V. Assuming the diff amp is ideal, compute the output voltage, V_{OUT}.

SOLUTION   The gain of the amplifier

$$A = \left(1 + \frac{25}{5}\right) = 6$$

Therefore, the output voltage is $6 \times 3 = 18$ V.

Differential Amplifier with Controlled Gain

The amplifier in Figure 5.14 is not a differential amplifier, because it does not satisfy the definition (Equation 5.1). In order to make it a diff amp, we may add a potentiometer and adjust it so that the circuit is balanced. In Figure 5.15 the pot R_p is added. The resistance below the wiper arm is αR_p, and the resistance above the wiper arm is $(1 - \alpha)R_p$. This is true because the sum of these comes to R_p. To calculate V_{OUT} in terms of V_1 and V_2 on the inputs, notice first that the voltage on node 2 is αV_2, by voltage division. The circuit analysis principle of superposition is used to compute the output voltage. By superposition,

$$V_{OUT} = V_{OUT1} + V_{OUT2}$$

where V_{OUT1} is the output voltage found when V_2 is set to zero, V_{OUT2} is the output voltage when V_1 is set to zero, and V_2 is considered the input voltage.

By superposition, V_{OUT} is computed when $V_2 = 0$, and V_{OUT1} is found from Equation (5.12) as

$$V_{OUT1} = (-R_f/R_i)V_1$$

and when $V_1 = 0$, V_{OUT2} is computed from Equation (5.17) as

$$V_{OUT2} = \alpha V_2\left(1 + \frac{R_f}{R_i}\right)$$

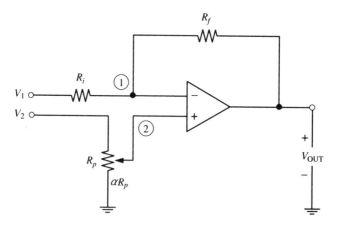

FIGURE 5.15
This is a diff amp when Equation (5.19) is satisfied.

where αV_2 is the voltage on node 2. The sum of V_{OUT1} and V_{OUT2} is then V_{OUT}, or

$$V_{OUT} = -\frac{R_f}{R_i} V_1 + \alpha V_2 \left(1 + \frac{R_f}{R_i}\right) \qquad \text{(unbalanced circuit)} \qquad \textbf{(5.18)}$$

To balance the circuit in Figure 5.15, we simply choose $\alpha = \alpha_B$ so that Equation (5.18) satisfies the definition of the diff amp, Equation (5.1). This is done by making the coefficients of Equation (5.18) add up to zero. That is, we set

$$\frac{R_f}{R_i} = \alpha_B \left(1 + \frac{R_f}{R_i}\right)$$

and solve for α_B:

$$\alpha_B = \frac{R_f}{R_f + R_i} \qquad \textbf{(5.19)}$$

Under the condition of balance, putting Equation (5.19) back into Equation (5.18) gives

$$V_{OUT} = -\frac{R_f}{R_i} (V_1 - V_2) \qquad \text{(balanced circuit)} \qquad \textbf{(5.20)}$$

Obviously, the differential gain A_d is

$$A_d = +\frac{R_f}{R_i} \qquad \textbf{(5.21)}$$

and the balanced circuit satisfies the definition of a diff amp. The balanced circuit is a diff amp with controlled gain. However, the input impedance is low. For example, the input impedance of the V_2 input equals R_p. To increase the input impedance, when a low gain value is undesirable, a buffer amp (Figure 5.13) can be connected to each input.

EXAMPLE 5.9 For the circuit in Figure 5.15, plot V_{OUT} versus V_1 when $R_f = 700 \ \Omega$, $R_i = 300 \ \Omega$, and $R_p = 10,000 \ \Omega$. Make separate plots for $\alpha = 0.1, 0.7,$ and 1, when $V_2 = 1$. Deduce from the plot the α for which the amplifier is balanced.

SOLUTION   The plot is obtained by substituting values in Equation (5.18):

$$V_{OUT} = -\frac{700}{300}\,V_1 + \alpha(1)\left(1 + \frac{700}{300}\right)$$

For the particular point $\alpha = 0.1$, $V_1 = 2$, we compute

$$V_{OUT} = -4.33\ \text{V}$$

Repeated calculation results in the plot in Figure 5.16. The balance condition is found by noting that balance occurs when $V_1 = V_2 = 1$ and the output is zero. The plot shows that this happens when $\alpha = 0.7$. That can also be verified by Equation (5.19). The calculation of Equation (5.18) is facilitated by the use of the calculator program given as Program A-4 in Appendix A.

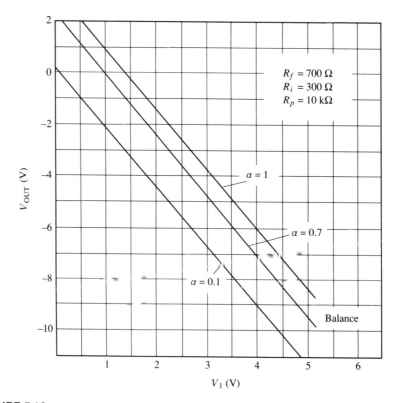

FIGURE 5.16
The output voltage of an amplifier in Figure 5.15.

Buffer Amplifier for a Diff Amp

In order to buffer both leads of a diff amp, such as that given in Figure 5.15, and to provide amplification at the same time, the circuit in Figure 5.17 may be used. Here, the diff amps are assumed to be ideal. Then the ideal diff amp voltage rule implies that

$$V_3 = V_{I1} \text{ and } V_4 = V_{I2} \tag{5.22}$$

Also, the current rule implies that, since no current goes into the input leads of the diff amps, the current through R_1 equals that through R_0 and that through R_2. Thus, KCL yields

$$\frac{V_3 - V_4}{R_0} = \frac{V_1 - V_2}{R_1 + R_2 + R_0} \tag{5.23}$$

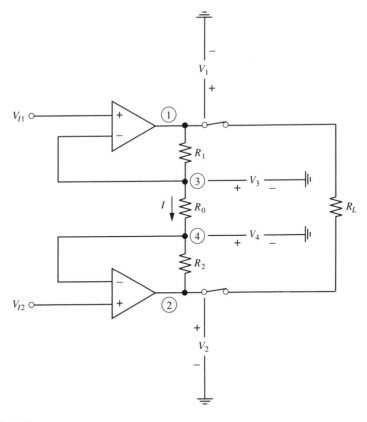

FIGURE 5.17
A buffer circuit for a diff amp.

Inserting Equation (5.23) into Equation (5.22) gives

$$(V_1 - V_2) = \frac{R_1 + R_2 + R_0}{R_0} (V_{I1} - V_{I2}) \qquad (5.24)$$

The gain of this amplifier is equal to the output differential voltage divided by the input:

$$\frac{R_1 + R_2 + R_0}{R_0}$$

Equation (5.24) shows that the output voltage does not depend on R_L so long as the ideal diff amps are operated in their linear range.

EXAMPLE 5.10   In Figure 5.17, $R_1 = 1$ kΩ, $R_2 = 2$ kΩ, and $R_0 = 3$ kΩ. Assuming the diff amps operate in their linear range, find V_1 when $V_{I1} = 1$ V and $V_{I2} = 2$ V.

SOLUTION   The voltage rule for diff amps yields $V_3 = V_{I1} = 1$ V, and likewise $V_4 = 2$ V. Thus, the current through R_0 is

$$I = \frac{1 - 2}{3000} = -0.333 \text{ mA}$$

This current also flows through R_1, since the op amp does not draw any current through its input lead. Then

$$\frac{V_1 - V_3}{R_1} = -0.333 \text{ mA} = \frac{V_1 - 1}{1000}$$

and $V_1 = 0.666$ V.

5.3 BIOPOTENTIAL MEASUREMENT INTERFERENCE

As mentioned earlier, the importance of diff amps is heightened by the fact that one of the major tasks in monitoring, diagnosing, and making measurements on medical patients is the measurement of potential differences that occur in the body, such as the ECG, EOG, and EEG measurements, and the potentials produced by skeletal muscles called electromyographic potentials (EMG). They are all measured as differences between sites on the surface of the body. In each case the instrument for doing this is the diff amp.

The situation in making a difference measurement on the body is shown in Figure 5.18. This illustrates a basic problem of such a measurement in the hospital environment: power-line, 60-cycle ($\sim$) interference. In such an environment, where thousands of pieces of electrical equipment are in use, the power requirements are high. Inevitably, patients are in close proximity to power buses and are therefore capacitively coupled to the power buses through the stray capacity between them and their bodies, which are essentially conductors. The amount of capacity can be estimated from the basic capacitance formula as

$$C = \epsilon_o \frac{A}{d}$$

where $\epsilon_o = 8.85 \times 10^{-12}$ F/m, A is area in square meters, and d is the distance in meters between the plates of area A. If one square meter of the body is coupled to power lines one meter away, a reasonable circumstance, then the stray capacitance is approximately

$$C = 8.85(10^{-12}) \frac{(1^2)}{1} = 8.85 \text{ pF}$$

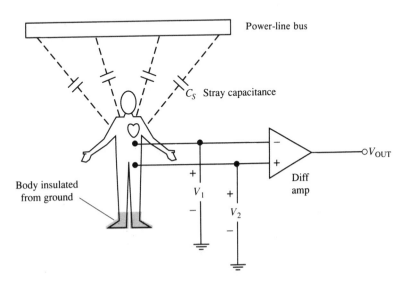

FIGURE 5.18
Power-line interference in biopotential measurements.

Therefore, we should expect stray capacity values between 1 and 10 pF to couple a patient to the power lines. Of course this value varies widely as the patient changes location and proximity to hardware; however, the calculation gives an order-of-magnitude estimate. It should give you a gut feeling for the amount of stray capacity you can expect from the power lines.

EXAMPLE 5.11   A patient is coupled by 5 pF stray capacity to a 60-$\sim$, 120-V power bus as indicated in Figure 5.18. A diff amp has a 10-MΩ driving point impedance at each lead. Compute the voltage V_2 and V_1.

SOLUTION   The equivalent circuit of Figure 5.19 in this case is for V_2. Note that the diagram for V_1 would be the same, except V_2 would be replaced by V_1.

$$V_2 = \frac{10^7}{10^7 - j5.305(10^8)}\ (120)$$

$$= \frac{120(10^7)}{5.306(10^8)\ \angle -88.9°} = 2.26\ \angle +88.9\ \text{V}$$

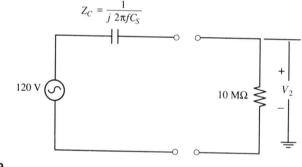

FIGURE 5.19

Thus, the 60-$\sim$ voltage, coupled by stray capacity, far exceeds the size of the biopotential, which is on the order of 1 mV.

This example shows that a relatively large proportion of the power-line voltage may exist at the patient leads of monitoring equipment. The voltage V_2 equals V_1. Therefore these are called common-mode voltages. In Figure 5.18, the output voltage would be the difference $V_{\text{OUT}} = A_d(V_2 - V_1) = 0$. This is one reason diff amps are used in this application. That is, the output of the diff amp due to the common-mode voltage interference is approximately zero. This, in the ideal case, eliminates that interference. However, imperfections in actual diff amps cause an output due to the common-mode voltage, as explained in the following section.

Common-Mode Rejection in a Diff Amp

In Example 5.11, it is shown that power-line interference may exceed the level of the signal being measured. This bad news is often cancelled by the fact that the interfacing signal appears equally intense at both input terminals of the diff amp, and is therefore called a *common-mode* signal. In this case the resulting output voltage is proportional to the difference of two equal voltages, which is zero. However, if the diff amp is not perfectly balanced, as is always the case in the real world, then the common-mode signal input will cause an output signal that then constitutes interference with the desired amplified signal. Since one of the functions of the diff amp is to reject the common-mode signal, we define a figure of merit, the *common-mode rejection ratio* (CMRR), which measures how well the rejection occurs.

In terms of the diff amp illustration in Figure 5.20, the common-mode rejection ratio CMRR is defined as the magnitude of the ratio of the differential voltage gain A_d to the common-mode voltage gain A_C. In the figure, A_d equals V_{OUT} divided by V_1 when node 2 is grounded, and V_1 is applied to node 1. Also, A_C equals V_{OUT} divided by V_1 when node 1 is connected to node 2, and V_1 is applied again. In formula this is

$$\text{CMRR} = \frac{|V_{OUT}| \text{ when } V_2 \text{ is grounded}}{|V_{OUT}| \text{ when } V_2 = V_1} \qquad (5.25)$$

In practice the CMRR is measured in the following steps:

1. Ground V_2, and apply a voltage V_1 to the upper terminal.
2. Measure the resulting V_{OUT}.
3. Lift V_2 from ground and short the two input leads of Figure 5.20, then apply the same value of V_1.
4. Measure the resulting V_{OUT}.
5. To compute CMRR, divide the results of step 2 by the result of step 4, and take the magnitude.

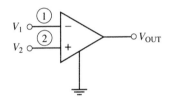

FIGURE 5.20
A diff amp.

The CMRR is a voltage ratio, and therefore in decibel units we may define CMRdB as

$$\text{CMRdB} = 20 \log \text{CMRR} \qquad \text{(in dB)}$$

Diff amp chips have a finite CMRR due to imperfections in manufacture, and the CMRR is given in the chip specifications. There is also a CMRR due to imbalance in the external circuit components. Even though the circuit is designed to be balanced, the balance is often upset by element tolerances and by environmental influences such as temperature, vibration, and humidity. The following example illustrates how to compute the CMRR due to diff amp circuit element imbalances.

EXAMPLE 5.12   Calculate the formula for the common-mode rejection ratio on the network in Figure 5.15.

SOLUTION   Applying the definition in Equation (5.25) to Equation (5.18), we get

$$\text{CMRR} = \frac{\left| -\dfrac{R_f}{R_i} V_1 \right|}{\left| \left(\dfrac{-R_f}{R_i} + \alpha \left(1 + \dfrac{R_f}{R_i} \right) \right) V_1 \right|}$$

The numerator of this equation is obtained when V_2 in Equation (5.18) is set to zero. The denominator comes from that equation when V_2 is set equal to V_1. The term V_1 then cancels in the numerator and denominator, so

$$\text{CMRR} = \frac{1}{\left| \alpha \left(\dfrac{R_i}{R_f} + 1 \right) - 1 \right|}$$

Here CMRR depends only on circuit elements. Since CMRR is a voltage ratio, in decibel units, CMRdB = 20 log CMRR, or

$$\text{CMRdB} = -20 \log \left| \alpha \left(\frac{R_i}{R_f} + 1 \right) - 1 \right| \qquad \textbf{(5.26)}$$

Equation (5.26) gives the CMRR of a circuit that is not a diff amp until it is balanced. For the balanced case, Equation (5.19) put into Equation (5.26) shows that CMRdB approaches minus infinity, assuming an ideal chip. A calculated example illustrates the effect of the external circuit components on the CMRdB.

EXAMPLE 5.13   In Figure 5.15, $R_f = 100 \ \Omega$ and $R_i = 10 \ \Omega$. Plot the common-mode rejection ratio CMRdB as a function of α in the potentiometer.

SOLUTION   Equation (5.26) becomes

$$\text{CMRdB} = -20 \log \left| \alpha \left(\frac{10}{100} + 1 \right) - 1 \right|$$

$$= -20 \log |1.1\alpha - 1|$$

To plot CMRdB versus α, take for example $\alpha = 0.6$. This makes CMRdB = 9.37 dB. The complete plot is shown in Figure 5.21. A program for computing Equation (5.26) is given as Program A-5 in Appendix A.

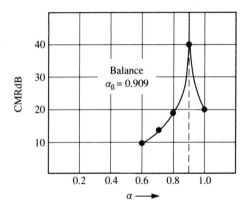

FIGURE 5.21
The common-mode voltage calculated in Example 5.13.

The plot in Figure 5.21 illustrates how the effect of small imbalances in a diff amp can spoil the common-mode rejection ratio. Practical amplifiers should have a CMRdB above 60. If the diff amp has a balance adjustment, as is the case in Figure 5.15, small changes in the adjustment of α can rapidly deteriorate the common-mode rejection ratio. In a medical instrument this would often appear as an increase in 60-$\sim$ hum.

5.4 TROUBLESHOOTING MEDICAL INSTRUMENTATION AMPLIFIERS

Integrated circuit diff amps usually come in dual in-line packages (DIP). They are susceptible to damage from external static voltage and excessive pin temperature, as well as from mechanical vibration. Component-level troubleshooting methods may be used to locate problems. Two basic methods for finding faults are voltage signal tracing and resistance measurements. To perform *signal tracing*, a dual-trace oscilloscope may be used to display the amplifier input signal on one channel and the output on the other channel. The gain may be deduced by comparing the two results. Comparing the measured gain with the calculated value may show a difference, and thus indicate a fault, either in the chip or in a passive circuit component ancillary to it.

To isolate the problem, a visual check of the components for discoloration or damage is a reasonable first step. The first voltage check should be on the power supply connection. Then the node voltages at the diff amp chip input should be checked. If the gain is too high, and the amplifier output is clipped, this could indicate a passive component failure.

With the power turned off, resistance measurements may be made with an ohmmeter. Removing the chip and doing a resistance measurement on the pins could locate a shorted diff amp. In general, the node resistance measurements of the amplifier under test can be compared to those of an identical amplifier, either in the same instrument or in a duplicate model known to work. Differences in a component resistance are evidence of a faulty component.

If possible, a defective soldered chip package should be replaced with a DIP socket. Plugging in a new chip avoids the need to solder a new chip, risking heat damage. However, if you choose to resolder the new chip, to make it more resistant to vibration, be careful to avoid overheating it. To do this, place a heat sink on the pin to be soldered, and solder as quickly as possible. If the component is critical, or expensive, it may be necessary to use low-temperature solder and a temperature-controlled soldering iron to avoid damage to the chip.

Troubleshooting Tip

When changing a soldered chip, replace it with a DIP socket if possible.

If 60-∿ noise on the output of a controlled-gain diff amp is excessive, it might be fixed by adjusting the balance potentiometer.

REFERENCES

Floyd, T. L. *Electronic Devices.* Columbus, OH: Charles E. Merrill, 1984.

Johnson, D. E., Hilburn, J. L., and Johnson, J. R. *Basic Electric Circuits Analysis.* Englewood Cliffs, NJ: Prentice-Hall, 1978.

Malvino, A. P. *Electronic Principles.* New York: McGraw-Hill, 1979.
"Operational Amplifier." Publication #012-01532. Haywood, CA: Pasco Scientific,
    1876 Sabre Street, 1983.
"Differential Amplifier." Cambridge, MA: Technical Education Research Center,
    575 Technology Square, 1972.

EXERCISES

1. An ideal differential amplifier is shown in Figure 5.22. The input voltage is 5 V d.c. Compute the output voltage V_{OUT}.

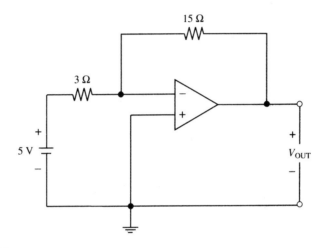

FIGURE 5.22

2. For the ideal operational amplifier shown in Figure 5.5(b), state the fundamental rules necessary to analyze a circuit containing it in terms of the voltages and currents indicated in the figure.

3. The circuit of Figure 5.23 is driven by a 10-V source. Calculate V_{OUT}. Assume the differential amplifier is ideal.

4. For the amplifier in Figure 5.24 using ideal components, compute:
   (a) The input impedance, Z_{IN}.
   (b) The gain, V_{OUT}/V_{IN}.
   (c) The output impedance, Z_{OUT}.

5. (a) What is the V_{OUT} in the circuit of Figure 5.25?
   (b) What is the input impedance R_{IN} seen by the ideal voltage source?

*6. In the differential amplifier shown in Figure 5.26, the voltages V_1 and V_2 are zero, and you are to calculate the Q-point bias voltage V_{B0} and the bias current I_{B0}. The circuit is symmetrical and has equal components on each

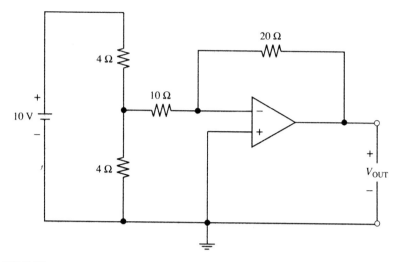

FIGURE 5.23

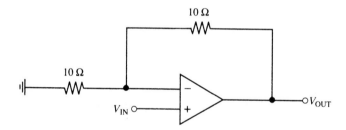

FIGURE 5.24

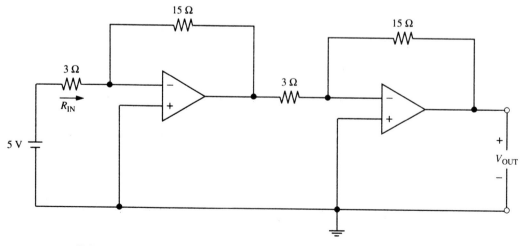

FIGURE 5.25

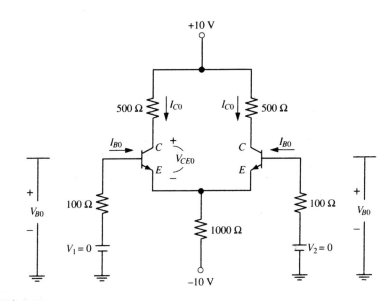

FIGURE 5.26

side of the center line. The current gain $\beta = 60$ in each transistor. The forward base to emitter voltage for the transistor $V_{BE} = 0.70$ V. The battery voltage $V_{BB} = 10$ V.

(a) Compute V_{B0} and I_{B0}.

(b) Compute V_{CE0} and I_{C0}. These points on the voltage-current characteristic of the transistor define the Q-point, when the sources V_1 and V_2 are both zero.

7. Compute the voltage output V_{OUT} of the amplifier in Figure 5.27.

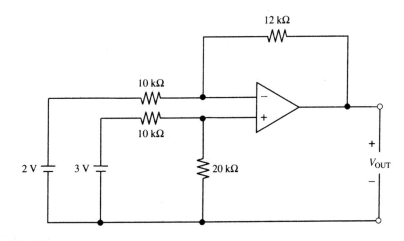

FIGURE 5.27

8. Compute the branch currents I_{OUT}, I_F, and I_L in the circuit of Figure 5.28. Assume the amplifier is linear.

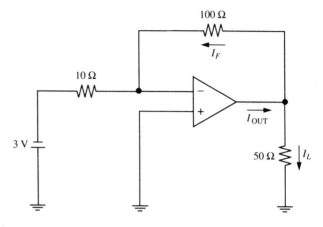

FIGURE 5.28

9. (a) Plot the current I_{OUT} as a function of R_L in Figure 5.29.
   (b) From this result, determine the output impedance looking to the left of terminals *x-x'*, Z_{OUT}.

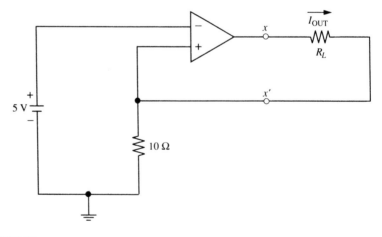

FIGURE 5.29

10. An ECG is being measured on a patient at two body sites by means of the differential amplifier shown in Figure 5.30. Because of proximity to the power bus in the hospital, the patient is capacitively coupled to the 200-V a.c. power line, having frequency 60 Hz. The capacitance between the patient and the power line is 3 pF.

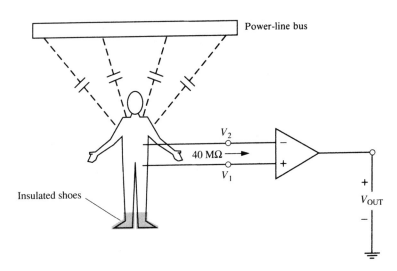

FIGURE 5.30

(a) Draw an equivalent circuit for calculation of V_2 due to capacitive coupling.
(b) Compute the voltage V_2.
(c) Compute the voltage V_1.

11. (a) In the circuit in Figure 5.31, $\alpha = 0.37$. When $V_1 = 2$ V and $V_2 = 1$ V, compute V_{OUT}, I_L, and I_{OUT}.
(b) For what value of α will the amplifier be balanced and act as a differential amplifier?

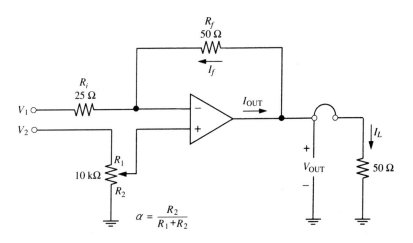

FIGURE 5.31

*12. In Figure 5.31 show that the amplifier is balanced and acts as a differential amplifier when the circuit components are chosen to satisfy the condition

$$\frac{R_f}{R_i} = \frac{R_2}{R_1}$$

13. In the circuit of Figure 5.32, the common-mode rejection ratio is measured by the following procedure: (a) Ground V_1, and apply $V_2 = 2$ V. (b) Raise V_1 from ground and connect to V_2, which equals 2 V. Compute the common-mode rejection ratio, CMRR, when $\alpha = 0.6$.

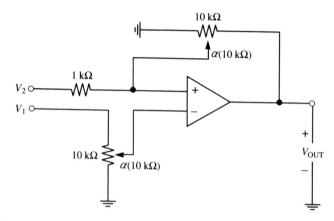

FIGURE 5.32

14. The output voltage of the nonideal differential amplifier is found to be

$$V_{OUT} = 10(V_1 - 1.03 V_2)$$

where V_1 and V_2 are the two input voltages. Compute the common-mode rejection ratio.

15. In the circuit in Figure 5.33, $V_A = 2$ V and $V_B = -3$ V. Assume the differential amplifiers are ideal, and compute V_3 and V_4.

16. In the circuit in Figure 5.33, $V_A = 10$ V and $V_B = 20$ V with reference to ground. The elements are ideal. Compute V_3 and V_4 when $R_1 = 10$ kΩ, $R_2 = 30$ kΩ, and $R_3 = 5$ kΩ.

17. The output voltage for a biopotential amplifier has been calculated to be

$$V_{OUT} = 25(1.003 V_1 - V_2)$$

where the voltages V_1 and V_2 are the inputs.

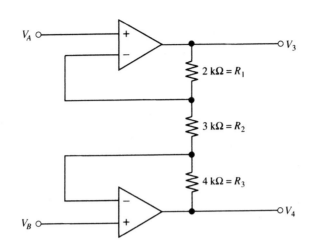

FIGURE 5.33

(a) Calculate the common-mode rejection ratio for this amplifier and express the answer in decibels.
(b) Compute the differential amplifier gain.

18. In the circuit of Figure 5.34, compute V_2, V_{OUT}, and I_2.

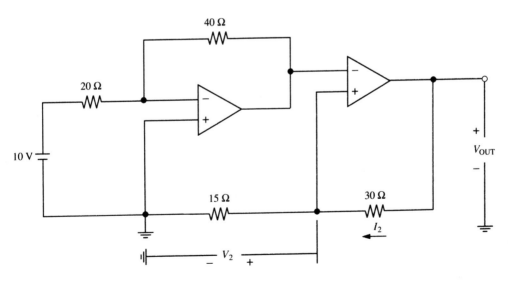

FIGURE 5.34

19. In Figure 5.3(b), compute V_{OUT} when $R_L = 500\ \Omega$, $r_b = 1000\ \Omega$, $V_{S1} = 3$ V, $\beta = 60$, and $V_{S2} = 5$ V. Also determine whether the amplifier is inverting or noninverting when V_{S1} is set to zero.

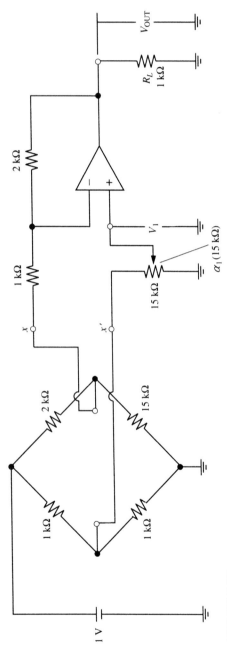

FIGURE 5.35

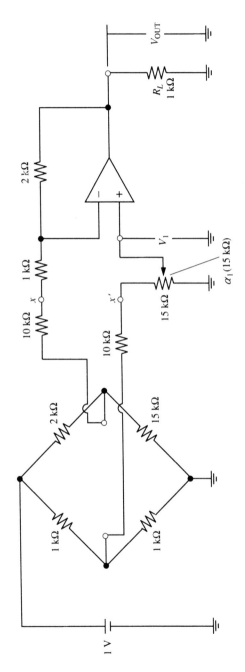

FIGURE 5.36

20. In Figure 5.35, the differential amplifier to the right of x-x' is balanced. The differential amplifier is ideal.

    (a) Find α_1, the fraction of the maximum wiper arm displacement from the bottom, for the balanced condition.
    (b) Find V_1 at the lower input node of the differential amplifier.
    (c) Find V_{OUT}.

21. In Figure 5.36, the differential amplifier to the right of x-x' is balanced. The differential amplifier is ideal.

    (a) Find α_1, the fraction of the maximum wiper arm displacement from the bottom for the balanced condition in the differential amplifier attached to points x-x'.
    (b) Find V_1 at the lower input node of the differential amplifier.
    (c) Find V_{OUT}.

*22. Derive the common-mode rejection ratio for the amplifier given in Figure 5.37 in terms of the resistors R_1, R_2, R_f, and R_i. Assume the diff amp chip has ideal properties. Show that

$$\mathrm{CMRR} = \frac{R_f(R_1 + R_2)}{|R_1 R_f - R_i R_2|}$$

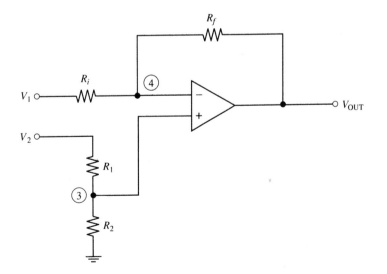

FIGURE 5.37
A diff amp when $R_f/R_i = R_2/R_1$.

23. The amplifier of Figure 5.37 is designed to be balanced and then to operate as a diff amp. The values chosen are $R_f = 20$ kΩ, $R_i = 1$ kΩ, $R_1 = 1$ kΩ,
$R_2 = 20$ kΩ. Calculate the CMRR if the resistor R_2 increases by 10% due to
temperature effects.

24. Repeat Exercise 23, but keep $R_2 = 20$ kΩ and increase R_1 by 10%. Then
compute CMRR.

PART II
Patient-Care Equipment

6. The Electrocardiograph and Unit-Level Trouble-shooting

7. The Electroencephalograph and Filtering

8. The Defibrillator and Step Response

9. The Pacemaker — A Digital Pulse Oscillator

10. Electrosurgical Units and Laser Surgery

11. Catheters and Blood Pressure Monitoring

12. Respiratory Equipment and Pulmonary Function Monitoring

13. The Central Station Monitor, Microprocessor-Based Equipment, and System-Level Trouble-shooting

6
The Electrocardiograph and Unit-Level Troubleshooting

The electrocardiograph is a widely used medical instrument that measures biopotential differences arising from electrical activity of the heart muscle. It usually uses surface electrodes, and it requires high-input-impedance differential amplifiers and compensation for common-mode voltage inputs. The electrocardiograph is designated with the initials ECG, as is the electrocardiogram, a record of the data. (The initials EKG, from the German translation, are also sometimes used.) In terms of the electrical signal, the ECG has a magnitude of about 1 mV at the electrode surface. In terms of signal processing, the significant features of the ECG data are the feature durations, polarities, and magnitudes.

6.1 THE ECG

The ECG is designed to measure and to record electrocardiograms, such as those illustrated in Figure 6.1 and described in Section 2.4 for the surface potential measured between two arms of a patient. The distinctive features, labeled *P*, *Q*, *R*, *S*, and *T*, vary considerably among subjects. Average amplitudes at the electrodes are given in Table 6.1 for these distinctive features at standard body site connections of the ECG. The ECG amplitude depends on the electrode connection sites, and on the size and physical condition of the patient, as will be explained in Section 6.2.

Important clinical variables from ECG waveforms include the magnitude and polarity of these features, as well as their relative time duration. Variations from these norms may indicate illness. For example, an extended *P-R* interval indicates prolonged conduction time of the atrioventricular

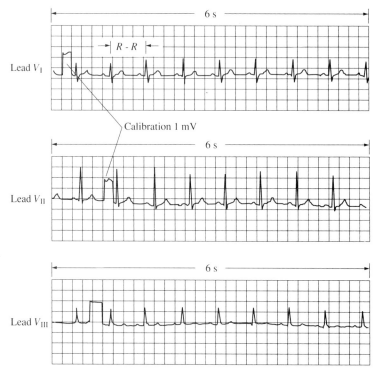

FIGURE 6.1
A normal ECG for the standard lead connections V_I, V_{II}, V_{III}. (Courtesy of Hewlett-Packard)

TABLE 6.1
Amplitudes of ECG Waves for Standard Lead Connections

| Wave | Lead voltage magnitudes [nominal (range)] | | |
	V_I (mV)	V_{II} (mV)	V_{III} (mV)
P	0.07 (0.01 to 0.12)	0.01 (0 to 0.19)	0.04 (0.0 to 0.13)
Q	0.03 (0 to 0.16)	0.03 (0 to 0.18)	0.04 (0 to 0.28)
R	0.53 (0.07 to 1.13)	0.71 (0.18 to 1.68)	0.38 (0.03 to 1.31)
S	0.10 (0 to 0.36)	0.12 (0 to 0.49)	0.12 (0 to 0.55)
T	0.22 (0.06 to 0.42)	0.26 (0.06 to 0.55)	0.05 (0.0 to 0.3)

(AV) node and may be diagnosed as an AV block. A widening of the *QRS* complex may be due to a bundle block, which may result from improper conduction in the nerve fiber in the bundle of His. An elevated *S-T* may indicate that a myocardial infarction has occurred, and a negative-polarity

T wave may be due to coronary insufficiency. Other distinctive features of the ECG important in disease diagnosis are *QRS* voltage amplitude; polarity, the time duration; the *R-R* interval, which is the reciprocal of the pulse rate; and the *T*-wave amplitude.

The pulse rate *BPM* is usually expressed in beats per minute (bpm), given by

$$BPM = \frac{60}{R\text{-}R} \qquad \text{(bpm)} \qquad\qquad \textbf{(6.1)}$$

where *R-R* is the period of the ECG in seconds. Normal heart rate is between 60 and 100 bpm at rest. An excessive rate is called *tachycardia*, and a rate below normal is called *bradycardia*. Abnormal waveforms indicative of these conditions appear in Figure 6.2. Heart fibrillation can be detected

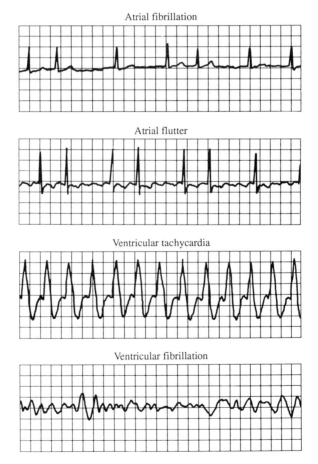

FIGURE 6.2
Abnormal cardiograms. [Courtesy of Nihon Kohden (America), Inc.]

by observation of the ECG. Ventricular fibrillation, a critical and potentially fatal condition, is indicated by loss of the *QRS* complex. The missing *QRS* means that the ventricle is not contracting and blood circulation is severely impaired. The ECG waveform of the fibrillating heart is illustrated in the figure as well. The waveform has distinctive high-frequency components that are used in automatic machine diagnosis of this condition. Atrial fibrillation, which is less serious, is indicated by a loss of the *P*-wave on the ECG. In this case, and in the case of atrial flutter, the *QRS* is still present and blood circulation is maintained.

Ectopic beats originate from a place other than the sinoatrial (SA) node. An ectopic beat in the ventricle causes an extra *R*-wave, indicative of a premature ventricular contraction (PVC). PVCs are easier to detect than ecotopic beats originating in the atrium, which are called premature atrial contractions (PACs). PVCs may be detected by monitoring the *R-R* interval of an ECG waveform.

The ECG Block Diagram

An ECG device, as illustrated in Figure 6.3, amplifies an ECG signal and displays it on an output unit. Representative specifications on the unit are as follows:

Input impedance	5 MΩ
Frequency response	±0.5 dB (0.14 Hz to 25 Hz)
	3 dB (to 100 Hz)

The ECG device processes the biopotential signal into a form suitable for the output unit. Often the data is presented graphically as in Figure 6.2, on a strip chart recorder:

Normal rate	25 mm/s
High rate	100 mm/s

In its path through the instrument, the biopotential from the surface electrodes passes through a defibrillator protection circuit. One configuration of this circuit consists of neon gas tubes that fire when a pulse from a defibrillator is present. The defibrillator pulse may exceed 1000 V, which has the capability of destroying the bioamplifier. Various combinations of the ECG leads can be selected for configurations we will describe in Section 6.2. A 1-mV calibration pulse is used to calibrate the bioamplifier by enabling the technician to observe the output and adjust the scale so that a known deflection corresponds to a 1-mV input signal. This calibration switch also provides a handy troubleshooting aid. If it works properly, it is clear that the electronics beyond it to the output is working, and that a failure, if pres-

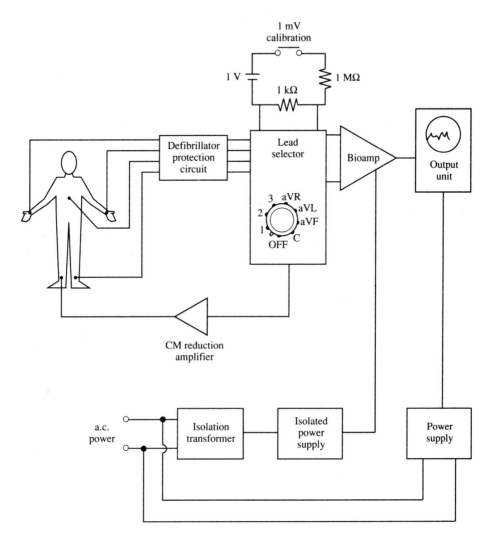

FIGURE 6.3
A simplified block diagram of an ECG.

ent, has occurred before it in the signal path. Troubleshooting tips for this section of the equipment appear in Box 1.

Since the patient leads of an ECG are connected through relatively low impedance electrodes, and are positioned on the skin across the heart, it is necessary to avoid the macroshock resulting from currents exceeding 10 mA. If the patient is wearing an external pacemaker, or the patient's heart is catheterized, a microshock hazard exists, and patient-level currents must

Box 1

SOURCES OF INTERFERENCE IN AN ECG TRACE

Possible Artifacts	Check the Following:
Base Line with No Wave Form	• Trace switch ON and gain control set high enough? Readjust as required. Select appropriate lead. • Lead wires and patient cable fully inserted into proper receptacle? • Cable or lead wires damaged? (Check with a lead continuity tester.)
Base Line Wander	• Patient moving excessively? Secure lead wires and cable to patient. • Caused by patient's respiration? Reposition electrodes. • Electrodes dry? Re-prep skin and apply fresh moist electrodes. • Static buildup around patient? Check with Engineering.
a.c. Noise	• Gain set too high? Readjust as required. • Unit in diagnostic mode? Select monitoring mode. • Electrodes dry? Re-prep skin and apply fresh moist electrodes. • Patient cable entwined with cables of other electrical devices? Separate patient cable from all other cables.

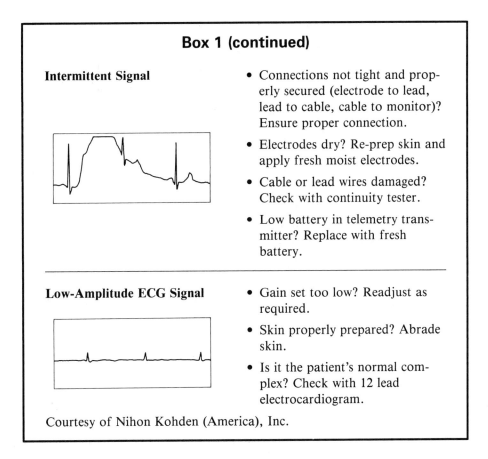

Box 1 (continued)

Intermittent Signal

- Connections not tight and properly secured (electrode to lead, lead to cable, cable to monitor)? Ensure proper connection.

- Electrodes dry? Re-prep skin and apply fresh moist electrodes.

- Cable or lead wires damaged? Check with continuity tester.

- Low battery in telemetry transmitter? Replace with fresh battery.

Low-Amplitude ECG Signal

- Gain set too low? Readjust as required.

- Skin properly prepared? Abrade skin.

- Is it the patient's normal complex? Check with 12 lead electrocardiogram.

Courtesy of Nihon Kohden (America), Inc.

be maintained below 10 μA. This is done by providing bias power to the amplifier through an isolation transformer, which drives an isolated power supply, as shown in Figure 6.3. Because the electronic power requirements are low, a rechargeable battery may also be used. The output unit, consisting of a paper chart recorder or a cathode-ray-tube screen, requires high power and often requires an electronic power supply. This power supply does not require the same degree of isolation as the bioamp because it normally does not contact the patient. Detailed circuitry that may be used in these blocks is described in subsequent sections.

A variation on the ECG instrumentation illustrated in Figure 6.4 uses a differential amplifier to measure the ECG of a fetus. The lead on the mother's chest referenced in a Wilson connection (see Section 6.2) measures her ECG, called M. The mother's ECG will be stronger and at a lower rate

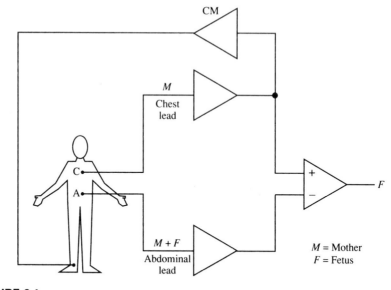

FIGURE 6.4
A block diagram of a fetal ECG.

than the ECG of the fetus. An electrode on the abdomen will measure both M and the fetus ECG, called F.

The differential amplifier then takes the difference $(M + F) - M = F$. Its output thus measures the ECG of the fetus, because the mother's ECG, M, is subtracted away.

Certain abnormalities of the heart, such as PVCs, may occur only when the body is under a physical stress such as exercise, which makes demands for higher cardiac output. To simulate these conditions in the clinical environment, and to obtain a record for diagnosis, stress testing ECG instrumentation, as illustrated in Figure 6.5, is used. The patient walks on a treadmill at a controlled rate, and vital parameters, including the ECG, blood pressure, and heart rate, are monitored and recorded. Signal processing in the instrumentation should be designed to eliminate, or compensate for, artifacts due to skeletal muscle contraction and electrode motion.

It is important to be aware of PVCs or other abnormal episodes in ill patients. To detect these, the ECG leads are attached permanently so that the patient can carry on normal activities. In the 1940s Norman Holter introduced the idea of recording the ECG on a tape recorder at slow speed and playing it back at high speed, so that 24 hours of ECG could be viewed in as little as 12 minutes by a trained observer. These devices are called Holter monitors. However, because use of the tape recorder is time-

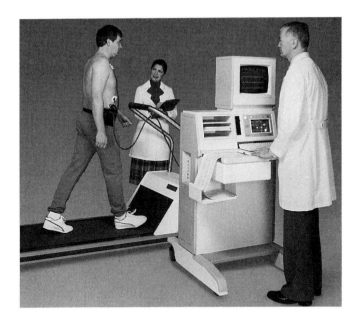

FIGURE 6.5
An ECG monitor for stress testing. (Courtesy of Quinton, Inc.)

consuming, and there are mechanical difficulties associated with it, hand-held computers have been developed that store only the critical episodes for review at a later time. These devices are small enough to be worn conveniently by the ambulatory patient, as illustrated in Figure 6.6. They contain a solid-state memory that receives data all day. The data may then be reviewed by the physician at a convenient time.

ECG hard-copy display devices often use a thermal stylus that leaves a trace on heat-sensitive paper, as illustrated in Figure 6.7(a). Modern units use dot-matrix displays. A temporary record for real-time viewing, using a liquid-crystal display surface (see Figure 6.7b), is convenient for battery-operated devices. The display has low power drain, so the batteries last a long time. A solid-state memory for storing ECG data for later analysis and interpretation is illustrated in Figure 6.7(c).

6.2 ECG LEAD CONNECTIONS

The process described in Section 2.3 gives rise to the electrocardiogram (ECG) voltages measured from the four human limbs, in either a standard connection, an augmented lead connection, or a Wilson lead connection, among others.

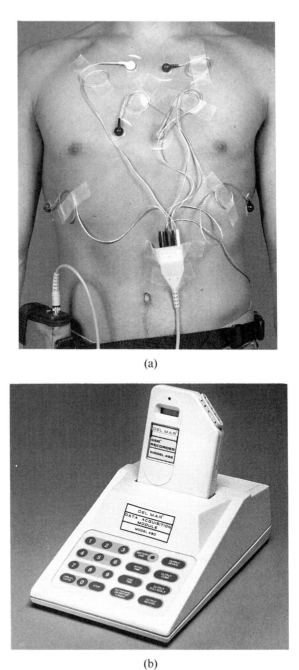

(a)

(b)

FIGURE 6.6
(a) A Holter monitor mounted on the belt with ECG leads attached. (Courtesy of Marquette Electronics) (b) A Holter recorder mounted in a reader for acquisition of recorded data. (Courtesy of Del Mar Avionics)

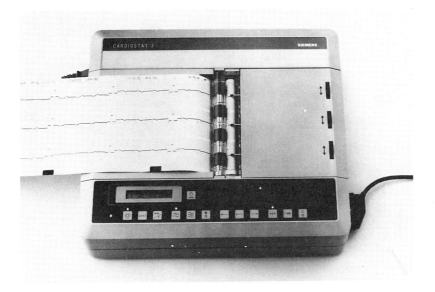

(a)

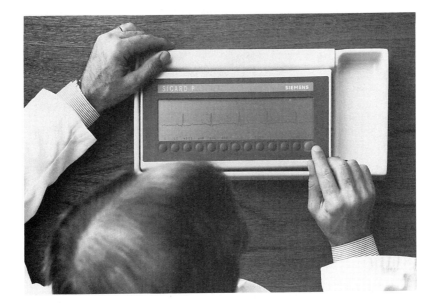

(b)

FIGURE 6.7
(a) A multichannel chart records several leads simultaneously. (b) ECG data is displayed on a large liquid-crystal unit that can store up to 20 ECGs for later analysis. (c) (next page) An interpretive ECG allows keyboard entry of patient data, storing up to 20 ECGs in memory for later retrieval and analysis. (Courtesy of Siemens, Inc.)

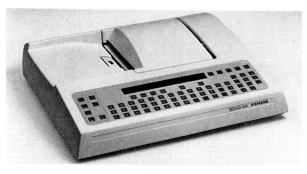

(c)

FIGURE 6.7 (continued)

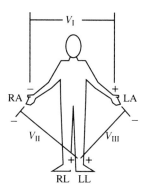

FIGURE 6.8
Standard ECG lead connections.

The standard biopotential polarities in Figure 6.8 show voltage V_I, the voltage drop from the left arm (LA) to the right arm (RA); V_{II}, the drop from the left leg (LL) to the right arm (RA); and lead voltage V_{III}, the drop from the left leg to the left arm. Kirchhoff's voltage law (KVL) applied to the figure yields

$$V_I = V_{II} - V_{III} \qquad (6.2)$$

Historically, the closed path RA to LA to LL and back to RA has been called the *Einthoven triangle*. It should be noted that the values in Table 6.1 are not consistent with Equation (6.2) because they are averages taken

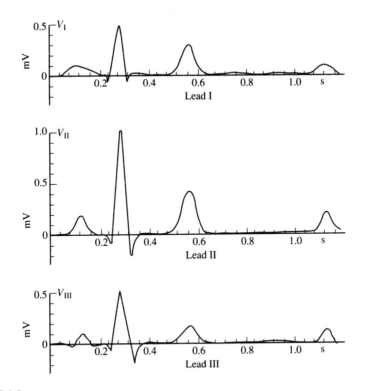

FIGURE 6.9
ECG lead voltage V_{III} is computed from V_I and V_{II}.

over a group of subjects. Equation (6.2) applies to the ECG waveforms taken at one time on one individual.

Example voltages as measured by the connection at lead I, V_I, and the lead II connection, V_{II}, are shown in Figure 6.9.

EXAMPLE 6.1 From the ECG lead I and lead II traces in Figure 6.9, compute the following:

(a) the *P-R* interval
(b) the *QRS* complex duration
(c) the heart rate
(d) the lead III, V_{III}, voltage as a function of time

SOLUTION The *P-R* time = 0.16 s; the *QRS* duration = 90 ms; the heart rate = 60 bpm. To compute V_{III} note that $V_{III} = V_{II} - V_I$ in Figure 6.8; V_{III} is plotted in Figure 6.9.

The ECG potentials are measured with color-coded leads according to the convention:

white – right arm
black – left arm
green – right leg
red – left leg
brown – chest

The standard voltage V_I is measured by connecting the left arm to the positive, noninverting terminal, and the right arm to the negative, inverting terminal of the differential amplifier. The common-mode, CM, voltage compensation is connected to the right leg as shown in Figure 6.10(a). Similarly, the lead connections for the standard voltage V_{II} and V_{III} are given in parts (b) and (c) of the figure.

Augmented ECG Lead Connections

For certain lead connections, a small increase in the ECG voltage can be realized by use of augmented lead connections, called augmented voltage right arm (aVR), augmented voltage left arm (aVL), and augmented voltage foot (aVF), illustrated in Figure 6.11. All resistors have the same value R, which is made small compared to the input resistance of the measurement amplifier. In order to calculate the augmented voltages from standard lead voltages, the following relations are obtained from Figure 6.11 by application of KVL:

$$aVR = -V_I - \frac{V_{III}}{2} \qquad (6.3)$$

$$aVL = V_I - \frac{V_{II}}{2} \qquad (6.4)$$

$$aVF = V_{II} - \frac{V_I}{2} \qquad (6.5)$$

EXAMPLE 6.2   From the standard lead ECG voltages V_I and V_{II} in Figure 6.9, compute the augmented lead ECG waveform aVF.

SOLUTION   Plotting Equation 6.5 in Figure 6.9 shows that aVF is larger than the voltage V_{III}, indicating an advantage of the aVF hookup in this case.

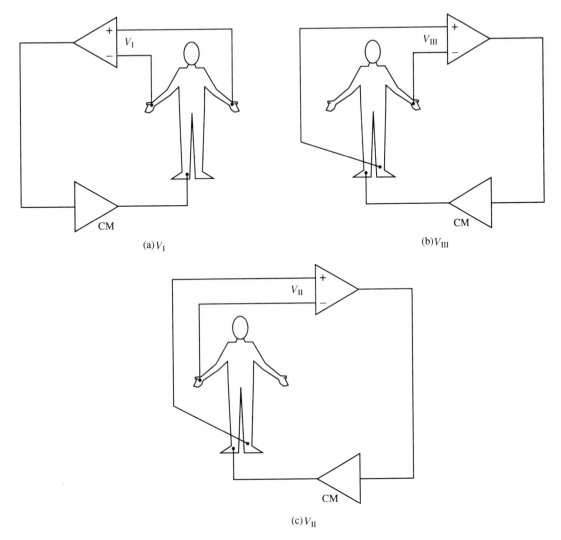

FIGURE 6.10
The standard ECG connections to the bioamplifier and common-mode reduction amplifier.

Chest Lead Connection

To make chest lead ECG measurements, the chest lead, *C*, is applied to the noninverting terminal of a differential amplifier, as shown in Figure 6.12. The reference is taken from the node of a wye connection of resistors, called the Wilson central terminal. The end-nodes of the Wilson connection are made to the right arm, left arm, and left leg, respectively.

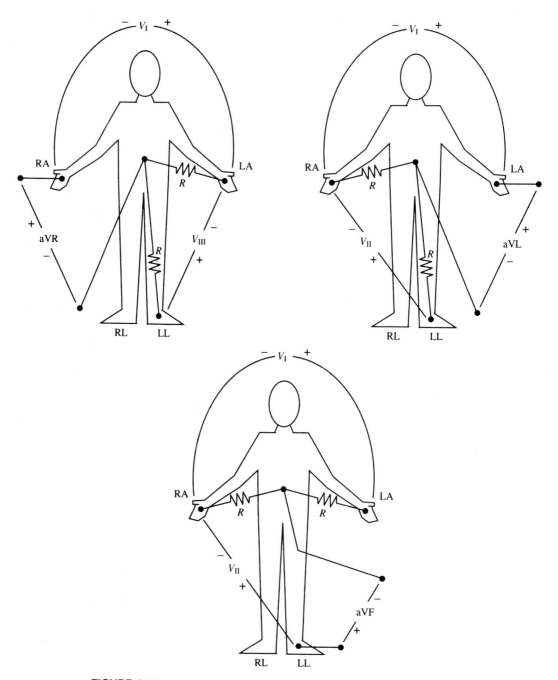

FIGURE 6.11
Augmented lead connections for an ECG.

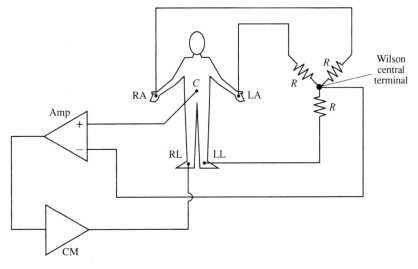

FIGURE 6.12
Chest lead connections to an ECG.

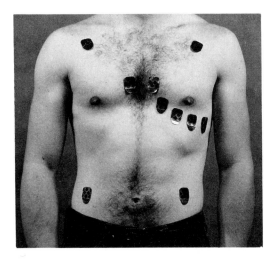

FIGURE 6.13
Chest lead electrode positions V_1 through V_6. The limb connections are made through the four corners of the torso. (Courtesy of Consolidated Medical Equipment, Inc.)

The shape of the ECG from the chest lead depends strongly on the anatomical position. Six chest voltages are measured as the voltage drops from the chest lead to the Wilson central terminal. The chest lead positions, shown in Figure 6.13 for these voltages, are:

V_1 – Fourth intercostal space, on the right sternal margin.
V_2 – Fourth intercostal space, on the left sternal margin.
V_3 – Midway between V_2 and V_4.
V_4 – Fifth intercostal space on the mid-clavicular line.
V_5 – Same level as V_4, on the anterior axillary line.
V_6 – Same level as V_4, on the mid-axillary line.

Example ECG wave shapes taken from these positions are shown in Figure 6.14. The R-wave is strongly negative in V_1 and V_2 positions, because the chest lead straddles the right and left sides of the heart there. V_6 is similar to the standard V_1 lead, because it is close to the left arm used in the V_1 measurement. The strong dependency of the chest voltages on position makes it possible to identify the regions of the heart that may be abnormal by observing the chest lead ECG. If, for example, leads V_1 and V_2 were to read normal while the others were abnormal, this would be evidence that the injured region is near the left side of the heart.

In order to select among the standard leads, the augmented leads, and the chest leads, the front panel of an ECG has a lead selector switch. This

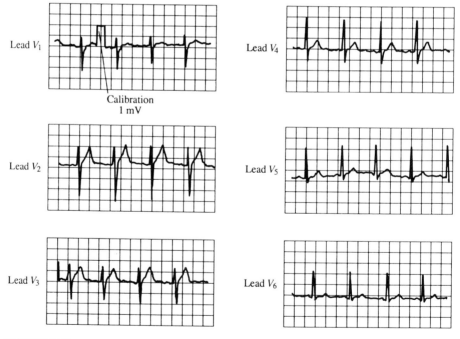

FIGURE 6.14
Dependency of the chest lead ECG waveforms upon position. (From 1500 A Electrocardiograph STM-108A Manual, Hewlett-Packard Company)

switch connects the patient leads to either the noninverting amplifier terminal (+), the inverting terminal (−), or the common-mode reduction circuit connection (CM), as indicated in Figure 6.15.

In order to diagnose the *P*-wave, it is an advantage to position the leads close to the atrium. This may be achieved with an *esophageal lead*, as shown in Figure 6.16. This lead is attached to a pill that is swallowed and then positioned in the esophagus next to the heart. X-ray may be used to aid in the exact positioning of the lead near the heart, as illustrated in Figure 6.17.

As discussed in Chapter 4, proper attachment of electrodes to the patient is crucial to accurate ECG waveforms. User errors or ECG operator errors are often traced to inadequate electrode gel application or poor connection. (See Troubleshooting Tips, Box 1.) Adhesive, pregelled electrodes (Figure 6.18) tend to standardize the collection and minimize the effects of patient movement. However, it is necessary to ensure that the expiration date of the electrodes is carefully observed, since the gel tends to dry out.

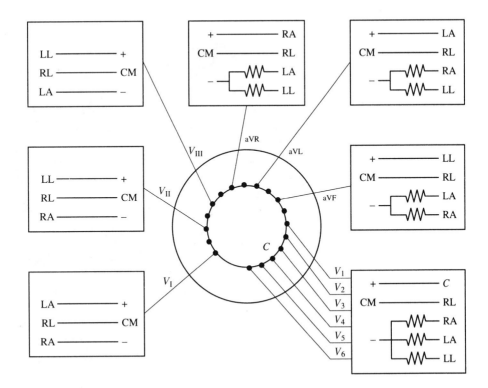

FIGURE 6.15
A lead selector switch schematic.

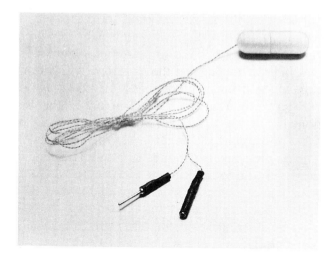

FIGURE 6.16
Esophageal lead with an attached pill electrode. (Courtesy of Consolidated Medical Equipment, Inc.)

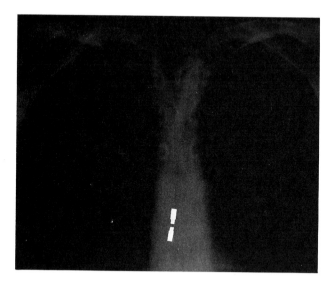

FIGURE 6.17
X-ray of an esophageal pill electrode in the esophagus near the heart. (Courtesy of Consolidated Medical Equipment, Inc.)

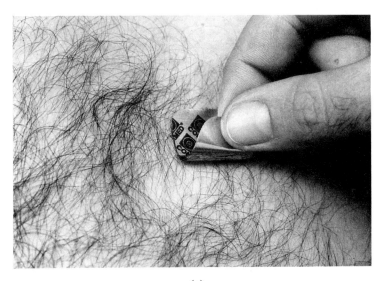

(a)

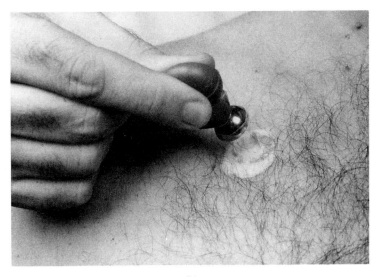

(b)

FIGURE 6.18
(a) An adhesive pregelled electrode applied to a hairy surface. (b) A suction-cup electrode with ample gel applied. (Courtesy of Consolidated Medical Equipment, Inc.)

6.3 COMMON-MODE VOLTAGE REDUCTION

The effects of the common-mode voltage (V_{CM}), such as excessive 60-$\sim$ hum, are discussed in Section 5.3. These effects are reduced by means of a buffered balanced amplifier, illustrated in Section 5.2, and by use of diff amps. In order to further reduce these effects, we employ feedback, which reduces the common-mode voltage on the body. A lower common-mode voltage then appears on the balanced circuit, as illustrated in Figure 6.19. This is a specific example of the common-mode rejection ratio (CMRR) reduction amplifier connected as shown in Figure 6.3 for an ECG. In its essential operation, this circuit amplifies V_{CM} and shifts it by 180° in phase. It then feeds it back to the body at such an amplitude that it tends to cancel the V_{CM} delivered through the stray capacity. The net effect is to reduce V_{CM} on the body.

Analysis of Figure 6.19 shows more precisely how this common-mode voltage is reduced. Kirchhoff's voltage law (KVL) applied to the source, C_S, and V_{CM} to ground, gives

$$V_S = \frac{I_S}{j\omega C_S} + V_{CM} \qquad (6.6)$$

Because the differential amplifiers are considered ideal, V_{CM} appears on both nodes 1 and 2. Therefore, the current through R_2 is zero, and V_{CM} appears on nodes 3 and 4. Applying the current law (KCL) on node 5 gives

$$\frac{V_{CM}}{R_4} + \frac{V_{CM}}{R_3} + \frac{V_{OUT}}{R_f} = 0 \qquad (6.7)$$

Also from Ohm's law on resistor R_{OUT}, we have

$$\frac{V_{CM} - V_{OUT}}{R_{OUT}} = I_S \qquad (6.8)$$

Algebraic manipulation of these equations is as follows: putting Equation (6.8) into Equation (6.6) yields

$$V_S = \frac{V_{CM} - V_{OUT}}{j\omega R_{OUT} C_S} + V_{CM}$$

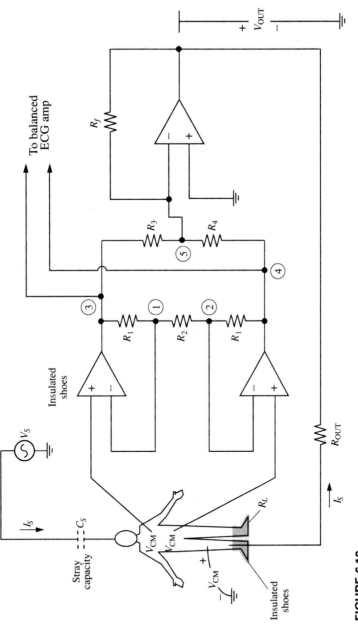

FIGURE 6.19
A common-mode voltage reduction circuit.

Solving this for V_{OUT} gives

$$V_{\text{OUT}} = V_{\text{CM}} - (V_S - V_{\text{CM}})j\omega R_{\text{OUT}}C_S$$

This equation into Equation (6.7) yields

$$V_{\text{CM}} = \frac{j2\pi f R_{\text{OUT}} C_S V_S}{\dfrac{R_f}{R_3} + \dfrac{R_f}{R_4} + 1 + j2\pi f R_{\text{OUT}} C_S} \tag{6.9}$$

where $\omega = 2\pi f$ is the frequency. Equation (6.9) shows that the common-mode voltage that appears on the body depends upon the resistor values in Figure 6.19 as well as frequency. The merit of knowing about this equation is that it allows you to determine exactly how R_f, C_S, R_{OUT}, and the other circuit parameters affect the value of V_{CM}. To study the effects of these parameters on V_{CM}, a computer program is given in Appendix A, Program A-6. The flow diagram is shown in Figure 6.20.

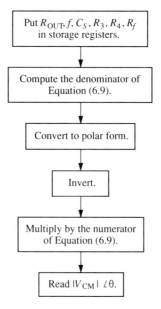

FIGURE 6.20
A flow diagram for Equation (6.9) for Program A-6, Appendix A.

Troubleshooting Tip

Failure of the circuit in Figure 6.19 will increase 60-$\sim$ hum and noise on all leads of the ECG.

A computer analysis of this circuit is illustrated in Exercises 15 and 16.

EXAMPLE 6.3 A patient is connected to a driven-right-leg feedback system and is insulated from ground. Sixty-$\sim$ power-line voltages are coupled to him through 2-pF stray capacity. This creates a common-mode voltage V_{CM} over his body. In Figure 6.19, take $R_1 = 10$ kΩ, $R_2 = 2$ kΩ, $R_3 = 30$ kΩ, $R_4 = 20$ kΩ, $R_f = 7$ MΩ, and $R_{OUT} = 7$ MΩ. Compute V_{CM}.

SOLUTION Using Equation (6.9), take $V_S = 120$ V:

$$V_{CM} = \frac{j2\pi 60(7)(10^6)(2)(10^{-12})(120)}{\dfrac{7(10^6)}{30(10^3)} + \dfrac{7(10^6)}{20(10^3)} + 1 + j2\pi 60(7)(10^6)(2)(10^{-12})}$$

or

$$V_{CM} = 1.084 \text{ mV}, \theta = 90°$$

Comparing this with Example 5.11, where no feedback was used, shows a large reduction in common-mode voltage due to the driven-right-leg system.

6.4 PUSH-PULL POWER AMPLIFIERS

The output unit of an ECG monitor, as well as many other medical instruments, requires sufficient electrical power to activate the display. Devices such as thermal styluses, paper chart recorder motors, cathode-ray tubes, and activation relays require efficient, relatively high power sources.

Power amplifiers generally use lumped element transistors, because a relatively large surface area is necessary to dissipate the heat generated in the chip due to high current required to develop the power. High power in integrated circuits is considered approximately greater than 0.1 W. The important figures of merit for the power amplifier are power gain, efficiency, input impedance, and output impedance. It is also important to consider impedance matching for maximum power transfer.

The basic circuit for a power amplifier using a silicon power transistor with a forward-biased emitter to base voltage $V_{BE} = 0.7$ V, and a *V-I* characteristic as illustrated, is given in Figure 6.21. The circuit operates as follows. When V_B is sufficiently positive, transistor $Q1$ is forward biased and conducts, while $Q2$ is reverse biased and remains OFF. KVL then yields

$$V_B = 0.7 + V_{OUT} \qquad (6.10)$$

Then when V_B is sufficiently negative, KVL through $Q2$ yields

$$V_B = -0.7 + V_{OUT} \qquad (6.11)$$

Also, when $-0.7 < V_B < 0.7$, both transistor base to emitter junctions are reverse biased, turning both the transistors OFF. In this case, $V_{OUT} \approx 0$ and $I_C \approx 0$. The resulting quiescent point, Q, is shown in Figure 6.21(b).

The V_{OUT}-V_B characteristic for the power amplifier plotted in Figure 6.22 from Equations (6.10) and (6.11) shows that the voltage gain of the amplifier is approximately 1 in the ideal case. A plot of the V_{OUT} resulting from V_B in Figure 6.22 clearly shows the crossover distortion near the dead region in the V_{OUT}-V_B curve. The maximum current that can pass

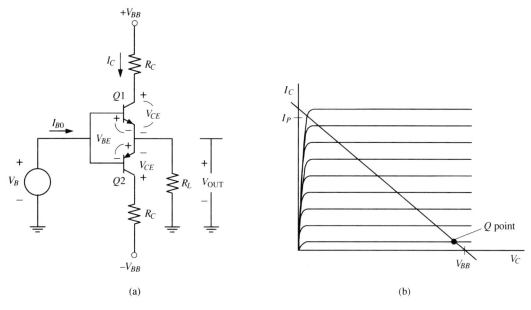

(a)   (b)

FIGURE 6.21
A push-pull power amplifier.

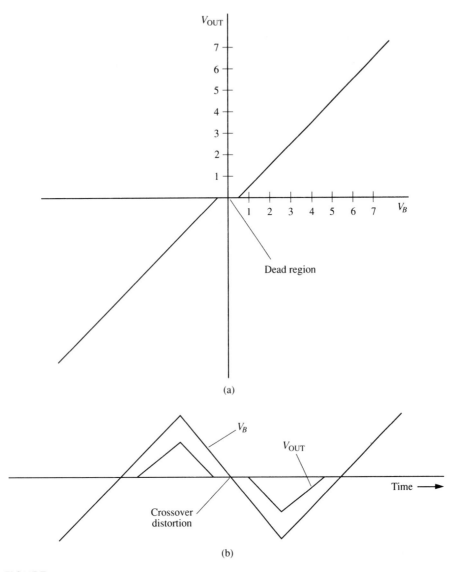

(a)

(b)

FIGURE 6.22
(a) The output voltage versus input voltage characteristic of a power amplifier. (b) The output and input voltages.

through the transistor occurs when the transistor is fully ON, and V_{CE} is approximately 0.2 V for a silicon transistor. That is,

$$I_{C\max} = \frac{V_{BB}}{R_C + R_L} \qquad (6.12)$$

when the transistor $Q1$ is fully ON. Under the approximation $I_E \approx I_C$ for a transistor with a current gain $\beta \gg 1$, we have a maximum output voltage of

$$V_{\text{OUTmax}} = \frac{R_L}{R_C + R_L} \, V_{BB} \qquad\qquad (6.13)$$

Likewise, the minimum voltage is

$$V_{\text{OUTmin}} = \frac{-R_L}{R_C + R_L} \, V_{BB} \qquad\qquad (6.14)$$

The input impedance of the amplifier is computed from the definition $Z_{\text{IN}} = V_B/I_B$. KVL applied to the base to emitter circuit, assuming $V_{BE} = 0.7$ V, gives

$$V_B = 0.7 + (1 + \beta)I_B R_L$$

Thus, when $V_B \gg 0.7$ V, we have

$$Z_{\text{IN}} \approx (1 + \beta)R_L \qquad\qquad (6.15)$$

It is now possible to calculate the power gain of the amplifier using the definition

$$G_P = \frac{P_{\text{OUT}}}{P_{\text{IN}}} \qquad\qquad (6.16)$$

First notice that

$$P_{\text{IN}} = \frac{V_B^2}{Z_{\text{IN}}}$$

Then using Equation (6.15),

$$P_{\text{IN}} = \frac{V_B^2}{(1 + \beta)R_L}$$

and

$$P_{\text{OUT}} = \frac{V_{\text{OUT}}^2}{R_L}$$

But for large voltage outputs $V_{OUT} \approx V_B$, and therefore Equation (6.16), using the above relations for P_{IN} and P_{OUT}, yields

$$G_{Pmax} \approx 1 + \beta \qquad (6.17)$$

where G_{Pmax} is the maximum value of the power gain of the amplifier. A basic limitation on the amount of power that a transistor can deliver is that the heat generated by circuit inefficiency must be dissipated. The higher the efficiency, the less heat generated, and the higher the power handling capability. The amplifier efficiency η is given by the definition

$$\eta = \frac{P_{OUT}}{P_{OUT} + P_{LOSS}} \qquad (6.18)$$

In Figure 6.21 the following power relationships hold, assuming d.c. voltages:

$$P_{OUT} = \frac{V_{OUT}^2}{R_L} \qquad (6.19)$$

The output power is considered to be that absorbed by R_L. The power absorbed by the transistor and R_C are considered loss:

$$P_{LOSS} = I_C^2 R_C + V_{CE} I_C \qquad (6.20)$$

When the top transistor in Figure 6.21 is conducting, KVL gives

$$V_{BB} = I_C R_C + V_{CE} + V_{OUT} \qquad (6.21)$$

For high current gain transistors ($\beta \gg 10$) we may approximate $I_C \approx I_L = V_{OUT}/R_L$. This into Equation (6.21) gives

$$V_{BB} = \frac{V_{OUT}}{R_L} R_C + V_{CE} + V_{OUT}$$

which may be solved for V_{CE} as

$$V_{CE} = V_{BB} - V_{OUT}\left(1 + \frac{R_C}{R_L}\right)$$

Substituting this equation for V_{CE} in Equation (6.20) results in

$$P_{\text{LOSS}} = \left(\frac{V_{\text{OUT}}}{R_L}\right)^2 R_C + \frac{V_{\text{OUT}}}{R_L}\left[V_{BB} - V_{\text{OUT}}\left(1 + \frac{R_C}{R_L}\right)\right]$$

This, along with Equation (6.19) into Equation (6.18), gives the efficiency:

$$\eta = \frac{\dfrac{V_{\text{OUT}}^2}{R_L}}{\dfrac{V_{\text{OUT}}^2}{R_L} + \left(\dfrac{V_{\text{OUT}}}{R_L}\right)^2 R_C + \dfrac{V_{\text{OUT}}}{R_L}\left[V_{BB} - V_{\text{OUT}}\left(1 + \dfrac{R_C}{R_L}\right)\right]}$$

This reduces to a simple equation for d.c. efficiency:

$$\eta = \frac{V_{\text{OUT}}}{V_{BB}} \qquad\qquad (6.22)$$

Under maximum power transfer conditions $R_C = R_L$ in Figure 6.21. The upper limit on V_L is then $V_{BB}/2$. The maximum d.c. efficiency is 50% under maximum power transfer conditions. Higher efficiency is possible as V_{OUT} gets closer to V_{BB}.

Maximum Power Transfer

The output terminals of an amplifier can be represented by its Thevenin equivalent, which consists of an open circuit voltage source in series with its "Thevenin" resistance. The "Thevenin" resistance is defined as the output resistance, R_{OUT}, of an amplifier or, in general, of a voltage source. An analysis of the power, P_L, delivered to a load, R_L, is obtained from Figure 6.23. By voltage division,

$$V_L = \frac{R_L}{R_{\text{OUT}} + R_L} V_{\text{OC}}$$

The power absorbed by the load, P_L, is equal to V_L^2/R_L, yielding from this equation

$$P_L = \frac{R_L}{(R_{\text{OUT}} + R_L)^2} V_{\text{OC}}^2 \qquad\qquad (6.23)$$

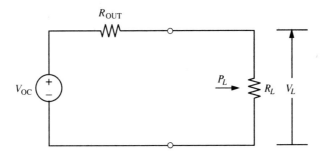

FIGURE 6.23
A Thevenin's equivalent voltage source loaded by R_L.

EXAMPLE 6.4 In Figure 6.23, let $R_{OUT} = 10\ \Omega$ and $V_{OC} = 10$ V, and plot the load power P_L versus the load resistance R_L.

SOLUTION Substitution of the values into Equation (6.23) results in

$$P_L = \frac{100R_L}{(10 + R_L)^2}$$

A plot of P_L for several values of R_L appears in Figure 6.24.

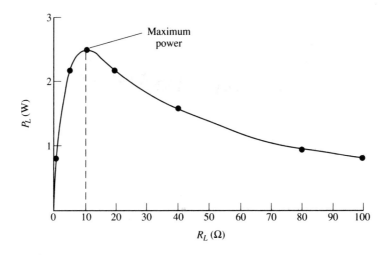

FIGURE 6.24
Maximum power is transferred when $R_L = R_{OUT}$.

This plot of the data shows that the maximum value, $P_{L\max} = 2.5$, occurs when $R_L = 10\ \Omega$. This is the same value as R_{OUT}. In general, it is true that maximum power is transferred to a resistive load in Figure 6.23 when R_L is chosen so that

$$R_L = R_{\text{OUT}} \tag{6.24}$$

A derivation using calculus is given in Box 2. It is also true that when a.c. impedances are involved, maximum power is transferred to a load Z_L when the output impedance of the source Z_{OUT} equals the complex conjugate of the load. That is,

$$Z_L = Z_{\text{OUT}}^* \tag{6.25}$$

where * indicates a complex conjugate. Recall that to form the complex conjugate of a number, we change the sign of the j everywhere it appears.

Box 2

CALCULUS FOR CLARITY

In general, the following analysis shows that maximum power transfer occurs when $R_L = R_{\text{OUT}}$ in Figure 6.23. A mathematical derivation of this fact goes as follows.

The maximum power occurs when $dP_L/dR_L = 0$. Thus, taking the derivative of Equation (6.23) yields

$$\frac{dP_L}{dR_L} = \frac{V_{\text{OC}}^2}{(R_{\text{OUT}} + R_L)^2} - \frac{2R_L V_{\text{OC}}^2}{(R_L + R_{\text{OUT}})^3} = 0$$

Rewriting this yields

$$\frac{R_L + R_{\text{OUT}} - 2R_L}{(R_L + R_{\text{OUT}})^3} = 0$$

Then we have $R_L = R_{\text{OUT}}$, which satisfies the condition for maximum power transfer.

A Push-Pull Amplifier with Crossover Compensation

In order to effectively eliminate the crossover distortion in a push-pull amplifier, an ideal noninverting amplifier may be inserted as shown in Figure 6.25. KCL applied to node 1, where the voltage is equal to V_{IN} by the voltage rule for ideal diff amps, yields the equation

$$\frac{V_{IN}}{R_i} + \frac{V_{IN} - V_L}{R_f} = 0$$

Solving for V_L then gives

$$V_L = V_{IN}\left(1 + \frac{R_f}{R_i}\right)$$

This shows that the output voltage V_L is linear with no crossover distortion, the voltage gain A_V being

$$A_V = 1 + \frac{R_f}{R_i} \qquad (6.26)$$

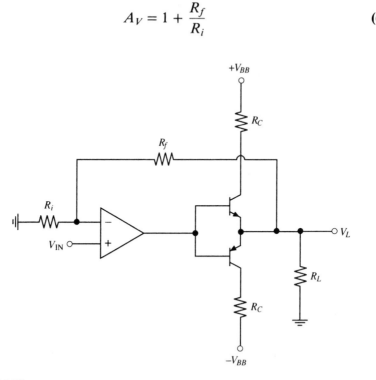

FIGURE 6.25
A power amplifier with crossover distortion compensation.

Since the input impedance of the operational amplifier is ideally infinite, it draws essentially zero current. Therefore, the input power is nearly zero, and the power gain approaches infinity.

A heuristic reason why the dead region is eliminated in the push-pull transistor pair is that in the dead region, the feedback resistance from the output of the operational amplifier to node 1 becomes large, which raises the gain and in turn raises the output voltage.

The d.c. efficiency of the amplifier is approximately given by Equation (6.22) since the argument leading to it is nearly unaffected by the presence of the operational amplifier in Figure 6.25. The power losses due to R_f, R_i, and the diff amp are assumed to be much smaller than those in the transistors and R_C.

Power Amplifier with Offset Control

The schematic for a power amplifier with crossover compensation and an offset control is shown in Figure 6.26. Such an amplifier is useful as the

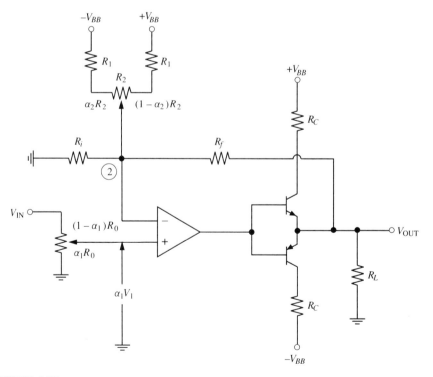

FIGURE 6.26
A power amplifier with an offset adjustment.

driver for an ECG chart recorder stylus, for example. The offset control, R_2, can be used to position the output stylus. Gain adjustment is achieved with R_0. To determine a formula for V_{OUT}, notice that the lower node voltage of the operational amplifier input is $\alpha_1 V_1$, and by the voltage rule for operational amplifiers, the voltage at node 2 is also $\alpha_1 V_1$, assuming ideal components. Applying KCL to the currents leaving node 2 gives

$$\frac{\alpha_1 V_1}{R_i} + \frac{\alpha_1 V_1 - (-V_{BB})}{\alpha_2 R_2 + R_1} + \frac{\alpha_1 V_1 - V_{BB}}{R_1 + (1 - \alpha_2) R_2} + \frac{\alpha_1 V_1 - V_{OUT}}{R_f} = 0$$

where V is the d.c. bias on the amplifier.

This equation is solved for V_{OUT} as follows:

$$V_{OUT} = \frac{R_f}{R_i}(\alpha_1 V_1) + R_f \frac{\alpha_1 V_1 + V_{BB}}{\alpha_2 R_2 + R_1} + R_f \frac{\alpha_1 V_1 - V_{BB}}{(1 - \alpha_2) R_2 + R_1} + \alpha_1 V_1$$

$$(6.27)$$

EXAMPLE 6.5   The power amplifier given by Figure 6.26 has the component values $R_f = 10$ kΩ, $R_i = 1$ kΩ, $R_1 = 2$ kΩ, $R_2 = 3$ kΩ, $\alpha_1 = 0.3$, and $\alpha_2 = 0.7$. The bias voltage $V_{BB} = 12$ V.

SOLUTION   These component values in Equation (6.27) give the values plotted in Figure 6.27 for V_{OUT} versus V_1. Program A-7 in Appendix A can be used for this calculation.

6.5 POWER SUPPLIES

Most patient-care instruments require a power supply to convert the 60-$\sim$ a.c. power-line voltage to a d.c. voltage. This is the case because most electronic circuits, including transistors, integrated circuits, and vacuum tubes, require a d.c. voltage for bias.

One of the simplest power supplies consists of a diode in series with a resistor. When the voltage across the combination forward-biases the diode, current flows. A reversal of the applied voltage then reverse-biases the diode and current stops. This describes a half-wave rectifier.

Practical single-phase power supplies often utilize a full-wave rectifier, shown in Figure 6.28. If V_{IN} is a sinusoidal voltage, then V_{AB} through an ideal transformer is

$$V_{AB} = \frac{N_2}{N_1} V_{IN}$$

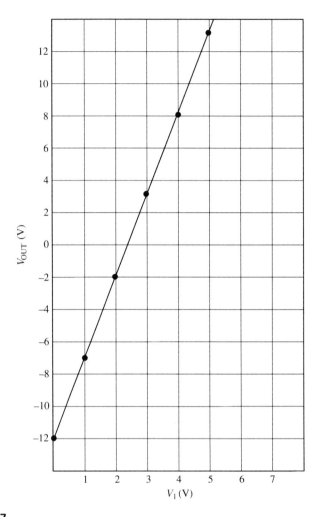

FIGURE 6.27
The output versus input voltage for Example 6.5.

When the voltage V_{AB} is positive, diodes 1 and 2 are forward biased, while diodes 3 and 4 are reverse biased. In this case,

$$V_{AB} = 2V_f + V_{OUT}$$

where V_f is the forward voltage of the diode, usually 0.7 V for silicon diodes. Combining the previous two equations gives us

$$V_{OUT} = \frac{N_2}{N_1} V_{IN} - 2V_f \qquad (V_{IN} \text{ positive}) \qquad \textbf{(6.28)}$$

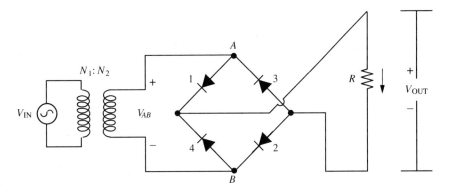

FIGURE 6.28
A full-wave power supply.

Likewise,

$$V_{\text{OUT}} = -\frac{N_2}{N_1} V_{\text{IN}} - 2V_f \qquad (V_{\text{IN}} \text{ negative}) \qquad \textbf{(6.29)}$$

EXAMPLE 6.6 The power supply in Figure 6.26 has $N_1{:}N_2 = 1{:}1$, and $V_f = 0.7$ V on silicon diodes. A 60-$\sim$ source voltage V_{IN} of 2 V peak is passed through the ideal transformer. Plot V_{OUT} versus V_{IN}.

SOLUTION In Equations (6.28) and (6.29), $V_{\text{IN}} = 2 \sin 377t$. A plot of V_{OUT} from these equations is shown in Figure 6.29. Because the V_{IN} is near V_f in magnitude, the crossover distortion is exaggerated in this example.

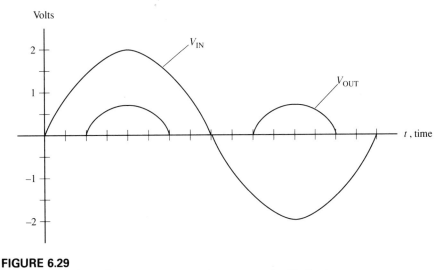

FIGURE 6.29
The output voltage from a power supply compared with the input.

In order to smooth the pulsating output voltage, V_{OUT} in Figure 6.29, a capacitor may be placed across R in Figure 6.28. The rise time of the current through the diodes is chosen to be short compared with the a.c. voltage period, while the fall time through the load resistor R is long compared with the a.c. voltage period. This is possible because the forward resistance of the diode can be made much less than R.

Power Supply Regulation

Because of the output impedance of a power supply, changes in the load current cause proportional changes in the output voltage. Power supply voltage regulation is required to reduce this effect. A sample voltage regulator of a d.c. power supply voltage is illustrated in Figure 6.30. The key element is the zener diode, whose *V-I* characteristics are given in Figure 6.31. The diode acts like an open circuit for negative voltages greater than V_Z, the zener breakdown voltage. When it is biased as a regulator, the voltage

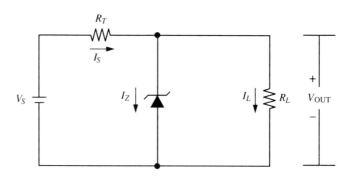

FIGURE 6.30
A regulating circuit using a zener diode.

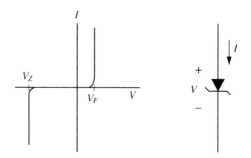

FIGURE 6.31
Zener diode voltage versus current characteristic.

across the diode is approximately V_Z and the current I_Z is determined by the external circuit.

In Figure 6.30 the output voltage $V_{OUT} = V_Z$ unless R_L decreases to the point that $I_L = I_S$, turning the zener diode OFF. In this case, $I_S = I_L$, making

$$\frac{V_S - V_Z}{R_T} = \frac{V_Z}{R_{Lmin}}$$

Solving for R_{Lmin},

$$R_{Lmin} = \frac{V_Z R_T}{V_S - V_Z} \qquad (6.30)$$

where R_{Lmin} is the minimum load resistance for which the zener regulates the output voltage.

EXAMPLE 6.7   A 10-V power supply has a 2-Ω output resistance. Find the largest load current that can be regulated to 7 V using the zener diode in Figure 6.30.

SOLUTION   The minimum load resistance, from Equation (6.30), is

$$R_{Lmin} = \frac{7(2)}{10 - 7} = 4.666 \ \Omega$$

The load current through this resistor is the largest load that can be regulated. That is,

$$I_{Lmax} = \frac{V_Z}{R_{Lmin}} = \frac{7}{4.666} = 1.5 \ A$$

6.6 UNIT-LEVEL TROUBLESHOOTING: ECGs

Troubleshooting of an ECG is done at the unit level. It is assumed that from a system-level perspective, all other possibilities have been eliminated, and it has been determined that there is a fault in the ECG instrument, including the patient leads and electrodes. Unless there is obvious physical damage, or overheating, the most likely source of symptoms will be on the display device.

The ECG trace, as indicated in Box 1, often reveals operator problems, such as maladjustment of the gain or poor connection of the electrodes to the patient. Dried-out electrode gel due to the use of out-of-date pregelled electrodes, or due to their being left on the patient too long, is an especially common problem. Visual inspection is usually sufficient to find this problem. Frayed or broken wires can be traced with an ohmmeter. A blank ECG trace can be caused by a blown fuse or an inoperative power supply. Suggested steps to take to remedy ECG trace artifacts are given in Box 1.

Proper placement of leads is especially important in ECGs such as the fetal monitor, the Holter monitor, and the stress tester. In the case of the fetal monitor, the site of the abdominal lead depends upon the position of the fetus. Both the Holter and stress-testing monitors have leads attached to ambulatory patients, and are thus subject to more movement, gel depletion, and abuse than usual.

After lead problem and operator errors have been eliminated as a source of trouble, circuit-board-level troubleshooting should be pursued with the aid of a block diagram, such as in Figure 6.3. The block diagram for a specific piece of equipment is available in the maintenance manual provided by the manufacturer. Referring to the figure, you would move logically from the input to the output, in a signal tracing procedure. To check the defibrillator protection circuit, you might interview the operator to determine if a defibrillator has recently been used. This problem would probably be specific to the channels being used, and could be further isolated with the lead selector switch shown in the figure. For example, if the defibrillator protection lead opens in the RA lead, the lead selector switch on positions 1 and 2 would yield a faulty trace. However, switch position 3 should be normal. This is verified by referring to Figure 6.8, and noting that the RA lead is not used when V_{III} is measured.

A failure in the CM reduction amplifier in the block diagram would increase the 60-$\sim$ hum on every channel of the ECG. Such a symptom could imply that the bioamp had a failure, or became unbalanced, and needed calibration. If 60-$\sim$ hum appears on only one channel, it is probable that the corresponding lead has lost its shielding or is improperly placed on the patient.

A distinction between a fault in the isolated power supply in the block diagram and a fault in the nonisolated power supply can be found by observing the output unit. If, for example, an output trace exists but there is no ECG signal, the isolated section of the power supply could be at fault.

Circuit-Board Swapping

After an instrument problem has been isolated by relating symptoms to the block diagram, the problem can be fixed by replacing the board containing the block. Circuit-board swapping should never be done blindly, however, or without careful investigation, as it is possible to damage an expensive circuit board in the process. For example, if the problem in the ECG is an overvoltage in the power supply that blows out components on the circuit board, then installing a new board could obviously damage it. To avoid this, check power supply voltages before considering circuit-board swapping.

Careful circuit-board swapping can be cost effective because it reduces equipment downtime. Furthermore, the old board can be easily shipped to the manufacturer, who can more economically trace the component problem and repair the board.

REFERENCES

Demarre, D. A., and Michaels, D. *Bioelectronic Measurements*. Englewood Cliffs, NJ: Prentice-Hall, 1983.

Hewlett-Packard Staff. *1500A/1511A Electrocardiographs STM 108A*. Waltham, MA: Hewlett-Packard, 1973.

Neuman, M. R. "Biopotential Amplifiers." Chapter 6 in *Medical Instrumentation*, edited by J. G. Webster. Boston: Houghton Mifflin, 1978.

Spach, M. S., *et al.* "Skin-Electrode Impedance and Its Effect on Recording Cardiac Potentials." *Circulation* 34 (1966): 649–656.

Yanof, H. M. *Biomedical Electronics*. 2nd ed. Philadelphia: F. A. Davis, 1972.

EXERCISES

1. The R-wave resulting from a standard lead connection has a peak amplitude $V_I = 0.2$ mV, and $V_{II} = 0.8$ mV. Compute the value corresponding to the V_{III}, R-wave peak amplitude.

2. The standard lead R-wave peak magnitude $V_I = 0.6$ mV and $V_{II} = 1.3$ mV. Compute the corresponding value of the augmented lead connection aVL.

3. The peak magnitude of the standard lead R-wave $V_I = 0.8$ mV, and $V_{III} = 2.0$ mV. Find the corresponding value of aVF.

4. At a certain point in time, an ECG wave has the values aVF = 0.7 mV and aVR = 0.3 mV. Find the corresponding value, V_I.

5. At the time that aVF = 0.6 mV and aVL = 0.8 mV, what is the value of V_{III}?

6. Solve Equations (6.3), (6.4), and (6.5) such that:
   (a) V_I is represented as a function of aVR, aVL, and aVF alone.
   (b) V_{II} is represented as a function of aVR, aVL, and aVF alone.
   (c) V_{III} is represented as a function of aVR, aVL, and aVF alone.

7. (a) In the amplifier in Figure 6.32, find the driving point impedance $Z_{aa'}$ at the primary of the transformer needed to match the amplifier such that the maximum power is delivered from the source to the amplifier. Assume ideal components.
   (b) Find the ratio $N_1:N_2$ required to produce this impedance.
   (c) If $V_S = 50$ V, compute V_2 for the ratio in part (b).
   (d) Compute V_L also for $V_S = 50$ V.

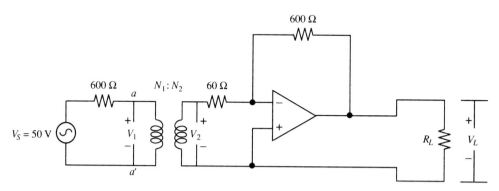

FIGURE 6.32

8. In Figure 6.32, let $V_S = 50$ V and $R_L = 10\ \Omega$, and compute the power absorbed by this load, P_L.

9. (a) Which ECG in Figure 6.33 would you expect to see after the patient exercises — (a) or (b)?
   (b) Suppose the ECG power cord is wrapped around the patient's arm. Sketch the change you would expect in Figure 6.33(b).

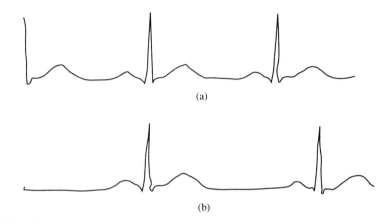

FIGURE 6.33

(c) Sketch from Figure 6.33(b) the change you would expect in the ECG if the muscles are tensed and relaxed vigorously.

(d) In order to minimize the effect you observe in part (b), would you increase or decrease the CMRR?

10. On the patient illustrated in Figure 6.34, three biopotentials referenced to ground are $V_a = 1$ mV, $V_b = 2$ mV, and $V_c = 0.5$ mV.

(a) Draw the equivalent circuit needed to compute V_R. Neglect the skin and electrode resistance in series with the 1-MΩ resistors.

(b) Compute V_R in volts.

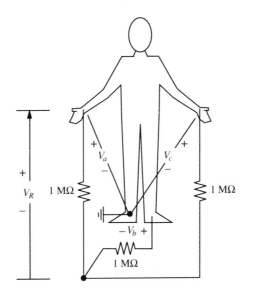

FIGURE 6.34

11. A patient is connected to a differential amplifier and is insulated from ground. Sixty-$\sim$ power voltages are coupled to him or her through 2-pF stray capacity. This creates a common-mode voltage V_{CM} over the patient's body. Using the circuit in Figure 6.35, compute the common-mode voltage V_{CM} measured from the body to ground. $V_S = 120$ V.

12. In Figure 6.36 the zener diode reverse breakdown voltage is 15 V.

(a) If $R_L \rightarrow \infty$ is an open circuit, find the zener diode current I_Z.

(b) What is the minimum value R_L for which the voltage across it will be regulated at 15 V?

13. (a) The diodes in Figure 6.37 are silicon with a 0.7 forward voltage. The input voltage v_{IN} is given by $5 \sin 2\pi\, 60t$. Sketch the output voltage waveform, v_{OUT}, accurately.

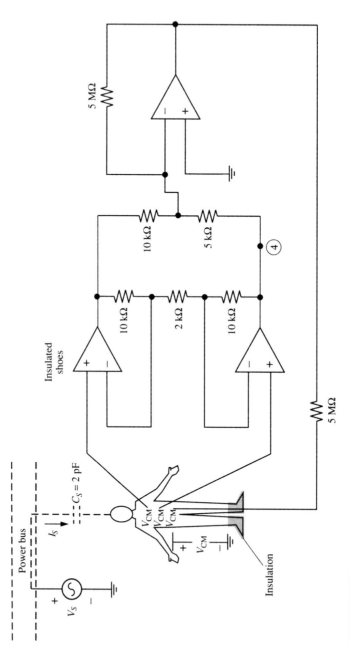

FIGURE 6.35

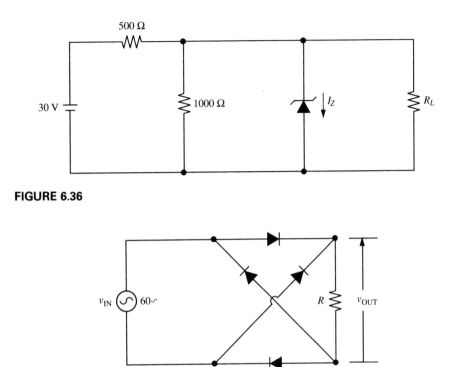

FIGURE 6.36

FIGURE 6.37

(b) A capacitor C is placed across the resistor to make a peak detector. What is the peak voltage for this circuit?

14. In the circuit in Figure 6.38, the differential amplifier integrated circuit IC is ideal and the transistors are silicon, with a forward voltage of 0.7 V.
    (a) Compute the voltage V_{OUT}.
    (b) Identify which transistor is ON, Q_1 or Q_2.
    (c) Compute the voltage V_C.
    (d) Compute the voltage V_{CE} for the ON transistor.
    (e) Consider the power out to be that absorbed by $R_L = 10\ \Omega$, and compute the circuit efficiency, taking into account the power absorbed in the transistor and collector resistors. Neglect the losses in the operational amplifiers and the offset circuit. Compute the efficiency with the formula

$$\eta = P_{OUT}/(P_{OUT} + P_{LOSS})$$

15. Beginning with the circuit and component values in Example 6.3, plot the magnitude of the common-mode voltage versus frequency.

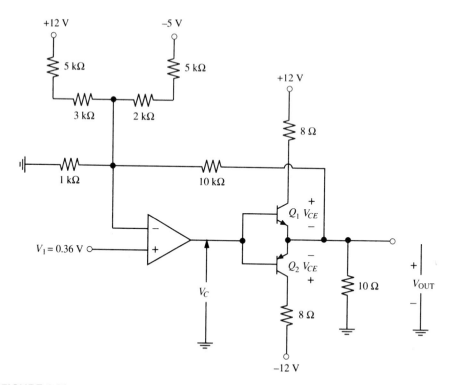

FIGURE 6.38

16. Beginning with the circuit and component values in Example 6.3:

(a) Plot the magnitude of the common-mode voltage, V_{CM}, versus the feedback resistance R_{OUT}.

(b) Plot the magnitude of V_{CM} versus the gain resistor, R_f.

(c) Plot the magnitude of V_{CM} versus R_3 when $R_3 = R_4$.

7

The Electroencephalograph and Filtering

7.1 THE EEG

The electroencephalograph (EEG) illustrated in Figure 7.1(a) is designed to measure the electrical activity of the brain, commonly called *brain waves*, by means of electrodes attached to the skull of a patient. The brain waves are the summation of neural depolarizations in the brain due to stimuli from the five senses as well as from the thought processes. On the surface of the brain, these voltages are on the order of 10 mV; but typical EEG electrodes measure the electrical activity propagated through skull bone and attenuated to levels from 1 to 100 μV, primarily in the frequency range from 0.5 to 3000 Hz. These potentials vary as a function of position over the surface of the skull, making it necessary for the EEG operator to select sets of electrodes grouped around the frontal, parietal, temporal, or occipital lobes of the brain. Figure 7.1(b) shows the receptacle for the electrode leads.

EEG Electrodes

In electroencephalography, electrodes are placed in standard positions on the skull in an arrangement referred to as the 10-20 system, a placement scheme devised by the International Federation of Societies of Electroencephalography. The electrodes in this arrangement are placed along a line drawn on the skull from the root of the nose, the *nasion*, to the *inion* ossification or bump on the occipital lobe. The first mark is placed 10% of the distance along this line, and others are arranged at 20% intervals, hence

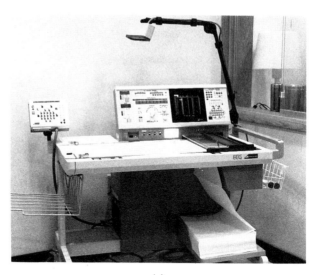

(a)

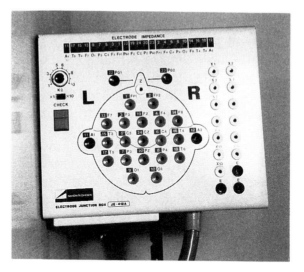

(b)

FIGURE 7.1
(a) AN EEG with a paper chart recorder for the data. (b) Detail of the lead receptacle box.

the name 10-20 system. A similar line is placed from one auricular (or ear) crease to the other. A third line goes around the circumference of the skull. A representative electrode arrangement placed at intersections of these lines is illustrated in Figure 7.2, where the first letter of the electrode designation

F stands for frontal lobe, C for central sulcus, P for parietal lobe, and O for occipital lobe on the skull. P_g is the nasopharyngeal point and A is on the ear lobe.

Electrode problems arise because of hair, which tends to increase the contact resistance. Surface electrodes may be made of silver, silver oxide disks from 1 to 3 mm in diameter. A conductive paste is used to lower the electrode resistance below 10 kΩ and to compensate for hair interference. The electrode may be covered with gauze and held with an adhesive such as collodion cement. To lower its resistance further, the skin may be abraded, but this introduces discomfort. Another method for reducing the electrode resistance employs a needle called a sphenoidal electrode, which breaks the skin and carries with it the danger of infection. The reference electrode may be attached to regions of negligible brain wave activity such as the ear lobe, or inserted into the nostrils. The nostril, or nasopharyngeal, electrode has a silver ball tip to reduce the contact resistance. If the skull is open during surgery, an electrocorticographic electrode, consisting of a cotton wick soaked in saline solution, may be placed on the brain to monitor electrical activity. Several different types of EEG electrodes are illustrated in Figure 7.3.

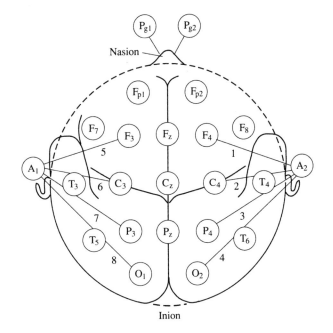

FIGURE 7.2
EEG electrode positions on the scalp (Craib and Perry, 1975).

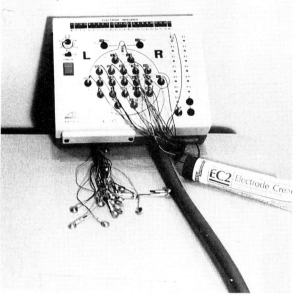

(a)

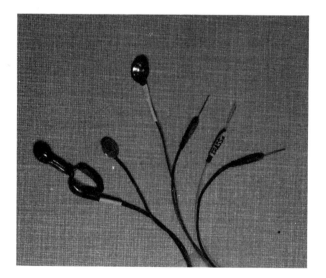

(b)

FIGURE 7.3
Examples of EEG electrodes. (a) Surface electrodes attached to the junction box. (b) Examples of needle, surface, and ear-clip electrodes.

An EEG Block Diagram

The signal path through the EEG is perhaps best understood by following Figure 7.4. The cable from the electrodes to the eight-channel selector has 21 leads and is vulnerable to breaks in the leads or shielding. It is also affected by 60-$\sim$ interference, as described in Section 5.3. The electrodes are attached to the EEG in Figure 7.1, for example, in groups of eight, called a *montage* of electrodes. A representative montage is illustrated in Figure 7.2. In that case, the right-brain electrodes are referenced to the right ear, which serves as a reference point, and the left-brain electrodes are referenced to the left ear. The brain wave activity in the ear lobe is very small, and it serves as an adequate reference point for EEG studies. It is often more comfortable for the patient to have the electrode attached to the ear rather than to the nostril.

Voltage measurements may also be taken between adjacent electrodes; this is called the *bipolar connection*. Or the measurements may be taken from one of the electrodes to a common point developed by a resistor circuit; this is called a *Wilson network*, or a unipolar connection, and is illustrated in Figure 7.5. In that case, each electrode is measured with respect to the same voltage. The voltage value at the reference usually cannot be computed because of insufficient data, but it is enough to know that each electrode is measured with respect to the same voltage.

The 60-$\sim$ interference is reduced by employing differential amplifiers with more than an 80-dB common-mode rejection ratio (CMRR), as discussed in Section 5.3, and by use of 60-$\sim$ notch filters, as we will describe in Section 7.2. The notch filter can introduce phase distortion and reduce the gain, but its effect is minimized by the fact that the most important EEG signals have frequencies below 30 Hz. For very precise or experimental measurements, it is sometimes best to place the EEG in a room covered by a ferrous metal screen, which will shield it from 60-$\sim$ radiation as well as any other frequency.

Because of the high internal impedance of the brain wave source, the input impedance of the differential amplifiers should exceed 10 MΩ to prevent loss of signal amplitude. The gain needs to be around 10^6 to produce voltages near 1 V, which are required to drive the display recorder or imaging scope.

According to Figure 7.4, the voltage output from the differential amplifiers may either be applied directly to the eight-channel display through the filter bank, or it may be stored as data on a tape recorder or in a computer memory for further processing.

The filter bank may contain high-pass, low-pass, or band-pass filters (see Section 7.2), and it enables the operator to select upper and lower fre-

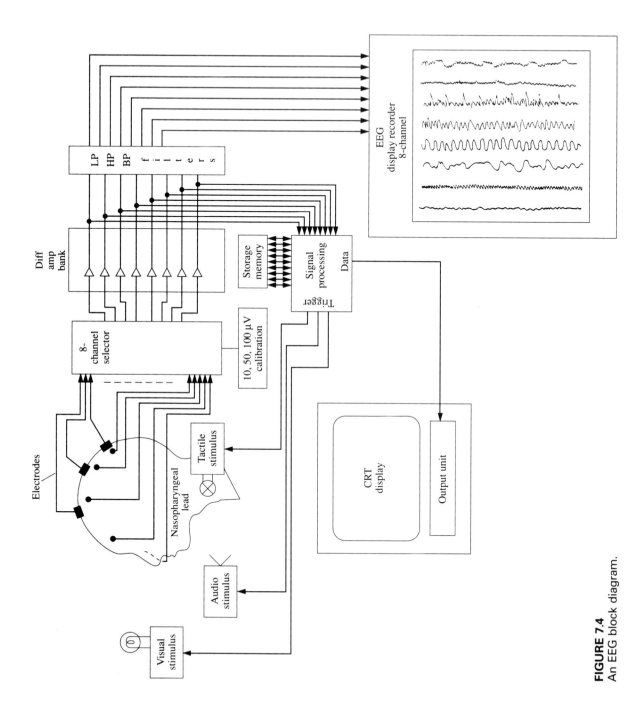

FIGURE 7.4
An EEG block diagram.

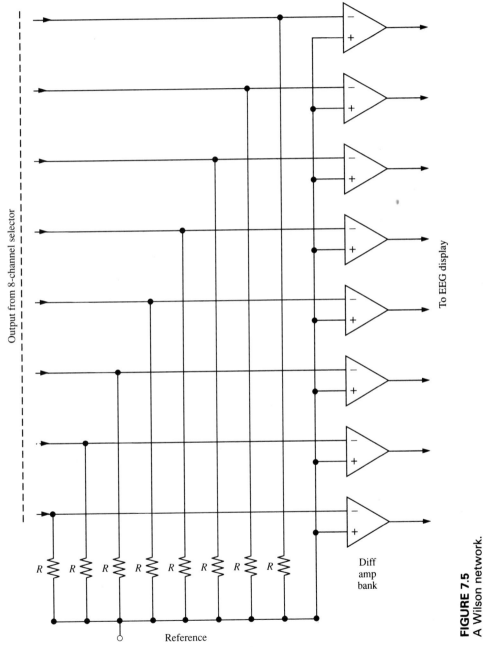

FIGURE 7.5
A Wilson network.

229

quency cutoffs. The appropriate filters are chosen in order to select frequency components of the brain wave significant in diagnosis of disease. The clinically significant bands are given approximately as follows:

delta: below 4 Hz
theta: 4 to 8 Hz
alpha: 8 to 13 Hz
beta: above 13 Hz

Electroencephalograms

The brain waves of normal individuals range from low-frequency, nearly periodic waves with a large delta component in deep sleep, to high-frequency, noncoherent beta waves measured on the frontal lobe channels during vigorous mental activity, as illustrated in Figure 7.6. A relaxed state is characterized by alpha waves from the occipital lobe channels. A visually evoked response is easily measured by opening and closing the eyes, as indicated in Figure 7.6. This figure illustrates the fact that brain waves in normal individuals vary significantly with electrode position and with mental state.

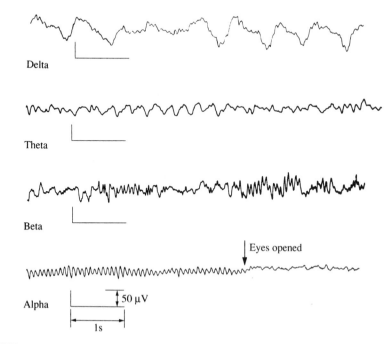

FIGURE 7.6
Example EEG waves. The vertical scale is 50 μV, and the horizontal scale is 1 s. The alpha wave is taken with eyes closed then opened where indicated by the arrow (Craib and Perry, 1975).

Box 1

TROUBLESHOOTING TIPS FOR EEGs

Abnormalities in the EEG waveform may be due to artifacts categorized as follows:

Artifacts due to electrode problems may result from

- Improper positioning
- Poor contact
- Poor electrode in the cap holding them
- Dried-out gel
- Oozing of tissue fluids in needle electrodes
- Frayed connections
- Sweating

Artifacts due to physiological interference may result from

- The heart ECG
- Tongue and facial movement
- Eye movement
- Skeletal muscle movement
- High scalp impedance
- Breathing

Artifacts due to electrical interference (EI) may result from:

- 60-$\sim$ common-mode interference
- Radio frequency interference due to use of an electrical surgical unit
- Defibrillation
- Presence of pacemakers and neural stimulators

Abnormal brain waves may indicate either a pathological state in the patient or the presence of some artifact introduced by the instrument. Such artifacts may be due to improper use of the instrument, especially at the electrode interface; or they may be due to instrumentation problems. Some examples are given in Box 1.

EEGs in Diagnosis

The purpose of the EEG is to help physicians diagnose disease. The pathological states or diseases most commonly diagnosed using the EEG are brain death, brain tumors, epilepsy, multiple sclerosis, and sleep disorders.

The advent of modern life-sustaining equipment, such as respirators, and the need for donor organs for transplant operations have changed the legal definition of death. The sustained absence of EEG signals is a clinical measure of brain death and can be used in deciding whether to transplant a heart, liver, or lung, or whether to shut down life-sustaining equipment such as a kidney dialyzer, a ventilator, or an artificial heart pump.

The EEG is widely used in diagnosing both generalized epilepsy and partial epilepsy. One form of generalized epilepsy is characterized by *grand mal* seizures, in which large electrical discharges are produced from the entire brain that last from a few seconds to several minutes. It may also be accompanied by skeletal muscle twitches and jerks. Evidence of grand mal seizures usually appears on all channels of the EEG. A less severe form of generalized epilepsy (but still "generalized" in that it affects the entire brain) is characterized by *petit mal* seizures, during which strong delta waves are produced for 1 to 20 seconds. Partial epilepsy affects only part of the brain and therefore is visible on fewer channels of the EEG.

It is important that patients with epilepsy have a warning that a seizure is about to occur, so that they can take medication and avoid injury or other inconveniences. Warnings of a seizure occur as vigorous electrical activity in particular foci in the brain, which would be recorded on the appropriate channel of an EEG. If the foci are in the temporal lobe, the patient would hear a sound; if in the occipital lobe, the patient would see flashes; and if in the motor area, the patient may experience muscle jerks. These are sensory warnings of an event that could develop into a grand mal seizure resulting in an extended stupor.

Transient signals due to epilepsy that do not result in physical seizures are important in diagnosis and treatment of the disease. To find such transients is tedious if not nearly impossible for a clinical technician unaided by instrumentation. One method of surveying large amounts of EEG data is to record it on magnetic tape at a low speed and play it back rapidly, at perhaps 60 times the original speed.

The availability of inexpensive minicomputers makes it feasible to search for particular patterns in the EEG, such as high-intensity bursts, and store them in memory for later review by a physician diagnosing their meaning. (See Figure 7.4.) Such techniques make ambulatory monitoring of epilepsy patients a technical possibility. Without computer storage and signal processing capability, the amount of data produced would overwhelm a human observer.

The effect of either visual, audio, or tactile stimuli upon the electroencephalogram of a patient is of clinical value in the diagnosis of disease.

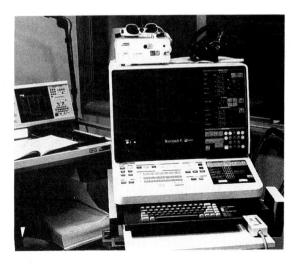

FIGURE 7.7
An EEG evoked response unit.

An instrument for evoking such responses is shown in Figure 7.7. In addition to the typical EEG display response to such stimulus-evoked responses, a measure of the time delay between the stimulus and response is of clinical value, and can be measured in the signal processing unit of the EEG illustrated in Figure 7.1.

7.2 FILTERS

There are many types of medical instruments in which it is necessary to select the frequency components of the input signal. For example, in the electroencephalograph, various brain states, such as the alert state, the sleep state, and the deep sleep state, produce distinctive frequency bands. In the EEG, theta waves in the frequency band 4 to 8 Hz indicate sleep, while beta waves in the frequency band 13 to 22 Hz indicate a high state of alertness. Filters may be used to direct these frequency bands to different channels to facilitate signal processing and disease diagnosis. In this case, filtering is essential to the diagnostic function of the instrument. In almost all monitoring, filtering is useful in reducing noise and often in reducing the effects of 60-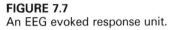 interference. In general, filters are used for either frequency selection or frequency rejection.

An ideal filter is one that passes the desired signal without either amplitude or phase distortion and completely rejects any unwanted or unnecessary signals.

Filters may be classified as either low-pass, high-pass, band-pass, or band-reject, as illustrated in Figure 7.8 in diagrams called *Bode plots*. Each filter has one or more cutoff frequencies, f_C, and a passband gain, often given in decibels (dB) as a function of frequency. The attenuation outside the passband as a function of frequency is called the filter roll-off and is often linear as a function of the logarithm of frequency (log f).

The figures of merit in filters are primarily measures of filter gain and frequency characteristics. The terms that specify these figures of merit are defined as follows:

Filter Gain. The filter gain, A_V, is the ratio of the output voltage of the filter to the input voltage. The gain is often expressed in decibels and is calculated from the formula $A_{\mathrm{dB}} = 20 \log A_V$.

High-Frequency Cutoff. The high-frequency cutoff, f_{CH}, is usually taken as higher frequency above which the gain remains 3 dB below the filter passband given.

Low-Frequency Cutoff. The low-frequency cutoff, f_{CL}, is the lower frequency below which the gain remains more than 3 dB below the filter passband gain.

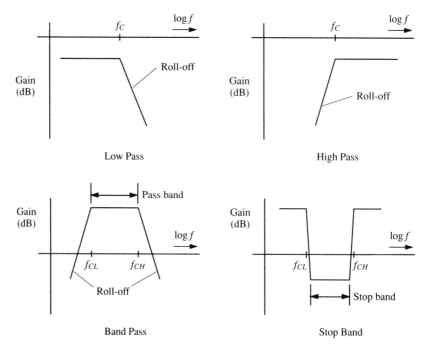

FIGURE 7.8
Filter Bode plots for low-pass, high-pass, band-pass, and stop-band filters.

Filter Bandwidth. The filter bandwidth, BW, is the difference between the low and high filter cutoff frequencies as calculated by the formula

$$BW = f_{CH} - f_{CL} \tag{7.1}$$

Band-Pass Filter Resonant Frequency. This resonant frequency, f_R, is the frequency midway between f_{CH} and f_{CL} on a logarithmic scale, given by the formula

$$\log f_R = (\log f_{CH} + \log f_{CL})/2$$
$$= \tfrac{1}{2} \log f_{CH} f_{CL}$$

Therefore, the resonant frequency is defined by the formula

$$f_R = \sqrt{f_{CH} f_{CL}} \tag{7.2}$$

Band-Pass Filter Quality. The filter with the highest quality, Q, is the one that gives the purest tone at the output. A mathematical definition consistent with this is given by the formula

$$Q = \frac{f_R}{BW} \tag{7.3}$$

since this indicates that the narrower the band of the filter, the higher the Q.

Bode Asymptote. A Bode asymptote is a straight line drawn on a semi-log plot of the filter gain A_{dB} versus the logarithm of the frequency. The line begins at a point defined by the filter passband gain and the cutoff frequency, either f_{CH} or f_{CL}. The line is then drawn to the asymptote of the high-frequency or low-frequency gain values, A_{dB}, as illustrated in Figure 7.10 for the low-pass case.

Filter Roll-off. The slope of the Bode asymptote on a semi-log scale is called the filter roll-off and is measured in decibels per octave (dB/octave). A frequency an *octave* above another is double that frequency. The units decibels per decade (dB/decade), where a *decade* frequency is ten times the initial frequency, are also often used to describe the roll-off.

Filter Order. The order N of the filter determines the slope of the filter roll-off. Ideally, the filter orders correspond to the formula

$$\text{Roll-off} = 6\,N \text{ dB/octave}$$

which is equivalent to $20\,N$ dB/decade. This formula generates a table of values as follows:

Filter order	Roll-off (dB/octave)
1	6
2	12
3	18
4	24

First-Order Filters

The order of a filter determines how sharply out-of-band signals are attenuated. We shall see examples of filters that show that first-order filters attenuate signals at the rate of 6 dB/octave, second-order filters at 12 dB/octave, third-order filters at 18 dB/octave, and so on.

The first case, Example 1.4 in Chapter 1, is a first-order, high-pass filter. A program for Equation 1.8 is given in Appendix A, Program A-8.

A plot of the gain for this filter, Figure 1.25, shows that the roll-off of this filter is 6 dB/octave. The cutoff frequency, f_C, defined as the frequency at which the gain is 0.707 times its maximum value, is $f_C = 1.59$ Hz. f_C is also known as the half-power frequency, since half the maximum power is attenuated at that frequency. This is an example of a first-order high-pass filter.

The second example is a low-pass filter that has the configuration of Figure 7.9. A calculation of the voltage gain A_V by voltage division gives

$$A_V = \frac{V_{\text{OUT}}}{V_{\text{IN}}} = \frac{\dfrac{1}{j\omega C}}{R + \dfrac{1}{j\omega C}}$$

$$= \frac{1}{1 + j2\pi fRC} \qquad (7.4)$$

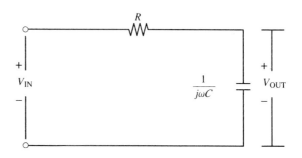

FIGURE 7.9
A first-order low-pass filter.

The program for Equation (7.4), Program A-9 in Appendix A, allows you to plot the frequency characteristics of this first-order low-pass filter.

EXAMPLE 7.1 In Figure 7.9, let $R = 100$ kΩ and $C = 1$ μF. Plot the gain, A_V, versus frequency and compute the cutoff frequency.

SOLUTION A_V computed for a particular frequency, 2 Hz, in Equation (7.4) yields

$$A_V = \frac{1}{1 + j2\pi(2)(10^5)(10^{-6})} = 0.62 \ \angle -51°$$

Converting to decibels,

$$A_V \text{ (dB)} = 20 \log(0.62) = -4.152 \text{ dB}$$

The computation of other values in the plot is facilitated with Program A-9 in Appendix A.

The plot as given in Figure 7.10 shows a roll-off of 6 dB/octave and a cutoff frequency f_C of 1.59 Hz.

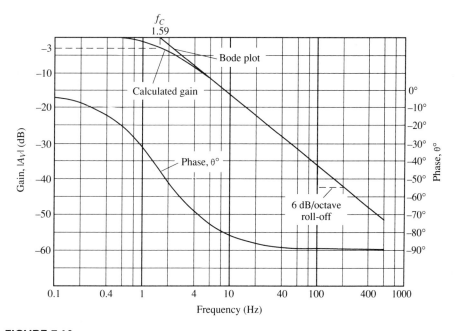

FIGURE 7.10
The gain magnitude and phase of the low-pass filter in Figure 7.9 when $R = 100$ kΩ and $C = 1$ μF.

f_C may also be computed from

$$f_C = \frac{1}{2\pi RC} \qquad (7.5)$$

The phase plot shows that phase distortion is greater than 45° for frequencies greater than 1.6 Hz, above the cutoff frequency. This phase distortion could, for example, cause the shape of a digital pulse to be altered.

The third example shows how the two filters dealt with above can be made into a band-pass filter. A first-order band-pass filter can be built as a low-pass filter followed by a high-pass filter, as in Figure 7.11. Since the input impedance of the ideal operational amplifier is infinite, while the output impedance is zero, the gain in this case is equal to the product of Equations (1.8) and (7.4), or

$$A_V = \left(\frac{1}{1 + j2\pi f C_1 R_1}\right)\left(\frac{1}{1 - j\dfrac{1}{2\pi f C_2 R_2}}\right) \qquad (7.6)$$

To achieve band-pass behavior it is necessary that the cutoff frequency for the high-pass section f_{CL} be less than the cutoff f_{CH} for the low-pass section. That is, $f_{CL} < f_{CH}$:

$$f_{CL} = \frac{1}{2\pi R_2 C_2} < \frac{1}{2\pi R_1 C_1} = f_{CH}$$

A program for Equation (7.6) is given as Program A-10 in Appendix A.

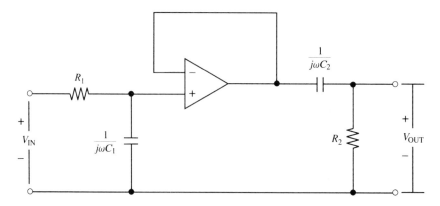

FIGURE 7.11
A first-order band-pass filter.

EXAMPLE 7.2 In Figure 7.11, let $R_1 = 5$ kΩ, $R_2 = 100$ kΩ, $C_1 = 1$ μF, and $C_2 = 1$ μF. Plot the filter gain versus frequency, and describe the resulting band-pass, first-order filter. Compute f_{CL} and f_{CH}.

SOLUTION The gain plot results from Equation (7.6). An example calculation for $f = 20$ Hz is

$$A_V = \left(\frac{1}{1 + j2\pi(20)(10^{-6})(5)(10^3)} \right) \left(\frac{1}{1 - j\dfrac{1}{2\pi(20)(10^{-6})(10^5)}} \right)$$

$$= 0.84 \angle -27.6°$$

In decibels the gain at 20 Hz is

$$A_V \text{ (dB)} = -1.51 \text{ dB}$$

The range of frequencies is plotted in Figure 7.12, which shows a bandwidth BW of 30.4 Hz and a roll-off of approximately 5.6 dB/octave. This filter is considered to be first-order since it has a roll-off of nearly 6 dB/octave.

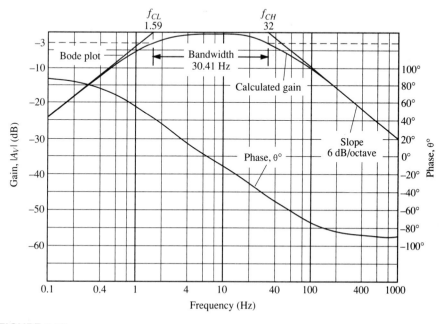

FIGURE 7.12
The gain and phase angle characteristic of the first-order band-pass filter in Example 7.2.

Phase distortion can be seen to increase on either side of the resonant frequency.

This filter uses a diff amp and therefore is an active filter. The diff amp provides a buffer between stages so that higher-order filters can be generated by placing stages in tandem (see Exercise 14, for example). Each buffer makes each stage independent and simplifies the gain formulas.

Higher-Order Active Filters

A second-order filter may be constructed using a differential amplifier from a circuit of the form in Figure 7.13, where Z_1, Z_2, Z_3, and Z_4 are complex-number impedances. Whether the filter is high-pass or low-pass depends upon the value of each impedance. Specific examples will be given below. In the general case, the gain of this filter is derived by applying node equations to node 1 and node 2. First, notice that $V_2 = V_{OUT}$, assuming an ideal diff amp. Then, at node 1, KCL gives

$$\frac{V_1 - V_{IN}}{Z_3} + \frac{V_1 - V_{OUT}}{Z_1} + \frac{V_1 - V_{OUT}}{Z_4} = 0 \qquad (7.7)$$

A second equation from KCL applied to node 2 is

$$\frac{V_{OUT} - V_1}{Z_4} + \frac{V_{OUT}}{Z_2} = 0$$

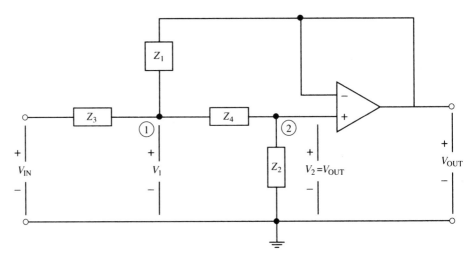

FIGURE 7.13
A generalized second-order filter.

To derive the gain from these two equations, solve this equation for V_1 and substitute it into Equation (7.7) as follows:

$$V_1 = V_{\text{OUT}} + \frac{Z_4}{Z_2} V_{\text{OUT}} \tag{7.8}$$

For convenience, Equation (7.7) is rearranged as follows:

$$V_1 \left(\frac{1}{Z_3} + \frac{1}{Z_1} + \frac{1}{Z_4} \right) - V_{\text{OUT}} \left(\frac{1}{Z_1} + \frac{1}{Z_4} \right) = \frac{V_{\text{IN}}}{Z_3}$$

Then, substituting Equation (7.8) into this yields

$$V_{\text{OUT}} \left[\left(1 + \frac{Z_4}{Z_2} \right) \left(\frac{1}{Z_3} + \frac{1}{Z_1} + \frac{1}{Z_4} \right) - \left(\frac{1}{Z_1} + \frac{1}{Z_4} \right) \right] = \frac{V_{\text{IN}}}{Z_3}$$

Rearranging this result then gives the gain $A_V = V_{\text{OUT}}/V_{\text{IN}}$ as follows:

$$A_V = \frac{1}{\left(1 + \dfrac{Z_4}{Z_2} \right) \left(1 + \dfrac{Z_3}{Z_1} + \dfrac{Z_3}{Z_4} \right) - \left(\dfrac{Z_3}{Z_1} + \dfrac{Z_3}{Z_4} \right)} \tag{7.9}$$

Equation (7.9) is the general form of the gain of the second-order filter. To get specific filters, the values of the impedances are appropriately substituted. This makes it easier to generate gain formulas for filters of the form given in Figure 7.13.

Second-Order Low-Pass Filters

A second-order low-pass filter uses impedances as indicated in Figure 7.14. This circuit becomes a Butterworth filter, with a 12 dB/octave roll-off, when $C_1 = 2C_2$. (Butterworth is the name of the person who did early work on this type of gain formula.) To obtain the gain formula, substitute the specific impedance values into the general Equation (7.9) as $Z_1 = 1/j\omega C_1$, $Z_2 = 1/j\omega C_2$, $Z_3 = R$, and $Z_4 = R$, where $\omega = 2\pi f$ is the radian frequency. Then for the second-order low-pass Butterworth filter,

$$A_V = \frac{1}{(1 + j2\pi f R C_2)(2 + j2\pi f R C_1) - (1 + j2\pi f R C_1)} \tag{7.10}$$

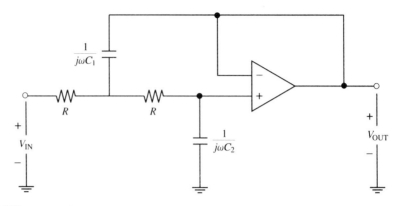

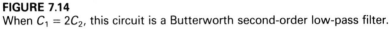

FIGURE 7.14
When $C_1 = 2C_2$, this circuit is a Butterworth second-order low-pass filter.

The cutoff frequency for this filter is given as

$$f_C = \frac{1}{2\pi R\sqrt{C_1 C_2}} \tag{7.11}$$

EXAMPLE 7.3   Work out a flow diagram for a programmable calculator used to compute Equation (7.10).

SOLUTION   In order to make studies of the effect of components on the filter gain, their values are put into storage registers. Appropriate use of polar to rectangular conversions leads to the flow diagrams in Figure 7.15. Specific programs for programmable calculators appear in Appendix A, Program A-11.

EXAMPLE 7.4   Use the program of Example 7.3 to plot the gain as a function of frequency in a second-order low-pass Butterworth filter in which $R = 15.9$ kΩ, $C_1 = 0.0141$ μF, and $C_2 = 0.007$ μF.

SOLUTION   A sample calculation of the gain Equation (7.10) for $f = 4000$ Hz is

$$A_V = 0.063 \ \angle -159° \ , \quad |A_V| = -24 \text{ dB}$$

A plot of the gain, computed using Program A-11 in Appendix A, is shown in Figure 7.16. There, f_C is found graphically to be $f_C = 1010$ Hz. The equation for f_C, Equation (7.11), yields

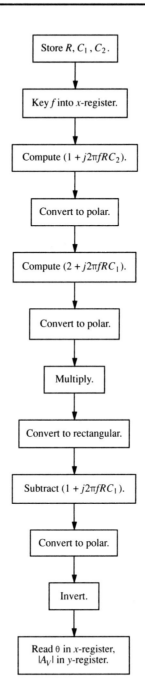

FIGURE 7.15
A flow diagram for calculating Equation (7.10), a low-pass second-order Butterworth filter gain.

$$f_C = \frac{1}{2\pi(1.59)(10^4)\sqrt{(0.0141(10^{-6})(0.007)(10^{-6})}}$$

$$= 1007.5 \text{ Hz}$$

The percentage difference between the graphically determined value and the calculated value is 0.25%.

This is clearly a low-pass filter. The plot in Figure 7.16 shows that the roll-off is 12 db/octave. The phase plot indicates the phase distortion as a function of frequency. Notice a 90° phase distortion at the cutoff frequency.

Second-Order High-Pass Filters

A second-order high-pass Butterworth-type filter results when the impedances are $Z_1 = R_1$, $Z_2 = R_2$, $Z_3 = 1/j\omega C$, and $Z_4 = 1/j\omega C$. The requirement for the Butterworth is that $R_2 = 2R_1$. The specific filter circuit is shown in Figure 7.17. The gain is obtained by plugging these impedance values into Equation (7.9) so that

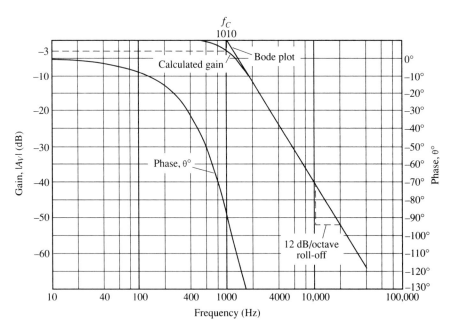

FIGURE 7.16
A graph of a second-order low-pass filter gain characteristic, as calculated in Example 7.4.

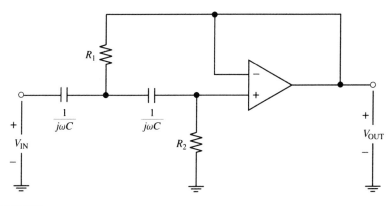

FIGURE 7.17
A second-order high-pass filter.

$$A_V = \frac{1}{\left(1 - j\,\dfrac{1}{2\pi fCR_2}\right)\left(2 - j\,\dfrac{1}{2\pi fCR_1}\right) - \left(1 - j\,\dfrac{1}{2\pi fCR_1}\right)} \qquad (7.12)$$

A flow diagram to facilitate plotting this equation as a function of frequency appears in Figure 7.18. A specific calculator program appears in Appendix A, Program A-12. Cutoff frequency f_C is derived by setting $|A_V| = 0.707$ in Equation (7.12). The result is

$$f_C = \frac{1}{2\pi C\sqrt{R_1 R_2}} \qquad (7.13)$$

EXAMPLE 7.5 Plot the gain versus frequency for the filter in Figure 7.17 when $C = 0.002\ \mu\text{F}$ and $R_1 = 9.3\ \text{k}\Omega$ for the Butterworth filter case.

SOLUTION To create a Butterworth filter, $R_2 = 2R_1 = 18.6\ \text{k}\Omega$. The plot results from calculations on Equation (7.12). For example, when $f = 6000$,

$$|A_V| = -3\ \text{dB}$$

A plot of the frequency characteristic in Figure 7.19 shows a roll-off of 12 dB/octave, characteristic of a second-order filter.

The cutoff frequency, f_C, measures 6050 Hz. The calculation of f_C by Equation (7.13) gives the value $f_C = 6050.5$, which verifies the graphically derived value of 6050 Hz.

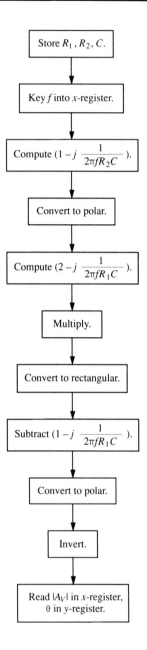

FIGURE 7.18
A flow diagram for calculating the gain of a second-order high-pass filter as given in Equation (7.12).

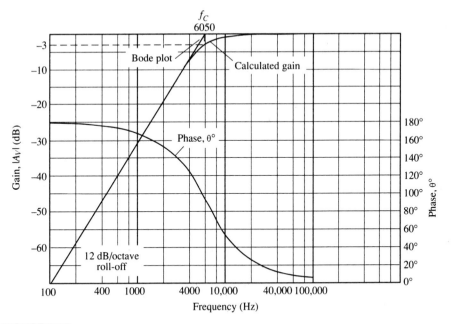

FIGURE 7.19
The gain and phase characteristic of a second-order high-pass filter as computed in Example 7.5.

Third-Order Low-Pass Filters

A third-order filter can be obtained by adding a stage to the second-order filters described previously. Since ideal operational amplifiers provide isolation between stages, the filter can be designed so that the gain of the second stage simply multiplies the gain of the first stage. The third-order filter results by adding a stage to Figure 7.14. Stage 1 drives the first-order stage 2, as shown in Figure 7.20.

The gain of stage 1, A_1, is given by Equation (7.10). The gain of stage 2 in Figure 7.20 is then

$$A_V = \frac{1/(j\omega C_3)}{R + 1/(j\omega C_3)}$$

$$= \frac{1}{1 + j\omega R C_3}$$

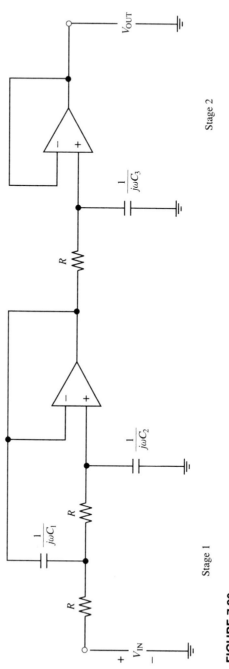

FIGURE 7.20
A third-order low-pass filter.

and the overall gain, $A_V = A_1 A_2$, is

$$A_V = \left(\frac{1}{(1 + j2\pi fRC_2)(2 + j2\pi fRC_1) - (1 + j2\pi fRC_1)} \right)$$

$$\times \frac{1}{(1 + j2\pi fRC_3)} \tag{7.14}$$

This gain follows a Butterworth filter response when

$$C_1 = 2C_3 \text{ and } C_3 = 2C_2 \tag{7.15}$$

A flow diagram for a computer program for calculating this gain as a function of frequency is shown in Figure 7.21. The specific program for a programmable calculator appears as Program A-13 in Appendix A.

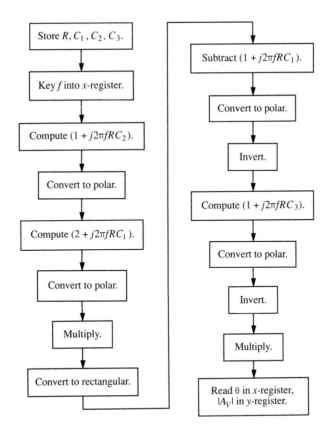

FIGURE 7.21
A flow diagram for calculating Equation (7.14), the gain of a third-order filter.

EXAMPLE 7.6 Show that a third-order filter results when $R = 15.9$ kΩ, $C_1 = 0.02$ μF, $C_2 = 0.005$ μF, and $C_3 = 0.01$ μF in Figure 7.20.

SOLUTION   The gain characteristic versus frequency is computed by Equation (7.14). For example, at $f = 2000$ Hz, we calculate

$$A_V = 0.124 \angle -209° \text{ , or } |A_V| = -18.13 \text{ dB}$$

A plot of A_V appears in Figure 7.22. This plot has an $f_C = 1001$ Hz, and a frequency and a roll-off of 18 dB/octave, as expected for a third-order filter.

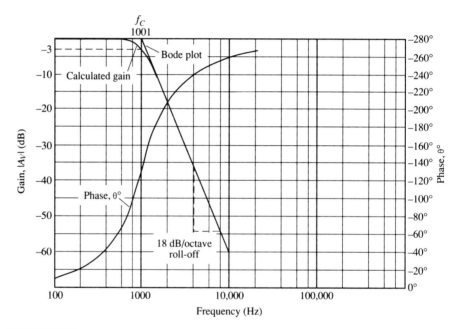

FIGURE 7.22
The gain characteristic of a third-order filter.

The critical frequency f_C may be computed from the formula

$$f_C = \frac{1}{2\pi R \sqrt[3]{C_1 C_2 C_3}}$$

The computed value of $f_C = 1000.8$ Hz compares well with the graphically derived value of 1001 Hz.

This example demonstrates that Figure 7.20 is, in fact, a third-order Butterworth filter when the condition of Equation (7.15) is satisfied. By a similar argument, we can design a third-order high-pass filter by combining the circuit in Figure 7.17 with that of a first-order high-pass filter connected in tandem.

Band-Reject Filters

There is probably no frequency that causes more interference in medical instrumentation than 60 ∿ a.c. A reason for this is that the power line carrying this frequency is in close proximity to patients and equipment. Other troublesome frequencies might be that of electrosurgical units (about 500 kHz) or ultrasonic frequencies (about 2 MHz). A narrow-band-reject filter may be used to reject these frequencies without introducing excessive distortion to complex signals passing through. For example, a 60-∿ band-reject filter can pass an ECG waveform containing frequencies up to 100 Hz through a band-reject filter tuned to 60 Hz. It will simply eliminate the 60-∿ frequency.

A band-reject filter containing a differential amplifier that measures the null voltage of a bridge circuit is shown in Figure 7.23.

The differential amplifier utilizing the three operational amplifiers has a gain of −1, since it is a balanced diff amp. Then

$$V_{\text{OUT}} = V_B - V_A$$

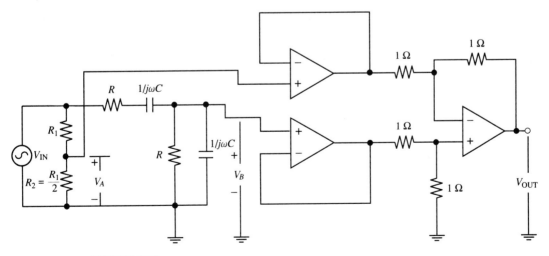

FIGURE 7.23
A band-reject filter isolated by a balanced diff amp.

The bridge network relates V_A and V_B to V_{IN} by the voltage division principle, so that

$$V_{\text{OUT}} = \left(-\frac{R_1/2}{R_1 + R_1/2} + \frac{\dfrac{R/j\omega C}{R + 1/j\omega C}}{R + 1/j\omega C + \dfrac{R/j\omega C}{R + 1/j\omega C}} \right) V_{\text{IN}}$$

Rearranging this equation gives

$$V_{\text{OUT}} = \left(-\frac{1}{3} + \frac{R/j\omega C}{(R + 1/j\omega C)^2 + R/j\omega C} \right) V_{\text{IN}}$$

The voltage gain $A_V = V_{\text{OUT}}/V_{\text{IN}}$ then becomes

$$A_V = -\frac{1}{3} + \frac{j2\pi f R C}{(1 + j2\pi f R C)^2 + j2\pi f R C} \qquad \textbf{(7.16)}$$

The flow diagram for a computer program for calculating this gain characteristic is given in Figure 7.24. A specific computer program appears in Appendix A, Program A-14.

EXAMPLE 7.7   A band-reject filter (Figure 7.23) uses resistors $R_1 = 10$ kΩ, $R_2 = 5$ kΩ, and $R = 2652.6$ Ω, while the value for $C = 1$ μF. Compute and plot the gain, A_V, as a function of frequency.

SOLUTION   Equation (7.16) is used to calculate the magnitude of the gain and phase of the band-reject filter. For example, when $f = 30$ Hz, we have

$$A_V = 0.149 \quad \text{at 30 Hz}$$

Converting this gain to dB gives

$$A_V \text{ (dB)} = 20 \log 0.149 = -16.5 \text{ dB}$$

The plot is formed by continuing these calculations for other frequency values. The calculation is facilitated by use of Program A-14 in Appendix A. A graph of A_V (dB) appears in Figure 7.25.

A plot of this data clearly shows that 60-$\sim$ frequencies are strongly rejected by this filter. At the notch frequency $f_N = 60$ Hz, 116 dB attenuation is calculated.

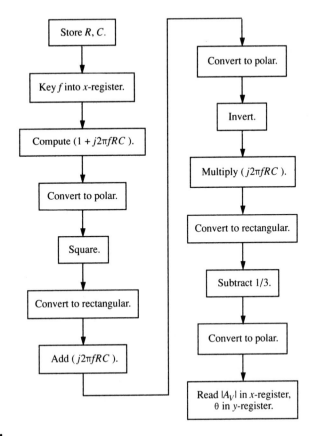

FIGURE 7.24
A flow diagram for calculating the band-reject filter characteristic of Equation (7.16).

This example verifies that the notch frequency f_N for the band-reject filter in Figure 7.23 is given by

$$f_N = \frac{1}{2\pi RC} \tag{7.17}$$

$$= \frac{1}{2\pi (2652.6)(10^{-6})} = 60 \text{ Hz}$$

A band-reject filter can be designed for other notch frequencies by use of Equation (7.17). The gain-phase characteristic is then computed by Equation (7.16).

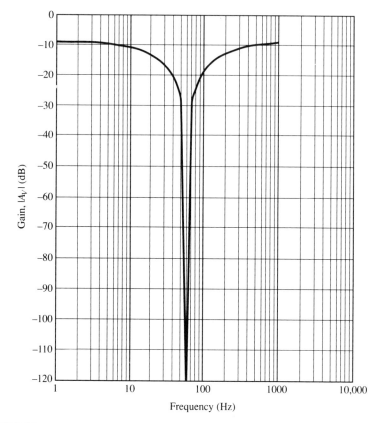

FIGURE 7.25
The gain characteristic of a 60-∿ band-reject filter as calculated in Example 7.7.

7.3 TROUBLESHOOTING AN EEG

Troubleshooting an EEG is similar in many ways to troubleshooting the other widely used surface-potential measurement device, the ECG. They both have common-mode interference problems. They both use multiple surface electrodes and leads. The procedures outlined in Section 6.6 for troubleshooting these problems in the ECG should be followed for the EEG. As with the ECG, also, an internal calibration control, illustrated in the block diagram (Figure 7.4) can be used to check the instrument electronics and to distinguish problems with it from those related to the electrodes.

Problems with the EEG are compounded by the fact that the signal levels are a thousand times smaller than the ECG potentials. Furthermore, there are multiple channels. A problem with one of the channels can be isolated to eliminate the possibility of problems with elements common to all channels, such as the power supply. To isolate a problem in the diff amp of a particular channel on the block diagram, and its corresponding electrode, the calibration switch can be used. If the channel under test can be calibrated with that switch, this would indicate that the electronics beyond it is working and that the problem would probably be in a lead.

A patient signal simulator can be built to test the evoked response timing. The visual stimulus can evoke a preset delay in the simulator, which may then be applied as a delayed signal on the EEG electrode. The stimulus and its response can then be recorded on the EEG display recorder in order to test the instrument-induced delays. Errors would indicate a fault in the output unit or in the strip chart speed.

The frequency response of filters can be checked by measuring the output of the filter due to a variable frequency input. The most vulnerable element in active filters is the diff-amp chip. Failure in the chip would cause a radical change in the frequency response. However, if the changes in frequency response are small, the problem may be a leaky capacitor, or aging, or thermal damage in the components.

REFERENCES

Carr, J. J., and Brown, J. M. "Instruments for Measuring Brain Parameters." Chapter 13 in *Introduction to Biomedical Equipment Technology*. New York: John Wiley & Sons, 1981.

Craib, A. R., and Perry, M. *Beckman EEG Handbook*. Brea, CA: Beckman Instruments, Inc., 1975.

Floyd, T. L. "Active Filters." Chapter 16 in *Electronic Devices*. 2nd ed. Columbus, OH: Merrill Publishing, 1988.

Kondraski, G. V. "Neurophysiological Measurements." Chapter 5 in *Biomedical Engineering and Instrumentation*, edited by J. D. Bronzino. Boston: Prindle, Weber & Schmidt, 1986.

EXERCISES

1. ECG electrodes are placed according to the 10-20 system on the skull illustrated in Figure 7.26. The skull has a radius of 10 cm. Compute the electrode locations relative to the root of the nose (nasion) and the occipital protuberance (inion). That is, find the arc lengths S_1, S_2, and S_3 in centimeters. Compute the distance between the electrodes.

2. Depressing the calibration switch on the EEG, illustrated in Figure 7.4, yields normal responses on all channels, yet the EEG display reads zero output.

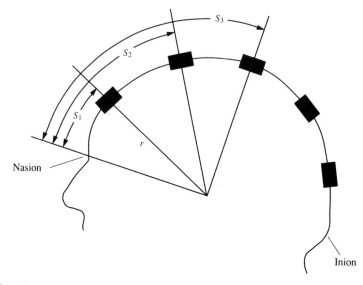

FIGURE 7.26

    (a) Identify the most likely problem.

    (b) Identify the modules of the EEG not checked out by this procedure.

3. Depressing the calibration switch gives normal responses on channels 1 through 8 of the ECG in Figure 7.4, except for a zero output on channel 4.

    (a) Identify the most likely problem with the equipment.

    (b) Identify the units that are not checked by this test.

4. A visual stimulus does not result in an evoked response in a normal patient, but all other EEG display functions are normal. What is a likely cause of the malfunction?

5. The upper cutoff frequency of a filter is 50 Hz and the lower cutoff frequency is 25 Hz. What is the resonant frequency?

6. A filter has a bandwidth of 60 Hz and a Q value of 10. What is its resonant frequency?

7. A first-order high-pass filter has a cutoff frequency of 150 Hz. Its midband gain is 0 dB. Sketch its Bode plot.

8. A low-pass Butterworth active filter has a cutoff frequency of 50 Hz, and the circuit illustrated in Figure 7.14. $R = 5$ kΩ. Compute the capacitors C_1 and C_2 that make this circuit a second-order filter.

9. Make an exact plot of the gain versus frequency of the filter specified in Exercise 8. Using semi-log paper, superimpose a Bode plot on this graph. Deter-

mine the roll-off of the filter. Calculate the percentage difference between the graphically determined cutoff frequency and the theoretical value.

10. A high-pass Butterworth second-order filter is to have a cutoff frequency $f_C = 12$ Hz. Using the circuit in Figure 7.17, let $R_1 = 7$ kΩ. Compute C and R_2 for this filter.

11. Make an exact plot of the gain versus frequency of the filter specified in Exercise 10. Determine the roll-off of this filter. Calculate the percentage difference between the graphically determined cutoff frequency and the theoretical value.

12. (a) Transform the circuit in Figure 7.27 into the phasor domain.
    (b) Derive the gain function $A_V(j\omega)$ as a function of frequency, f.
    (c) Let $R = 0.795$ kΩ and $C = 20$ μF, and compute the values of the magnitude and phase angle of A_V for the frequencies 0.01, 0.1, 2, 10, and 100 Hz.
    (d) Plot the gain A in dB as a function of frequency on a semi-log scale. Plot the phase angle on the same scale. Find the cutoff frequency f_C and the roll-off in units of dB/octave.
    (e) Name the type and order of this filter.

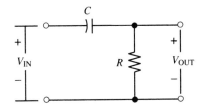

FIGURE 7.27

13. A band-pass filter has a gain as a function of frequency as given in Figure 7.28.
    (a) Find the roll-off of the filter in dB/octave.
    (b) Determine the bandwidth, BW, between the three dB cutoff frequencies.
    (c) Find the quality, Q, of the filter.

14. Derive the gain formed for the three-stage filters given in Figure 7.29 in terms of frequency f, R, and C.
    (a) Compute the gain function $A(j\omega)$ in magnitude and phase for the frequencies 0.01, 0.1, 1, 2, 10, and 100 Hz when $C = 20$ μF and $R = 0.795$ kΩ.
    (b) Plot the gain function A as a magnitude and as a phase function.
    (c) Graphically find the cutoff frequency f_C and the roll-off in units of dB/decade.
    (d) What order filter is this?

15. (a) Compute the gain function $A(j\omega)$ magnitude as a function of frequency in Figure 7.30.

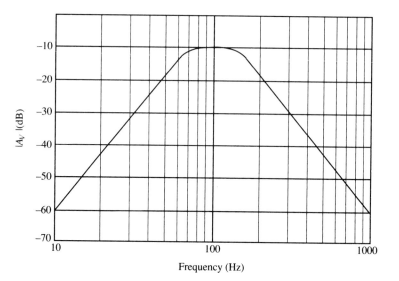

FIGURE 7.28

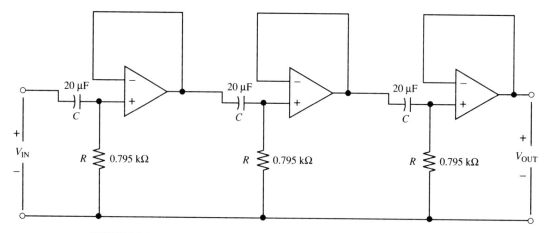

FIGURE 7.29

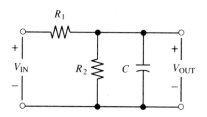

FIGURE 7.30

(b) Let $R_1 = 100$ kΩ, $R_2 = 500$ kΩ, and $C = 1$ μF. Compute the value of A_V at 1.2 Hz, and convert to dB units.

(c) Make a Bode plot for this circuit.

16. (a) In Figure 7.31, compute the magnitude of the gain function $A = V_{OUT}/V_{IN}$ for the frequencies 10, 30, 50, 60, 70, 80, 100, and 500 Hz. Choose R and C to make a 120-Hz notch.

(b) Identify the type of filter.

(c) Why is this type of filter especially useful in ECG and EEG equipment?

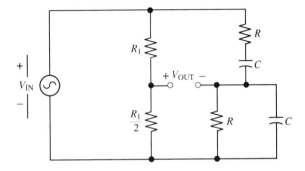

FIGURE 7.31

17. A low-pass filter at a particular frequency has the phasor domain schematic given in Figure 7.32. The numbers are values of the element impedances or source voltages. Compute the output voltage V_{OUT} in magnitude and phase.

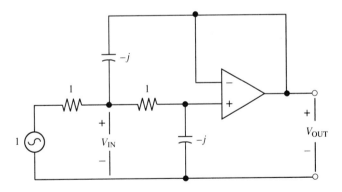

FIGURE 7.32

18. Design a third-order filter that passes an alpha wave of an EEG while it rejects the beta wave. Using semi-log paper, make an exact plot of the gain of this filter versus frequency.

19. A third-order high-pass filter for beta waves has a cutoff frequency of 13 Hz. By how many decibels are the theta waves rejected?

8 The Defibrillator and Step Response

8.1 THE DEFIBRILLATOR

In the United States, hundreds of thousands of persons die of sudden cardiac arrest each year. If they could be treated with a defibrillator within one minute of the attack, 80% would have an increased chance of survival. However, if this treatment is delayed by only ten minutes, the statistic falls from 80% to 15%, thus illustrating how important the defibrillator is, and how important it is to have it available to the general population.

A defibrillator is an electronic device that creates a sustained myocardial depolarization of a patient's heart in order to stop ventricular fibrillation or atrial fibrillation. These fibrillations occur because ectopic, or out-of-place, stimulus sites take place in the heart and cause a disorganized cardiac muscle contraction. When this fibrillation happens to the ventricles, it causes a drastically reduced cardiac output of blood flow and results in death in a few minutes. An atrial fibrillation causes reduced cardiac output but is usually not fatal. The d.c. defibrillator is effective in treating both conditions.

In Chapter 2 we indicated that 1 to 10 A of current can cause a sustained myocardial contraction. The early a.c. defibrillators proved unreliable and have since been replaced with more effective units, such as the d.c. defibrillator and biphasic units, which deliver d.c. pulses alternatively in opposite directions. A d.c. defibrillator is designed to deliver 50 to 400 joules (J), or watt-seconds (W-s), of energy through the thorax. The energy required depends upon the size of the patient and his or her skin resistance. The voltages required vary from 1000 to 6000 V, depending upon the duration of the d.c. pulse used. For example, if a 2000-V, 5-ms pulse is reduced in voltage, the duration must be extended to maintain the same energy delivery to the patient. The current level delivered by a defibrillator varies from 1 to 20 A. If the defibrillator pulse is applied directly to the heart during open-heart surgery, or with an implanted defibrillator, the energy level is reduced to 15 to 50 J.

All defibrillators must have a mechanism for adjusting the energy level, by controlling either the amplitude or the duration of the defibrillator pulse. A schematic of the d.c. defibrillator like that introduced by Bernard Lown in 1962 is given in Figure 8.1. When the switch is in the charge position, current flows through the diode in one direction and charges the capacitor to its peak value, V_P. The voltage V_P can be varied by changing the setting on the varactor. The energy stored in the capacitor and available for defibrillation, W_A, is

$$W_A = \tfrac{1}{2}CV_P^2 \tag{8.1}$$

Therefore the energy available from the defibrillator is varied by the varactor setting.

The defibrillator pulse is delivered by placing paddles covered with an electrode electrolyte gel against the skin of the patient and placing the switch in the discharge position. The paddles have a metal surface from 8 to 10 cm in diameter for adult patients. They may be placed either in the *anterior-anterior* position so that the current flows through the heart, or in the *anterior-posterior* so that the current flows from the back to the chest through the heart. In the anterior-anterior position, one paddle is placed above the apex of the heart and the other is placed on the sternum. This causes the current to flow from the bottom to the top of the heart.

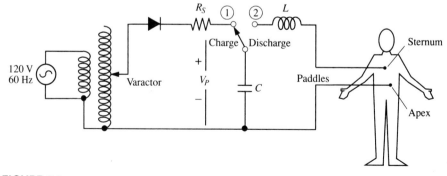

FIGURE 8.1
Schematic of a d.c. defibrillator.

The discharge switch is usually mounted on the paddle. It is important that the attendants using the defibrillator avoid having the defibrillation pulse pass through their own bodies. For example, electrode gel on the paddle handle could provide a path for the defibrillation pulse through one arm of the attendant through the heart to the other arm. An attendant touching the patient is likewise in danger of a shock.

Because of the reduced surface resistance, the defibrillator pulse may be delivered to the open heart using paddles from 4 to 5 cm in diameter, and the voltage levels may be reduced by one third. For pediatric patients, the external paddles are approximately 5 cm in diameter and energy levels of about 50 J are delivered.

Defibrillation is indeed a hazardous procedure, since it involves stopping the heart; and if applied incorrectly, it could induce fibrillations in a normal heart. Therefore, it is essential that a diagnosis be made by trained specialists to ensure that the patient needs the treatment before it is initiated. In order to reduce this risk, and to make the defibrillator available for more cardiac arrest victims more quickly, diagnostic circuitry is used to assess that a fibrillation is in fact occurring before the defibrillation pulse is applied to a patient. This then makes it safe for attendants with less training to use the defibrillator.

Figure 8.2 shows the generic block diagram of a defibrillator capable of diagnosing fibrillation. An ECG instrument is attached to the patient.

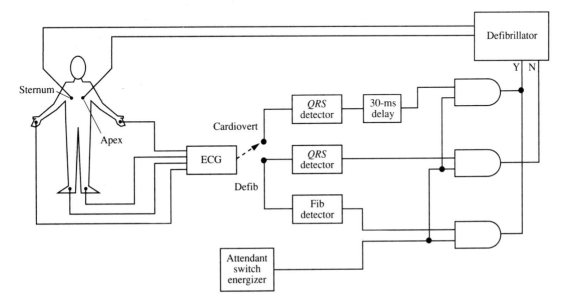

FIGURE 8.2
Defibrillator/cardioverter block diagram.

If ventricular fibrillation is suspected, the switch is placed in the defibrillator position. A *QRS* detector consists of a threshold circuit that would pass an *R*-wave if such a wave is present. When the attendant energizes the switch to deliver a defibrillation pulse, the signal passes through a logical AND gate, which is a digital circuit that provides an output signal only when an appropriate input appears on the two input nodes simultaneously. In this case the two inputs are the *R*-wave from the *QRS* detector and a signal from the attendant's switch. If both are present, the defibrillator is inhibited and will not deliver the pulse. A defibrillator pulse is delivered only if the fibrillation detector produces an output at the same time that the attendant energizes the switch. The fibrillation detector searches the ECG signal for frequency components above 150 Hz. If they are present, fibrillation is probable. Under this condition, when the attendant energizes the switch the defibrillation voltage would actually be delivered to the patient.

A second mode of operation, *cardioversion*, is used, for example, when an atrial fibrillation is diagnosed. After a diagnosis is made by specialists, treatment may be initiated. The ECG signal in the instrument is delivered to a *QRS* detector. The signal is used to time the delivery of the defibrillation pulse with a delay of 30 ms. At this time, the ventricles will be in a uniform state of depolarization, and the normal beat will not be disturbed. If the pulse were applied during the *T*-wave between 50 and 150 ms after the *QRS* complex, for example, while the heart is in the process of repolarizing, it would be possible to introduce a fibrillation into the heart. Therefore the 30-ms delay allows the attendant to defibrillate the atrium with a low risk of inducing a ventricular fibrillation. Coming within 30 ms of the *R*-wave, the defibrillation pulse will occur before the period of ventricular vulnerability to fibrillation, namely during the *T*-wave.

Such diagnostic circuitry has been further developed to make it possible to permanently implant a defibrillator and attach it to a patient's diseased heart. If the heart fibrillates, a defibrillator pulse is automatically applied to the surface of the heart.

Example Defibrillators

Commercially available defibrillators typically have specifications with the following ranges:

Weight	7 to 50 lbs (typically 30)
Maximum delivered energy	320 to 450 J
Charge time	1 to 22 s
Battery capability	20 to 80 discharges
Battery recharge time	1 to 16 h

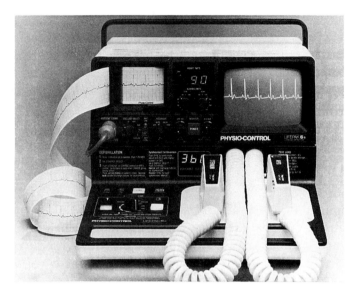

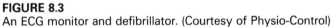

FIGURE 8.3
An ECG monitor and defibrillator. (Courtesy of Physio-Control)

A physio-control defibrillator and cardioverter unit is illustrated in Figure 8.3.

Because the defibrillator delivers therapeutic current to critically ill patients, reliability is crucial. The unit is tested as often as every day in many hospitals. Also, to facilitate testing it immediately before use, test circuits are built into the unit, as shown in Figure 8.3. The test procedure requires (1) turning on the line power, (2) setting the energy selector to maximum, (3) charging the unit, and (4) discharging the paddles into their holders, as placed in the illustration. The defibrillator is automatically discharged into a 50-Ω load connected to the paddle holders in the defibrillator. An indicator light then verifies that the proper energy was discharged into the test load.

Defibrillation of a patient is performed by personnel trained and authorized to use the defibrillator. After a diagnosis is made using an ECG, an electrode gel is applied to the paddles. The defibrillator is then recharged to the proper energy level. The paddles may then be placed on the sternum and apex, respectively, of the patient's chest. Both discharge buttons on the paddles are engaged to defibrillate the patient. The paddles are usually isolated electrically from ground so that ground loops are eliminated that could injure the patient or attendants. Clearly marked paddles are shown on the defibrillator in Figure 8.4.

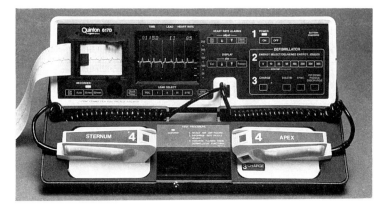

FIGURE 8.4
A defibrillator with built-in testing capability. (Courtesy of Quinton, Inc.)

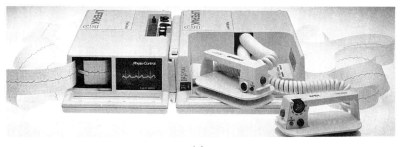

(a)

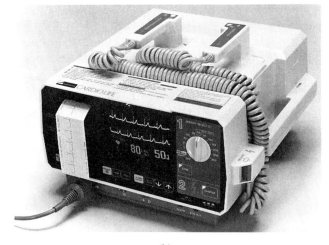

(b)

FIGURE 8.5
(a) A portable defibrillator. (Courtesy of Physio-Control) (b) A portable defibrillator. (Courtesy of Nihon Kohden of America, Inc.)

Cardioversion is done on the unit in Figure 8.3 with the use of the ECG. The amplitude of the ECG is increased until a marker appears on the R-wave. This assures the user that the instrument will synchronize to the R-wave. To perform cardioversion, the user selects the cardioversion mode on the instrument by pushing the SYNC switch. The defibrillator is then charged to the proper energy level, and the defibrillator pulse is delivered to the patient approximately 30 ms after the R-wave peak, as explained earlier.

A defibrillator designed especially for portability is illustrated in Figure 8.5(a), with the paddles removed from their holders. An alternative model is shown in part (b) of the figure.

8.2 DEFIBRILLATOR ENERGY DELIVERY

Proper distribution of energy is crucial in the use of a defibrillator, since energy that is directed to body tissue other than the heart can cause discomfort or injury to the patient. Most important, energy absorbed by the skin at the paddle can cause burns, since it is there that the current density is highest and the I^2R heat losses are concentrated. This resistance can be reduced by proper application of electrode gel and proper pressure (approximately 30 lb), variables that depend on the operator. Hence, improper operator technique can cause injury to the patient.

To quantify the energy delivery, we may consider a defibrillator that produces a square pulse. Such a circuit has been constructed using digital circuits that shunt out the defibrillator capacitor as it discharges so as to square up the pulse. The square wave may also serve as a first-order approximation to a Lown-type defibrillator pulse, precisely computed in Section 8.3. An equivalent circuit representing the square pulse defibrillator is shown in Figure 8.6, where R_D is the internal resistance of the defibrillator, R_E is the electrode-skin resistance, and R_T is the thorax resistance. The energy in the pulse, W_D, equals the instantaneous power times the pulse duration T_D. That is,

$$W_D = T_D V_D I_D \tag{8.2}$$

The total circuit resistance is

$$R_{\text{TOT}} = R_D + 2R_E + R_T \tag{8.3}$$

The resistance between the cables attached to the patient is

$$2R_E + R_T$$

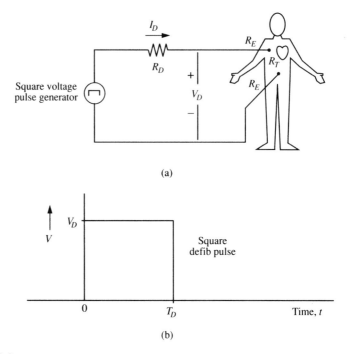

FIGURE 8.6
An idealized square-wave defibrillator.

Therefore,

$$W_D = \frac{V_D^2}{2R_E + R_T} T_D \tag{8.4}$$

$$= I_D^2 T_D(2R_E + R_T)$$

where

$$I_D = \frac{V_D}{2R_E + R_T}$$

Since the current is equal through each of the resistances, the energy in each resistance is as follows:

Energy loss in the defibrillator:

$$W_L = I_D^2 R_D T_D \tag{8.5}$$

Energy loss in each electrode and skin:

$$W_E = I_D^2 R_E T_D \tag{8.6}$$

Energy delivered to the thorax:

$$W_T = I_D^2 R_T T_D \tag{8.7}$$

Energy available from the capacitor:

$$W_A = I_D^2 R_{\text{TOT}} T_D \tag{8.8}$$

The available energy is given by

$$W_A = W_T + 2W_E + W_L$$

Putting Equations (8.5), (8.6), and (8.7) into this yields

$$W_A = (R_T + 2R_E + R_D) I_D^2 T_D$$

Multiplying the right side by R_T/R_T and using Equation (8.8) yields

$$W_T = \frac{R_T}{R_T + 2R_E + R_D} W_A \tag{8.9}$$

Thus, the energy delivered to the thorax, W_T, is diminished from the available energy by the effects of both R_E and R_D.

EXAMPLE 8.1   A defibrillator produces a square pulse of 3000 V with a duration of 5 ms. The instrument resistance $R_D = 10 \ \Omega$, the skin-electrode resistance $R_E = 30 \ \Omega$, and the thorax resistance $R_T = 30 \ \Omega$. Compute the energy delivered to the patient's thorax when the defibrillator is connected as in Figure 8.6(a).

SOLUTION   The current from the defibrillator during the pulse is given by the voltage divided by the sum of the resistances as

$$I_D = \frac{3000}{10 + 2(30) + 30} = 30 \text{ A}$$

The energy absorbed by the thorax from Equation (8.7) is

$$W_T = (30^2)(30)(5 \times 10^{-3}) = 135 \text{ J}$$

EXAMPLE 8.2   For the case in Example 8.1, calculate the energy absorbed by the two electrodes.

SOLUTION   From Equation (8.6),

$$W_E = 2(30)^2(30)(5 \times 10^{-3}) = 270 \text{ J}$$

Notice that in these examples, more energy is absorbed by the skin at the electrodes than is delivered to the thorax. If the resistance is reduced by half, either by use of a larger electrode, by better contact with electrode gel, or by increased pressure on the electrode, the energy absorbed by the skin would be reduced. This illustrates how proper electrode use and design can reduce the likelihood of tissue injury due to use of a defibrillator.

8.3 ANALYSIS OF THE DEFIBRILLATOR VOLTAGE WAVEFORM

The basic defibrillator circuit, shown in Figure 8.1, contains a step source. The step source consists of a charged capacitor suddenly connected to an inductor in series with a resistance, when the switch is moved from position 1 to position 2. Analysis of a circuit to a step source requires that you find the step response of the network. The proliferation of digital signals made up of a series of steps from LO state to HI state and vice versa makes it imperative that you understand the method of analysis for step response of systems.

The method of step analysis of electronic circuits is similar in broad outline to that of finding the response of an electrical circuit to a sinusoidal signal, but it is quite different in details such as the form of the equations. In a.c. analysis, you will recall that we employ complex numbers called phasors, having a real part and an imaginary part, characterized by the $j\omega$. To do step response, the $j\omega$ is replaced by a Laplace variable, s.

The Laplace method of circuit analysis is developed in various circuit analysis texts (see Hayt and Kemmerly, 1978). A derivation of the Laplace method is beyond the scope of this text, but the procedure for using it is as simple as a.c. analysis. Since the method greatly enhances your ability to analyze and understand modern medical equipment, the procedure for use of the method is given in Appendix B. We discuss its application to the d.c. defibrillator in the following section.

The Lown Voltage Waveform of a Defibrillator

It is important in the analysis of the circuit in Figure 8.1 for the output voltage waveform of the defibrillator to consider the energy state of the two energy-storage elements, the capacitor and the inductor, at the instant the discharge switch is thrown from position 1 to position 2 in the equivalent circuit. The Lown defibrillator is a step-response device. The capacitor C in the figure is first charged to a voltage V_P by placing the switch in position 1. To deliver a defibrillation pulse the switch is suddenly moved from position 1 to position 2. A step-response voltage then appears momentarily across the defibrillator paddles. In this section that voltage will be analyzed.

An equivalent circuit of the Lown defibrillator is given in Figure 8.7(a), where R_D is the resistance of the inductor including the internal resistance of the defibrillator, R_E is the skin-electrode resistance, and R_T is the thorax resistance. The total resistance, R_{TOT}, is given by Equation (8.3).

Assume in Figure 8.7(a) that the switch is thrown from position 1 to position 2 at $t = 0$, after having been in position 1 long enough to completely

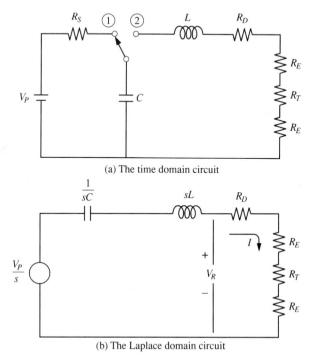

(a) The time domain circuit

(b) The Laplace domain circuit

FIGURE 8.7
A defibrillator attached to the body.

change the capacitor voltage V_P. Therefore the initial voltage on the capacitor will be V_P. V_P will remain on the capacitor immediately after $t = 0$ because it represents the energy stored in the capacitor by Equation (8.1). Energy, you will recall, has inertia and cannot change its level immediately. Likewise, the current will be zero through the inductor the instant after the switch is closed because it represents the energy, $Li^2/2$, stored in the inductor. Therefore the initial inductor current $i_0 = 0$ in this case. This makes the voltage source in series with the inductor in the Laplace equivalent circuit equal to zero. Therefore, the Laplace equivalent circuit of the Lown defibrillator is as shown in Figure 8.7(b).

A method of analyzing the step response of a circuit such as this is the *Laplace method*, and it is outlined in Appendix B. The equivalent circuit of the defibrillator as given here in the time domain can be transformed into the *Laplace domain*. In the Laplace domain, the circuit elements as expressed in the time domain are replaced by their equivalent *Laplace impedances*.

This is analogous to what you do when you transform the circuit into the phasor domain in ordinary a.c. circuit analysis. Notice that, in the equivalent circuit, the impedances describing the defibrillator in the Laplace domain are very similar to phasor impedances, except the $j\omega$ is replaced by s, the Laplace variable. Furthermore, as illustrated in Appendix B, the Laplace domain equivalent circuit can be analyzed using Kirchhoff's laws and Ohm's law.

The voltage waveform of a Lown defibrillator as illustrated in Figure 8.1 can be analyzed using the Laplace techniques described in the appendix. To use the Laplace method it is first necessary to transform Figure 8.7(a) into the Laplace domain by using the Laplace equivalents given in Appendix B, Figures B.3, B.4, and B.5.

The resulting Laplace equivalent circuit, shown in Figure 8.7(b), can be analyzed by voltage division. The voltage across the resistors, V_R, is

$$V_R = \left(\frac{R_{\text{TOT}}}{R_{\text{TOT}} + sL + \dfrac{1}{sC}} \right) \frac{V_P}{s}$$

Algebraic manipulation puts this equation into the form

$$V_R = \left(\frac{V_P(R_{\text{TOT}}/L)}{s^2 + (R_{\text{TOT}}/L)s + \dfrac{1}{LC}} \right)$$

This equation is further manipulated to put it in a form so that the Laplace table can be used to give the voltage v_R as a function of time. To this end the square in the denominator is completed by adding and subtracting $(R_{TOT}/2L)^2$ so that

$$V_R = \frac{V_P(R_{TOT}/L)}{\left[s^2 + \dfrac{R_{TOT}}{L}s + \left(\dfrac{R_{TOT}}{2L}\right)^2\right] - \left(\dfrac{R_{TOT}}{2L}\right)^2 + \dfrac{1}{LC}}$$

The term in the large parentheses is now a perfect square, so this equation becomes

$$V_R = \frac{V_P(R_{TOT}/L)}{\left(s + \dfrac{R_{TOT}}{2L}\right)^2 + \dfrac{1}{LC} - \left(\dfrac{R_{TOT}}{2L}\right)^2} \qquad (8.10)$$

This equation has different time-domain equivalents depending on the conditions:

$$\left(\frac{R_{TOT}}{2L}\right)^2 < \frac{1}{LC} \qquad \text{(underdamped)} \qquad (8.11)$$

$$\left(\frac{R_{TOT}}{2L}\right)^2 > \frac{1}{LC} \qquad \text{(overdamped)} \qquad (8.12)$$

$$\left(\frac{R_{TOT}}{2L}\right)^2 = \frac{1}{LC} \qquad \text{(critical damped)} \qquad (8.13)$$

Case I (Underdamped)

The Equation (8.10) for V_R is in a form that can be transformed directly into the time domain. The corresponding voltage v_R is obtained from transform #4 of the Laplace table, Table B.1 in Appendix B. Using $\alpha = R_{TOT}/2L$, and $K = V_P R_{TOT}/L$, we have

$$v_R = \frac{V_P R_{TOT}}{\omega L} e^{-(R_{TOT}/2L)t} \sin \omega t \qquad (8.14)$$

where

$$\omega = \sqrt{\frac{1}{LC} - \left(\frac{R_{TOT}}{2L}\right)^2} \qquad (8.15)$$

The reason for the underdamped condition, Equation (8.11), now becomes clear. Otherwise ω would be an imaginary number, and the Laplace transform #4 would not be applicable. Equation (8.14) therefore represents the defibrillator voltage in the underdamped case.

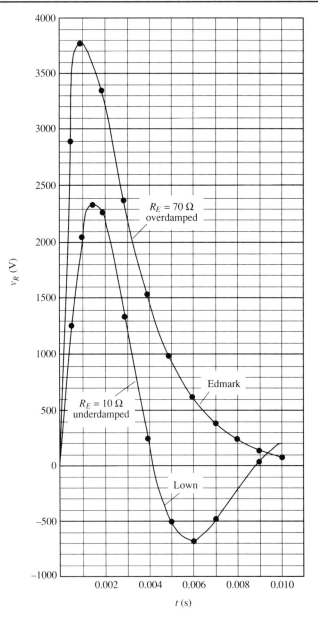

FIGURE 8.8
A Lown defibrillator waveform.

EXAMPLE 8.5 A defibrillator illustrated in Figure 8.7(a) has an inductance $L = 0.1$ H, $C = 16$ μF, an electrode-skin resistance $R_E = 10$ Ω, an internal resistance $R_D = 20$ Ω, and a thorax resistance $R_T = 20$ Ω. Compute the required charging voltage for the capacitor and the voltage v_R as a function of time. Plot a curve of the results.

SOLUTION The required charging voltage is obtained from Equation (8.1):

$$200 = (\tfrac{1}{2})(16 \times 10^{-6})V_P^2$$

Solving for V_P shows it to be 5000 V.

To compute v_R, we first determine whether the circuit is overdamped or underdamped by testing Equation (8.11) for $R_{TOT} = 20 + 10 + 10 + 20 = 60$ Ω. Is $[60/(2)(0.1)]^2 < 1/(0.1)(16 \times 10^{-6})$? The answer is yes, and we conclude that the circuit is underdamped. Thus the output voltage is given in Equation (8.14), where

$$\alpha = R_{TOT}/2L = 60/[2(0.1)] = 300$$

and

$$\omega = \sqrt{1/[0.1(16 \times 10^{-6})] - 300^2} = 731.4$$

Then

$$v_R = \{60(5000)/[0.1(731.4)]\}e^{-300t}\sin 731.4t)$$

A plot of v_R versus t is given in Figure 8.8 for this underdamped case. Notice the voltage tends to oscillate, but the oscillations are damped to a relatively low magnitude. This calculation is facilitated by use of Program A-15 in Appendix A.

Case II (Overdamped)

In the overdamped case it is convenient to rewrite Equation (8.10) as

$$V_R = \cfrac{(R_{TOT}/L)V_P}{\left\{s + \left[\dfrac{R_{TOT}}{2L} + \sqrt{\left(\dfrac{R_{TOT}}{2L}\right)^2 - \dfrac{1}{LC}}\right]\right\}\left\{s + \left[\dfrac{R_{TOT}}{2L} - \sqrt{\left(\dfrac{R_{TOT}}{2L}\right)^2 - \dfrac{1}{LC}}\right]\right\}}$$

Notice that condition (8.12) guarantees that the number under the square root sign is positive, so that the numbers remain real. The appropriate Laplace transform in Table B.1, Appendix B, is #2, where

$$K = (R_{\text{TOT}}/L)V_P$$

$$\alpha = \frac{R_{\text{TOT}}}{2L} + \sqrt{\left(\frac{R_{\text{TOT}}}{2L}\right)^2 - \frac{1}{LC}} \qquad (8.16)$$

$$\gamma = \frac{R_{\text{TOT}}}{2L} - \sqrt{\left(\frac{R_{\text{TOT}}}{2L}\right)^2 - \frac{1}{LC}} \qquad (8.17)$$

Thus v_R as a function of time, according to the table, is

$$v_R = \frac{R_{\text{TOT}}}{L} V_P \frac{e^{-\alpha t} - e^{-\gamma t}}{\gamma - \alpha} \qquad (8.18)$$

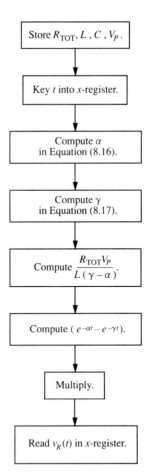

FIGURE 8.9
Flow diagram for the overdamped defibrillator case.

This equation can be used to calculate v_R. Such a calculation is facilitated with a computer program, Program A-16 (in Appendix A), whose flow diagram is given in Figure 8.9.

EXAMPLE 8.6 Increase the skin resistance R_E in Example 8.5 to $R_E = 70\ \Omega$ for each electrode. Show that the defibrillator now becomes overdamped, and compute the voltage at the electrodes $v_R(t)$.

SOLUTION To test the overdamped condition, Equation (8.12), first note

$$R_{\text{TOT}} = 20 + 2(70) + 20 = 180$$

Then,

$$\left(\frac{180}{2(0.1)}\right)^2 > \frac{1}{0.1(16)(10^{-6})}$$

This inequality is calculated as $8.1 \times 10^5 > 6.25 \times 10^5$ to verify that the defibrillator is overdamped in this case. To compute $v_R(t)$, use Equation (8.18). A plot of the overdamped case is given in Figure 8.8.

8.4 TROUBLESHOOTING DEFIBRILLATORS

Symptoms of defibrillator problems usually show up during routine testing procedures. Since it is an emergency-care device, capable of inflicting a fatal shock on a patient or an attendant, procedures for its use must be fail-safe. Safety of the defibrillator is ensured by frequent testing and by proper training of the operators.

The defibrillator block diagram in Figure 8.2 uses the signal from an ECG monitor. An outline for troubleshooting this module is given in Section 3.5. Test procedures that reveal problems in the blocks beyond the ECG are usually found with a defibrillator analyzer. This device provides a 50-Ω resistance discharge path for the defibrillator paddles that simulates the torso resistance. The defibrillator electrodes are placed on the metal test pads. Energy levels of discharges into the test pads are measured up to 1000 J. The waveform of this discharge may be displayed on an oscilloscope. The defibrillator analyzer generates an R-wave of an ECG pattern at approximately 60 bpm, and it then displays the time between the leading edge of the R-wave and the cardioverter discharge. This measurement detects failures in the QRS detector and the 30-ms delay circuit in the block diagram.

In the defibrillator mode, the R-wave would be used along with the energize switch to ensure that the defibrillator properly inhibits unnecessary defibrillator pulses. The tester may also simulate a fibrillation waveform to ensure that a defibrillator discharge can be activated by the attendant switch as necessary. Any errors in the waveform or energy level would indicate problems in the defibrillator itself.

The wearing element that would yield low-energy output is the battery pack. The battery voltage should be tested under loaded conditions. In accordance with manufacturer specification, it should be periodically fully discharged (sometimes called "deep discharged"). After recharging, the battery will be capable of delivering its rated energy. Otherwise, polarization on the battery terminals could limit its performance.

REFERENCES

Association for the Advancement of Medical Instrumentation (AAMI). *Essential Standards for Biomedical Equipment Safety and Performance.* Arlington, VA: AAMI, 1985.

Babbs, C. F., and Bourland, J. D. "Defibrillators." Chapter 3 in *Therapeutic Medical Devices, Application and Design*, edited by A. M. Cook and J. G. Webster. Englewood Cliffs, NJ: Prentice-Hall, 1982.

Feinberg, B. N. *Applied Clinical Engineering.* Englewood Cliffs, NJ: Prentice-Hall, 1986.

Hayt, W. H., and Kemmerly, J. E. *Engineering Circuit Analysis.* New York: McGraw-Hill, 1978.

Lown, B., Amarasingham, R., and Neuman, J. "New Method for Terminating Cardiac Arrhythmias." *New England Journal of Medicine* 182 (1962): 548–555.

Mirowski, M., *et al.* "Termination of Malignant Ventricular Arrhythmias with an Implantable Automatic Defibrillator in Human Beings." *New England Journal of Medicine* 303 (1980): 322–324.

Spooner, R. B. *Hospital Electrical Safety Simplified.* Research Triangle Park, NC: Instrument Society of America, 1980.

Tacker, W. A. "Electrical Defibrillators." In *Encyclopedia of Medical Devices and Instrumentation, Vol. 2*, edited by J. G. Webster. New York: John Wiley & Sons, 1988.

Van Valkenburg, M. E. *Network Analysis.* Englewood Cliffs, NJ: Prentice-Hall, 1955.

EXERCISES

1. In the defibrillator of Figure 8.7, R_{TOT} is the total resistance made up of the internal resistance of the defibrillator R_D, the electrode-skin resistance R_E, and the thorax resistance R_T. If $R_D = 10 \ \Omega$, $R_E = 20 \ \Omega$, and $R_T = 15 \ \Omega$, compute the total resistance, R_{TOT}.

2. An idealization of the waveform measured across the defibrillator electrodes described in Exercise 1 is given in Figure 8.10. Use the resistance values given in Exercise 1.

(a) Compute the total energy delivered by the defibrillator to the patient and the attached paddles.

(b) Compute the current waveform delivered by the defibrillator through the electrodes.

(c) Compute the energy absorbed in each of the skin electrodes, R_E.

(d) Compute the energy absorbed in the thorax of the patient, R_T.

(e) Compute the percentage of the total defibrillator energy that is absorbed by the thorax. Based upon the result, evaluate the effectiveness of the equipment, and make recommendations for improving the defibrillation procedures.

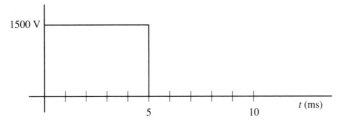

FIGURE 8.10

3. The voltage pulse delivered to two defibrillator paddles attached to a patient is given in Figure 8.10. The thorax resistance $R_T = 50\ \Omega$. What must the electrode-skin resistance be at each electrode in order that 100 J of energy will be delivered to the thorax of the patient? Assume $R_D = 5\ \Omega$.

4. In a certain defibrillator, the voltage in Figure 8.10 across the skin electrodes delivers 200 J of energy.

(a) How much energy does it deliver if the pulse height is reduced to half?

(b) How much energy does it deliver if the pulse height is reduced to half but the duration of the pulse is doubled?

5. In the defibrillator of Figure 8.7, what size capacitor is necessary to make 400 J of energy available for defibrillation when the charging voltage equals 3000 V?

6. The defibrillator in Figure 8.7 has a 50-μF capacitor. What must the range of charging voltages be in order to make from 50 to 400 J of energy available to the defibrillator?

*7. In Figure 8.11, the switch is closed at $t = 0$. The initial charge on the capacitor is zero. Compute the output voltage v_{OUT} versus time. (Refer to Appendix B.)

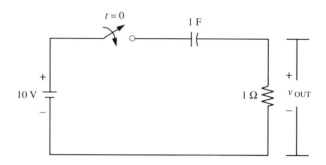

FIGURE 8.11

*8. In Figure 8.12, the switch on the battery is closed at $t = 0$.

(a) Write the Laplace domain equivalent of this circuit on the diagram.
(b) Calculate V_R as a function of the Laplace variable s, and L, R, and V_I.
(c) Find the resistor voltage v_R as a function of time for values $L = 2$ H, $R = 3$ Ω, and $V_I = 10$ V.

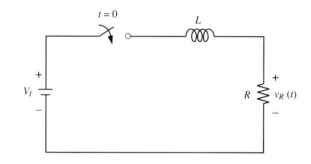

FIGURE 8.12

*9. In Figure 8.13, use Laplace transforms to show that the current is given by

$$i = \frac{V_F - v_I}{R} e^{-t/RC} \text{ for } t > 0$$

where v_I is the voltage on the capacitor at $t = 0$. (See Appendix B.)

10. A defibrillator whose schematic is shown in Figure 8.7 has an inductance $L = 0.2$ H, with a 15-Ω internal resistance. The electrode-skin resistance is 20 Ω, and the thorax resistance $R_T = 15$ Ω. The capacitor is $C = 18$ μF. It is desired to have 300 J of energy available in the charged capacitor.

(a) Compute the voltage on the fully charged capacitor.
(b) Compute the voltage v_R for $t > 0$ when the capacitor is discharged at $t = 0$. Plot the result on a scale of voltage versus time.

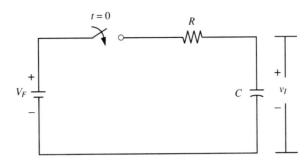

FIGURE 8.13

(c) On the same axis, plot the voltage across the thorax.
(d) What is the peak current through the thorax?

11. Use the relationships defining the conditions on damping to explain why the resistance for critical damping is given by

$$R_C = 2\sqrt{\frac{L}{C}}$$

in Figure 8.7. The critical resistance R_C is defined as the value of the resistance below which the defibrillator is underdamped, and above which it is overdamped when discharging.

12. (a) In Exercise 10, compute the critical resistance, R_C.
(b) What is the minimum value of the skin-electrode resistance for which the defibrillator is overdamped?

13. (a) In the defibrillator in Figure 8.7, the circuit values are equal to those given in Exercise 10 except $R_S = 100 \ \Omega$. For this case compute and plot the voltage across the thorax as a function of time.
(b) Compute and plot the current delivered by the defibrillator to the thorax.

9

The Pacemaker — A Digital Pulse Oscillator

A pacemaker is a prosthetic device for the heart, first conceived in 1932 by Albert S. Hymen, an American cardiologist. In 1952 the pacemaker was used clinically by Paul M. Zoll as an external device. With the advent of solid-state circuitry in the early 1960s, it was made into a battery-operated prosthesis that was implantable into the patient. Credit for the implantable pacemaker is given to the American physicians William Chardack and Andrew Gage and to the engineer Wilson Greatbatch. Other heart prostheses, or spare parts, include coronary bypass vessels and artificial heart valves. An especially innovative recent heart prosthesis is the artificial heart, the best known example of which is the Jarvik-7, designed by Robert K. Jarvik and implanted into Barney Clark by William DeVries in 1982. Another implantable artificial heart was developed in 1985 at Penn State University by a team headed by William Pierce.

A pacemaker is a prosthesis specifically for the sinoatrial (SA) node of the heart. The SA node may become ineffective for several reasons, among them: (1) the SA node tissue or atrium may become diseased; or (2) the path of the heart depolarization—specifically, the atrioventricular (AV) node from the atrium to the ventricles—may become diseased, producing a heart block. Furthermore, bradycardia, a slowing of the heart rate generally to below 50 or 60 beats per minute (bpm), may develop because of aging or other reasons. These diseases may be treated either with a pacemaker or with medicine, depending upon the case. In the case that the SA node fails to pace the heart properly, the ventricles may beat at their own self-paced rate, normally about 40 bpm. At this heart rate, a patient may survive, but may not be able to function normally.

9.1 PROPERTIES OF THE PACEMAKER

Because the pacemaker is battery-operated and surgically implanted, battery lifetime is one of the most important considerations. The lifetime is determined primarily by the stimulus requirements, as well as the current drain caused by the pacemaker circuitry. The use of complementary metal-oxide semiconductor (CMOS) integrated circuits has dramatically reduced the current drain, but the stimulus requirements are determined by physiology and cannot be reduced effectively. In this section, we will discuss how increased stimulus demand shortens the pacemaker battery lifetime.

As is usually the case with physiological stimuli, there is a curve of stimulus intensity versus duration associated with the physiological response of heart depolarization. Figure 9.1 shows the stimulus voltage, V_S, at the tissue-electrode interface. It has a stimulus duration T_D, measured in milliseconds. Such curves depend upon the electrode-heart resistance, R_H, which may range from 100 to 1400 Ω; the curve in Figure 9.1 is typical. The value of R_H may change over time because of tissue scarring at the electrode-tissue interface. In order to produce a stimulus pulse, it is necessary to deliver energy to the electrode with a pacemaker circuit as shown in the block diagram in Figure 9.2.

A pacemaker in its simplest configuration is essentially a battery-operated digital pulse generator. A digital pulse of the form shown in Figure 9.3 has a voltage V_S that may be made variable to allow adjustments

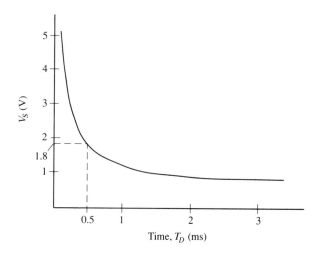

FIGURE 9.1
Pacemaker stimulation threshold versus pulse width.

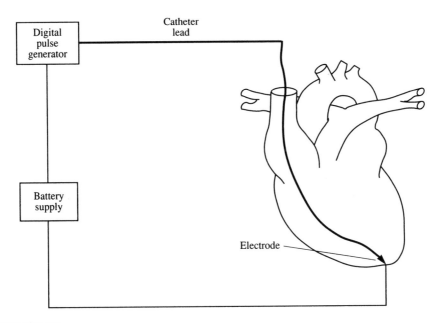

FIGURE 9.2
A pacemaker block diagram.

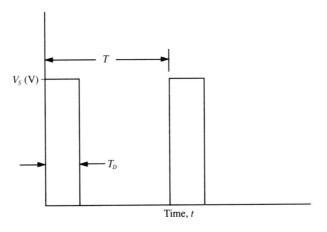

FIGURE 9.3
A pacemaker pulse.

in the energy, E_P, delivered by the pacemaker to the heart during each pulse. During the pulse duration, T_D, the stimulus voltage drives energy into the heart. When the pulse is OFF, it causes an energy drain given by $V_S I_D T$, where T is the time period between successive pulses, and I_D is the current drain on the battery when the pulse is OFF. Therefore, the energy delivered by the pacemaker during each pulse is given as

$$E_P = \frac{V_S^2}{R_H} T_D + V_S I_D T \qquad \text{(in J/pulse)} \qquad \textbf{(9.1)}$$

EXAMPLE 9.1   Using Figure 9.1, compute the energy per pulse when the pacemaker pulse width is 0.5 ms, the circuit-current drain is 1 μA, the heart-electrode resistance is 200 Ω, and the heart rate is 70 bpm.

SOLUTION   From Figure 9.1, $V_S = 1.8$ V. Also, $T = (60/70)$ s. Then, from Equation (9.1),

$$E_P = \frac{1.8^2}{200} 0.5(10^{-3}) + 1.8(10^{-6}) \frac{60}{70}$$

Thus the energy used for each pulse is

$$E_P = 9.643 \ \mu\text{J/pulse}$$

Pacemaker Batteries

Battery-operated equipment is convenient in many applications other than pacemakers because it can be used without a power cord, and it is safer because leakage currents are not usually present. The disadvantage is that batteries are relatively large and of limited energy-storage capability. Even so, the energy demand of the pacemaker is such that batteries with lifetimes between five and ten years are available. Mercury cells with two-year lifetimes, used in pacemakers in the past, have been made obsolete by lithium iodide cells which can last as long as 15 years before they need to be replaced. Nuclear pacemaker batteries have been used to extend battery lifetimes to over 20 years, even for dual-chamber pacemakers that use higher amounts of battery power. Nuclear batteries pose an environmental hazard, however, because in an accident the radioactive material could be released into the environment. Nuclear batteries are being considered for artificial implanted hearts also, because of the potential for high energy storage, but this research is only beginning. Rechargeable batteries are not widely used for low-power pacemaker application, since their shelf life is no longer than that of a lithium iodide pacemaker battery in normal use.

The lifetime of a storage battery depends on both its ampere-hour (A-H) rating and its shelf life. Shelf life is limited self-discharge of the battery due to internal leakage currents, particle migration, formation of insulating layers, and internal shorts. An illustrative example of a battery A-H rating versus its current drain is given in Figure 9.4. At high current drain, polarization of the metal electrolyte boundary increases the internal resistance of the battery and decreases the A-H rating.

Implantable batteries are usually encased in metal. If they become too hot, such as when shorted, the case may rupture. Pacemaker design should ensure that the case is strong enough to contain such a rupture and prevent toxic materials from entering the body of the patient.

EXAMPLE 9.2 Compute the energy in joules stored in a lithium iodide battery having a rating of 1 A-H and a terminal voltage of 1.8 V.

SOLUTION Battery energy = (1 A-H)(1.8 V)(3600 s/h) = 6480 J. In doing the dimensional analysis here, recall that the dimensions of volts are joules per coulomb (J/C).

EXAMPLE 9.3 Using the pulse and data from Example 9.1, compute the lifetime of the battery in Example 9.2.

SOLUTION The energy in each pulse is 9.643 μJ and the pulse period $T = 60/70 = 0.857$ s. The battery lifetime is then

$$\frac{6480 \text{ J}}{9.643 \text{ } \mu\text{J}} \, 0.857 \text{ s} = 5.759(10^8) \text{ s}$$

Converting this to years gives

$$5.759(10^8 \text{ s})\left(\frac{1 \text{ h}}{3600 \text{ s}}\right)\left(\frac{1 \text{ day}}{24 \text{ h}}\right)\left(\frac{1 \text{ yr}}{365 \text{ day}}\right) = 18.26 \text{ yr}$$

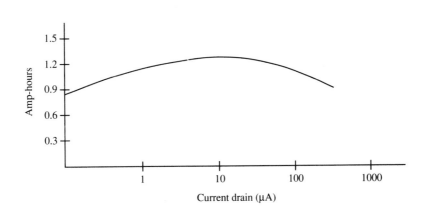

FIGURE 9.4
A typical ampere-hour rating of a lithium iodide battery as a function of battery current.

The calculation in Examples 9.1, 9.2, and 9.3 is summarized with the following formula:

$$\text{Lifetime} = \frac{(A\text{-}H)V_S T(1.142)(10^{-4})}{\dfrac{V_S^2}{R_H} T_D + V_S I_D T} \qquad \text{(in yr)} \qquad (9.2)$$

Also, the pulse rate, *BPM*, is given by

$$BPM = \frac{60}{T}$$

where *T* is given in seconds and the units of *BPM* are pulses (or beats) per minute (bpm).

It is clear from Equation (9.2) that the battery lifetime is inversely proportional to the *BPM* and the T_D pulse duration. Thus, increasing the stimulus pulse rate or the pulse duration will reduce the battery lifetime.

Illustrative Pacemaker Characteristics

The pacemaker consists of three major components illustrated in Figure 9.2: the lead wire, the electronic pulsing circuit, and the battery.

The lead can cause a failure due to metal fatigue, introduced by the motion and beating of the heart. To avoid such fatigue, the lead may be constructed by winding platinum ribbon around polyester yarn. Each lead may have three such wires for redundancy.

The pacemaker electrode must make a secure contact with the heart for several years. To ensure this, two methods of implantation are used under the following classifications: (1) *endocardial* lead, in which the pacemaker lead is inserted through a major vein through a catheter guide into the right ventricle of the heart; and (2) *epicardial* lead, in which the pacemaker electrode is sutured to the external wall of the heart during open-heart surgery (see Figure 9.5), and a wire electrode is thereby secured into the tissue.

For endocardial lead implantation the electrode may be attached with tines as illustrated in Figure 9.6(a). The tines are pushed into the Purkinje muscle fibers of the ventricle and latch themselves in place. The porous electrode tip minimizes motion between the tip and the tissue so as to reduce the scar tissue buildup. This tends to keep the contact resistance low. The electrode may also be held in place with a helical wire that is screwed into the tissues with a twisting motion, as illustrated in Figure 9.6(b). In this case a *bipolar* electrode a few centimeters behind the contact electrode serves as

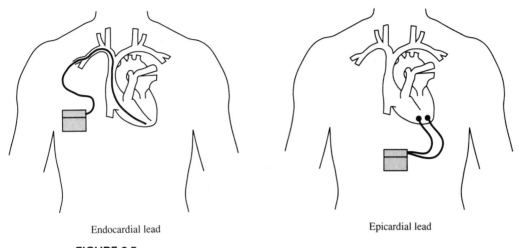

Endocardial lead   Epicardial lead

FIGURE 9.5
Placement of implantable pacemakers. (From Cardiac Pacemakers, Inc.)

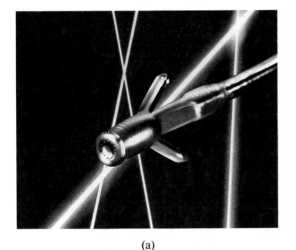

(a)

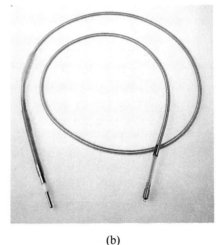

(b)

FIGURE 9.6
Illustrative pacemaker leads. (Courtesy of Telectronics Inc.)

a return path for current to the pacemaker. A pacemaker with a bipolar lead is shown in Figure 9.7. In the *unipolar* pacemaker lead, the second electrode is eliminated, and the return conductive path to the pacemaker is made through body fluids. A unipolar lead electrode may also be held in place by either sutures, tines, or a helical wire.

The electrode-muscle contact can change after a time because of (1) polarization by ionic current flow; (2) tissue and scar growth; or (3) mechanical

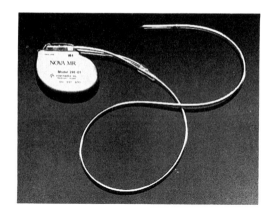

FIGURE 9.7
A pacemaker with a bipolar lead. (Courtesy of Intermedics, Inc.)

motion of the heart. A symptom of such change may be an increased electrode impedance. The problem may be fixed by increasing the pulse voltage from the pacemaker or by lengthening its duration. Loss of contact altogether may require surgical reimplantation.

In order to reduce the effects of polarization on the electrode, a biphasic pulse is sometimes used. Such a pulse is produced by the voltage generator set to be positive on one cycle and negative on the next. Each successive pulse tends to cancel the polarization effects of the previous one.

The typical ranges of parameters found in pacemakers are given in Table 9.1.

TABLE 9.1
Ranges of Pacemaker Parameters

Rate	25–155 bpm
Sensitivity	0.7–5.5 mV
Pulse width	0.1–2.3 ms
Pulse amplitude	2.5–10 V
Battery capacity	0.44–3.2 A-H
Longevity	3.5–18 yr
End-of-life indicator	2–10% drop in pulse rate
Size	22–80 cm^3
Weight	33–98 g
Encapsulization	Silicon rubber, titanium, stainless steel

9.2 PROGRAMMABLE PACEMAKERS

The implantable pacemaker considered above is presented as a battery-powered, digital pulse generator, and it may be considered an asynchronous type of unit. Other types of pacemaker include the *R*-wave synchronous, *R*-wave inhibited, and *P*-wave synchronous pacemakers. The *asynchronous* pacemaker produces a pulse at a preset rate, for example 70 bpm, and delivers pulses to the heart regardless of the heart's natural beating tendency and independent of the *QRS* complex. This pacemaker does not increase the heart rate in response to the body demand for more blood during exertion. However, a *P-wave synchronous* pacemaker does. The SA node depolarization responds to body demands through the vagus nerve and hormones transported in the blood. In a *P*-wave synchronous pacemaker, the SA node triggers the pacer, which in turn drives the ventricle. It is used when the AV node is blocked because of disease. As shown in Figure 9.8(d), this pacemaker requires two leads. The atrial lead feeds the atrial pulse back to a sensing amplifier. The driver, connected to the ventricle, delivers the pacing pulse. The *R-wave inhibited* pacemaker also allows the heart to pace at its normal rhythm when it is able to. However, if the *R*-wave is missing for a preset period of time, the pacer will supply a stimulus. Therefore, if the pulse rate falls below a predetermined minimum, the pacemaker will turn on and provide the heart a stimulus. For this reason it is called a *demand* pacemaker.

Another type of demand pacemaker uses a piezoelectric sensor shielded inside the pacemaker casing. When this sensor is slightly stressed or bent by the patient's body activity, the pacemaker will automatically increase or decrease its rate. According to Medtronic, Inc., their model will react to a movement of one-millionth of an inch. It will change heart rates to as high as 150 bpm during vigorous activity or as low as 60 bpm during rest periods.

A *programmable* pacemaker is one that can be altered both in its block diagram and in the size and rate of the pulse it delivers. A pacemaker that can be reconfigured into four different block diagrams, after having been implanted, is illustrated in Figure 9.8. A magnet may be placed over the pacemaker on the skin of the patient in order to activate a reed switch, which switches the pacemaker into one of the four configurations shown.

Another kind of programming is done to alter the delivered stimulus and the pacemaker sensitivity to feedback signals.

A programmable pacemaker is shown in Figure 9.9. The telemetric programmer may be placed over the pacemaker to select pulse rates ranging from 30 to 155 bpm, feedback sensitivities from 0.7 to 4.5 V, pulse amplitudes from 2.5 to 10 V, and pulse widths from 0.25 to 1 ms, among other parameters. A hard copy of the programming record is provided by the printer shown.

When temporary heart pacing is needed, an external pacemaker, illustrated in Figure 9.10, may be used. Since this device is not implanted, there is no need for extensive surgery. A temporary pacing lead (Figure 9.11) uses a balloon tip, so that the flow of blood will carry the pacing electrode into the heart when the balloon is inflated.

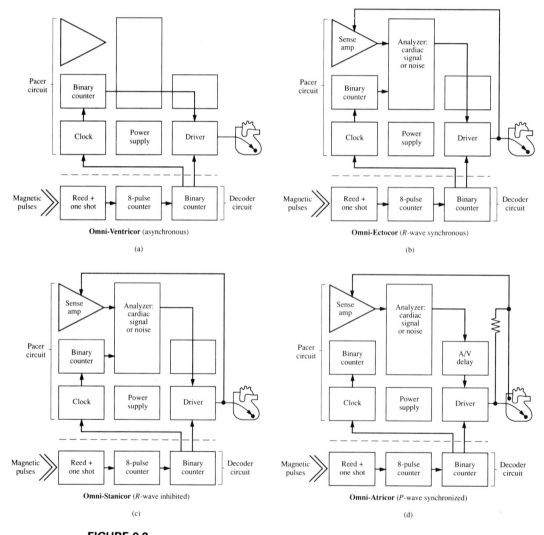

FIGURE 9.8
A programmable pacemaker block diagram. (Courtesy of Telectronics Inc.)

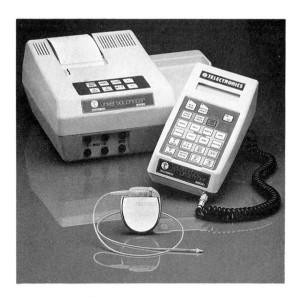

FIGURE 9.9
A pacemaker programming unit. (Courtesy of
Telectronics Inc.)

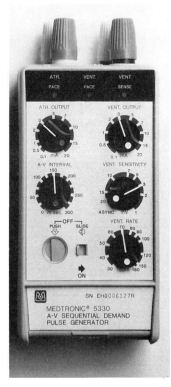

FIGURE 9.10
An external programmable pacemaker that may be applied to the
ventricle or the atrium of the heart. (Courtesy of Medtronic, Inc.
©1979 Medtronic, Inc. Reprinted by permission)

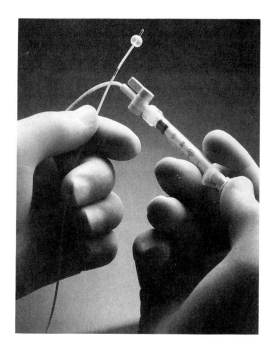

FIGURE 9.11
A balloon-tip, temporary pacing lead, Model 6404. The hypodermic needle is used to inflate the balloon through a catheter lumen, or channel. (Courtesy of Medtronic, Inc. ©1985 Medtronic, Inc. Reprinted by permission)

9.3 DIGITAL PULSE OSCILLATORS

To provide a pacing pulse such as is illustrated in Figure 9.3, an electronic digital pulse oscillator is required. Digital circuits process pulses that exist in either of two states, one or zero. In order to build circuits to generate such digital pulses, the use of integrated circuit diff amps is most convenient and economical when fabricated by large-scale integrated (LSI) circuit techniques. In this section, the basic circuits for producing these signals are analyzed, and calculation software is developed. One of the simplest building blocks of these digital oscillators is the comparator circuit.

A Comparator Circuit

A simple comparator circuit consists of an ideal diff amp with one input grounded, as shown in Figure 9.12. When the input voltage V_{IN} is higher than ground, the output voltage V_{OUT} is driven into negative saturation, $-|V_{SAT}|$. Then, when V_{IN} goes below ground, the output voltage becomes

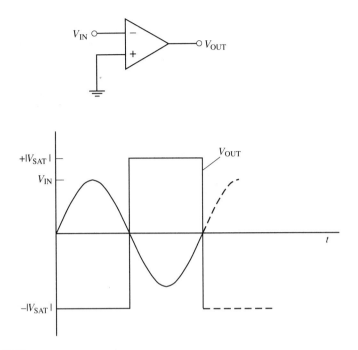

FIGURE 9.12
A comparator with a sine-wave input.

$V_{OUT} = |V_{SAT}|$, the positive saturation voltage of the op amp. In the case illustrated in Figure 9.12, the sinusoidal input produces a square-wave output whose wave is independent of the amplitude of the input, V_{IN}.

In order to introduce protection against noise when there is no input, a positive feedback is added to the circuit by the resistors R_1 and R_2, as illustrated in Figure 9.13(a). Again, assuming an ideal diff amp whenever $V_{IN} > V_R$, the output $V_{OUT} = -|V_{SAT}|$, and when $V_{IN} < V_R$, the value of $V_{OUT} = +|V_{SAT}|$. This fact results in the transfer function graphically illustrated in Figure 9.13(b). V_R has two different values. When $V_{OUT} = +|V_{SAT}|$, since $I_2 = 0$ in an ideal diff amp,

$$V_{R1} = \frac{R_1}{R_1 + R_2} |V_{SAT}| \tag{9.3a}$$

But when $V_{OUT} = -|V_{SAT}|$,

$$V_{R2} = \frac{-R_1}{R_1 + R_2} |V_{SAT}| \tag{9.3b}$$

V_{IN} switches the output voltage when $V_{IN} = V_{R1}$ as V_{IN} ascends from a large negative value, and it switches when $V_{IN} = V_{R2}$ as it descends from a large positive value. The difference between these two trigger values is called *hysteresis voltage*. In a sense the trigger voltage depends upon the "history" of V_{IN}. Mathematically, the hysteresis voltage V_H is defined as the difference between these trigger voltages. That is,

$$V_H = V_{R1} - V_{R2} \qquad (9.4)$$

Equations (9.3a) and (9.3b) into this equation yield

$$V_H = \frac{2R_1 |V_{SAT}|}{R_1 + R_2} \qquad (9.5)$$

One way of describing the hysteresis voltage is to say that $V_H/2$ is the minimum noise voltage that will trigger the comparator when the intended input voltage is zero. Another way of describing the hysteresis is to say that it is the difference between the triggering voltage of a positive-going input, V_{R1}, and the triggering voltage of the negative-going input, V_{R2}. From Equation

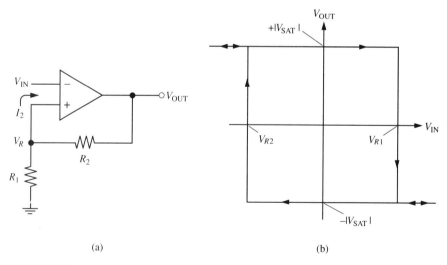

(a)   (b)

FIGURE 9.13
A comparator with hysteresis.

(9.5), it is clear that the hysteresis voltage is adjustable by selecting values for R_1 and R_2.

A Threshold Detector Analysis

In order to adjust the value at which the voltage level detector is caused to change V_{OUT} from $-|V_{\text{SAT}}|$ to $+|V_{\text{SAT}}|$, a bias network is introduced by the potentiometer R_P in Figure 9.14. Here, α is the fraction of the resistance below the adjustable wiper arm of the potentiometer, R_P. Then, to derive an equation from the transfer characteristic V_{OUT} versus V_{IN}, Kirchhoff's laws and the rules for ideal diff amps are employed. KCL at node 2 gives

$$\frac{V_R - V_{\text{OUT}}}{R_2} + \frac{V_R - V_1}{R_1} = 0 \tag{9.6}$$

where V_R is the voltage drop from the noninverting node to ground. KCL at node 1 gives

$$\frac{V_1 - V_R}{R_1} + \frac{V_1 + V_B}{\alpha R_P} + \frac{V_1 - V_B}{(1 - \alpha)R_P} = 0 \tag{9.7}$$

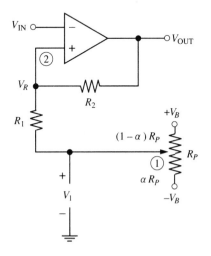

FIGURE 9.14
An adjustable threshold detector.

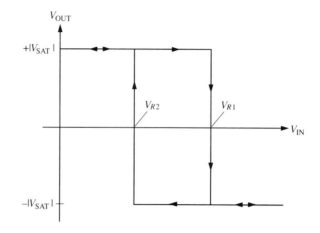

FIGURE 9.15
The output voltage characteristic of the adjustable threshold detector.

These are two independent equations having two unknown variables, V_1 and V_R. They may be solved for V_R to give

$$V_R = \frac{\dfrac{R_1 V_{OUT}}{R_1 + R_2} - \dfrac{R_1 R_2 V_B (1 - 2\alpha)}{[\alpha(1 - \alpha)R_P + R_1](R_1 + R_2)}}{1 - \dfrac{R_2 R_P \alpha(1 - \alpha)}{[\alpha(1 - \alpha)R_P + R_1](R_1 + R_2)}} \qquad \textbf{(9.8)}$$

From Equation (9.8), it is possible to compute V_R for any set of circuit components R_1, R_2, R_P, α. The value of the output voltage V_{OUT} is either $|V_{SAT}|$ or $-|V_{SAT}|$. Thus, the form of the transfer function is given in Figure 9.15. V_{R1} is computed by inserting $V_{OUT} = |V_{SAT}|$ into Equation (9.8), and V_{R2} results when $V_{OUT} = -|V_{SAT}|$. A calculator program for computing Equation (9.8) is given as Program A-17 in Appendix A. The threshold voltage, V_{TH}, of the detector is the average of the two values of V_R and is given by

$$V_{TH} = \frac{V_{R1} + V_{R2}}{2}$$

EXAMPLE 9.4 Find V_{R1} and V_{R2} for all values of α when $R_1 = 1$ kΩ, $R_2 = 47$ kΩ, $R_P = 10$ kΩ, $V_B = 12$, and $|V_{SAT}| = 12$ V.

SOLUTION   Insert the values given in the example into Equation (9.8). First take $\alpha = 0.4$ and $V_{OUT} = +12$ V $= |V_{SAT}|$. Then the calculated value of $V_{R1} = -1.42$. Next take $\alpha = 0.4$ and $V_{OUT} = -12$ V. Then the calculated value of $V_{R2} = -3.05$. Continuing with this procedure yields the plot of V_{R1} and V_{R2} versus α in Figure 9.16.

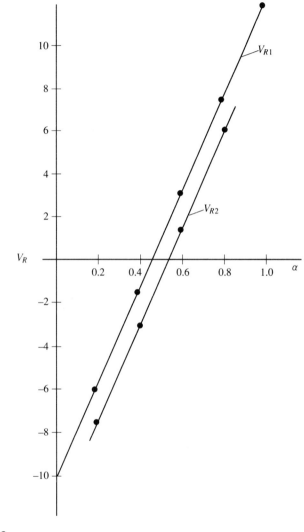

FIGURE 9.16
Threshold levels as a function of α.

Notice that the value of V_H from Equation (9.4) depends on α also.

Square-Wave Generator

Because of the need to provide digital clock signals to a pacemaker as well as most other medical electronic equipment, it is important to understand a square-wave generator and to be able to analyze it. Such a generator produces a wave as shown in Figure 9.17. Its period is T, and the negative and positive pulse both have the same duration, T_D. One circuit for producing square waves is obtained by adding a capacitor, C, and a resistor, R, to a voltage level detector, as illustrated in Figure 9.18. The added capacitor is on node 1. Because the differential gain of the ideal diff amp is very high, the voltage V_{OUT} will be either $|V_{SAT}|$ or $-|V_{SAT}|$, where $|V_{SAT}|$ is the

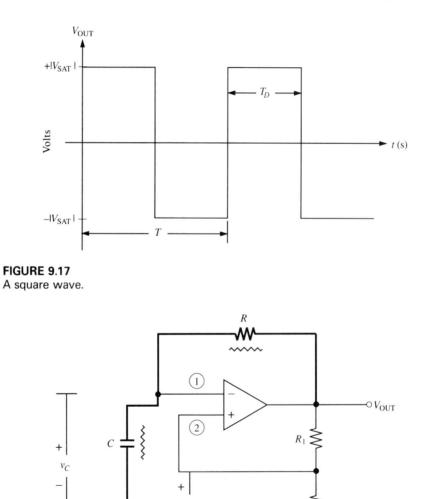

FIGURE 9.17
A square wave.

FIGURE 9.18
A square-wave generator.

saturation voltage of the operational amplifier. The feedback voltage fraction, α, is defined as

$$\alpha = \frac{R_2}{R_1 + R_2} \tag{9.9}$$

Thus,

$$V_R = \alpha V_{\text{OUT}}$$

The voltage across the capacitor, v_C, is given by the capacitor charging equation for the *RC* circuit, which holds because the current into the ideal diff amp input terminal is essentially zero. The lowercase "v" is used to indicate that this is a continuously changing function of time. The capacitor charging circuit is shown in Figure 9.19. The capacitor voltage, as proved in Appendix B, is given by the charging equation

$$v_C = [V_F + (V_I - V_F)e^{-t/RC}] \tag{9.10}$$

where V_I is the initial voltage on the capacitor, and V_F is the final voltage approached as the capacitor charges. In this case $V_F = V_{\text{OUT}}$. To plot the voltage v_C, suppose $V_{\text{OUT}} = -|V_{\text{SAT}}|$, and therefore, $V_I = -\alpha|V_{\text{SAT}}|$ at $t = 0$. As v_C tries to go more negative than $-\alpha|V_{\text{SAT}}|$, the output voltage will switch to $+|V_{\text{SAT}}|$. $|V_{\text{SAT}}|$ then becomes equal to V_{OUT}, the charging voltage applied to the capacitor. Thus we have the charging equation, Equation (9.10), as

$$v_C = |V_{\text{SAT}}| + (-\alpha|V_{\text{SAT}}| - |V_{\text{SAT}}|)e^{-t/RC} \tag{9.11}$$

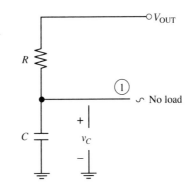

FIGURE 9.19
The capacitor charging circuit.

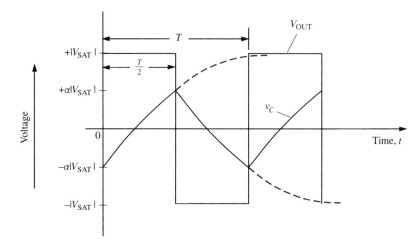

FIGURE 9.20
The capacitor charging voltage, and output voltage versus time.

This equation holds as long as $v_C < \alpha|V_{SAT}|$, above which voltage the node 1 on the diff amp in Figure 9.18 becomes positive relative to node 2, and the charging voltage on the capacitor V_{OUT} is forced to equal $-|V_{SAT}|$. A sketch of the resulting waveform across the capacitor, v_C, is given in Figure 9.20. The charging phase of the capacitor is summarized as follows: At t just greater than zero ($t > 0$), the capacitor charges from $-\alpha|V_{SAT}|$ toward the voltage $|V_{SAT}|$. However, when $v_C = \alpha|V_{SAT}|$, before it reaches its final value, V_{OUT} switches to $-|V_{SAT}|$ and the capacitor begins to discharge again.

By use of a discussion similar to that used to explain Equation (9.11), we can show that the equation describing v_C in the time period $T/2 < t < T$ is given by

$$v_C = -|V_{SAT}| + (\alpha|V_{SAT}| + |V_{SAT}|)e^{-(t-T/2)RC} \qquad (9.12)$$

EXAMPLE 9.5   Plot the voltage v_C in the time period $0 < t < T/2$ when $R = 1$ kΩ, $C = 1$ μF, $|V_{SAT}| = 10$ V, $R_1 = 1$ kΩ, and $R_2 = 1$ kΩ. Also find the period T graphically and plot V_{OUT}.

SOLUTION   Equation (9.9) gives $\alpha = 0.5$. Then from Equation (9.11) we have

$$v_C = 10 + [-0.5(10) - 10]e^{-t/0.001}$$
$$= 10 - 15e^{-t/0.001}$$

For example, a calculation of this equation at $t = 0.25$ ms yields $v_C = -1.68$ V. A complete plot of v_C versus time is given in Figure 9.21. The half period $T/2$ is the time it takes for the voltage v_C to rise from $V_{SAT} = -5$ to $V_{SAT} = +5$. From Figure 9.21, we see that $T/2 = 1.1$ ms, or $T = 2.2$ ms. Thus the output voltage V_{OUT} is a square wave going between $+10$ V and -10 V with a period $T = 2.2$ ms.

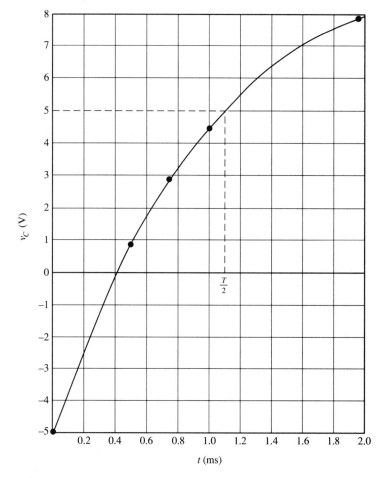

FIGURE 9.21
A plot of capacitor voltage versus time.

A formula for the period of the square-wave oscillator can be derived directly from Equation (9.11). Notice that when $t = T/2$, $v_C = \alpha|V_{SAT}|$, and then

$$\alpha|V_{SAT}| = |V_{SAT}| + (-\alpha|V_{SAT}| - |V_{SAT}|)e^{-T/2RC}$$

Cancelling the $|V_{SAT}|$, we have

$$\frac{1-\alpha}{1+\alpha} = e^{-T/2RC}$$

Taking the natural logarithm of both sides gives

$$T = -2RC\ln\frac{1-\alpha}{1+\alpha} \qquad\qquad (9.13)$$

The implication of this equation is that the period of the square-wave generator can be adjusted by changing α or the RC time constant. Notice also that the peak amplitude of V_{OUT} is always equal to $|V_{SAT}|$.

EXAMPLE 9.6   Check the period in Example 9.5, using Equation (9.13).

SOLUTION $T = -2(10^{-3})\ln[(1 - 0.5)/(1 + 0.5)] = 2.197$ ms. This result is close to the estimate, 2.2 ms, from Figure 9.21.

Monostable Multivibrator

The square-wave generator is sometimes called an *A-stable multivibrator*. This means it is not stable in either state but periodically switches between the output voltages $|V_{SAT}|$ and $-|V_{SAT}|$. Another circuit, illustrated in Figure 9.22, is stable in only one state and is called a *monostable multivibrator*.

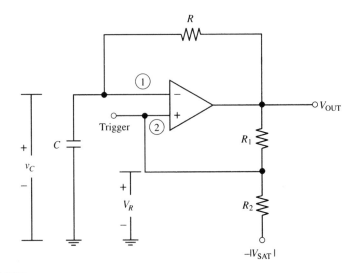

FIGURE 9.22
A monostable multivibrator.

A monostable multivibrator circuit can be used to produce a digital pulse of a specified duration, T_D. This circuit may be made temporarily unstable, which is to say, it may be *triggered* by applying an appropriate voltage to node 2 when the circuit is stable. If the monostable multivibrator is triggered periodically, a pulse train, such as is shown in Figure 9.3, is produced. Furthermore, if that period is on the order of one second, the pulse could be used in a pacemaker for a human heart.

The monostable multivibrator can be made by replacing one of the ground connections of Figure 9.18 with a negative voltage source of value approximately $-|V_{SAT}|$ as shown in Figure 9.22. After all transients have passed on this circuit, the output voltage $V_{OUT} = -|V_{SAT}|$ in value. When this is true, the voltage at nodes 1 and 2 is also equal to $-|V_{SAT}|$. No currents flow in this case, and the circuit is in a stable state. Suppose, then, at time $t = 0$, a positive trigger voltage is applied to node 2. Since the capacitor holds node 1 temporarily at $-|V_{SAT}|$, the output voltage V_{OUT} of the diff amp will immediately switch to $+|V_{SAT}|$. This will cause the capacitor to charge according to Equation (9.10) such that

$$v_C = |V_{SAT}| + (-|V_{SAT}| - |V_{SAT}|)e^{-t/RC} \qquad (9.14)$$

The voltage v_C is illustrated in Figure 9.23 along with the corresponding output voltage, V_{OUT}. The capacitor continues to charge according to Equation (9.14) until $v_C = V_R$ and the node 1 voltage tends to exceed the

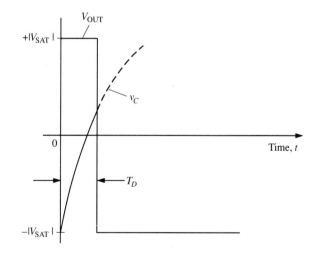

FIGURE 9.23
The output voltage, V_{OUT}, and capacitor charging voltage, v_C, versus time.

node 2 voltage. This forces the output V_{OUT} back to the stable point $-|V_{SAT}|$. In the meantime, while $V_{OUT} = |V_{SAT}|$,

$$V_R = \frac{[|V_{SAT}| - (-|V_{SAT}|)] R_2}{R_1 + R_2} - |V_{SAT}|$$

That is,

$$V_R = \frac{R_2 - R_1}{R_2 + R_1} |V_{SAT}|$$

The time T_D that it takes for v_C to become equal to V_R is computed by putting $V_R = v_C$ into Equation (9.14) and making $t = T_D$ as follows:

$$\frac{R_2 - R_1}{R_2 + R_1} |V_{SAT}| = |V_{SAT}|(1 - 2e^{-T_D/RC})$$

Solving this equation gives

$$2e^{-T_D/RC} = \frac{R_1 - R_2}{R_1 + R_2} + 1 = \frac{2R_1}{R_1 + R_2}$$

Taking the natural logarithm of both sides yields

$$T_D = -RC \ln\left(\frac{R_1}{R_1 + R_2}\right) \qquad\qquad \textbf{(9.15)}$$

From this equation, we see that the output voltage duration T_D can be computed from, and is seen to depend on, the RC time constant of the monostable multivibrator and the resistors R_1 and R_2.

In summary, after a positive trigger is applied to node 2 (Figure 9.22), an output pulse of peak-to-peak value $2|V_{SAT}|$ and duration T_D is produced.

Positive-Edge Triggered Multivibrator

The multivibrator in Figure 9.22 is appended with a positive-edge trigger circuit in Figure 9.24. A positive step at the trigger input will pass through the capacitor and the diode and will raise the voltage at the lower node of the diff amp. The capacitor C_C should be chosen so as to make five time constants equal to T_D. Otherwise, the trigger would still be present after T_D has passed and a second pulse would be erroneously generated. Thus we choose

$$5(R_1 \| R_2)C_C = T_D \qquad\qquad \textbf{(9.16)}$$

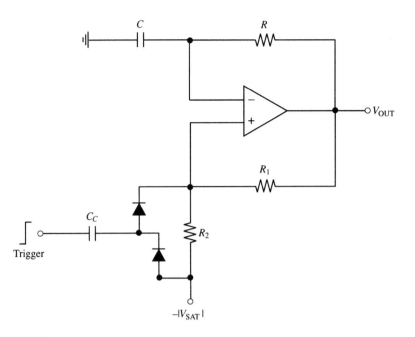

FIGURE 9.24
A positive-edge triggered monostable multivibrator.

EXAMPLE 9.7 The monostable multivibrator in Figure 9.24 has components $R = 721\ \Omega$, $C = 1\ \mu F$, $R_1 = 1.2\ k\Omega$, and $R_2 = 1\ k\Omega$. Compute the duration of the output pulse.

SOLUTION From Equation (9.15),

$$T_D = -721(10^{-6})\ln\frac{1200}{2200}$$

Thus $T_D = 0.437$ ms.

EXAMPLE 9.8 Choose a coupling capacitor C_C such that five time constants equal the pulse duration in Example 9.7.

SOLUTION Let $T_D = 0.437(10^{-3})$ in Equation (9.16). Then C_C (1200/ 2.2)5 = 0.437 (10^{-3}). Thus $C_C = 0.160\ \mu F$.

An Illustrative Pacemaker Circuit

Using the square-wave oscillator to provide positive-edge triggers to the monostable multivibrator results in the practical pacemaker circuit illustrated in Figure 9.25. The first diff amp circuit is a square-wave oscillator.

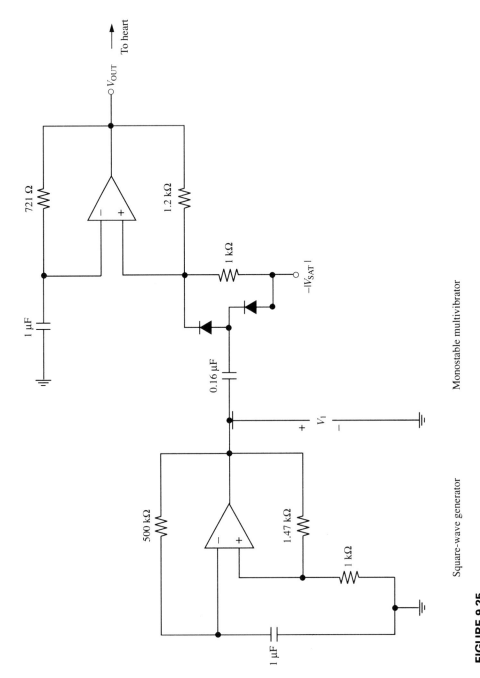

Square-wave generator   Monostable multivibrator

FIGURE 9.25
An illustrative pacemaker circuit.

The positive edges are passed by the 0.16-μF capacitor and trigger the monostable multivibrator formed by the second diff amp. The period of the pacemaker is given by Equation (9.13) since this measures the period between positive-edge triggers. The pulse duration rate then is given by Equation (9.15). This duration would not be greatly affected by the loading of the heart tissue. In modern pacemakers, such a circuit would be fabricated on a single large-scale integrated (LSI) circuit.

EXAMPLE 9.9   Sketch the output pulse of the pacemaker circuit given in Figure 9.25, when $|V_{\text{SAT}}| = 6$ V.

SOLUTION   The waveform is given in Figure 9.3. The pulse duration $T_D = 0.437$ ms from Example 9.7. The pulse period T is computed from Equation (9.13). For this equation, $\alpha = 1/2.47 = 0.405$, using Equation (9.9):

$$T = -2[500,000(10^{-6})]\ln[(1 - 0.405)/(1 + 0.405)]$$

$T = 0.859$ s. This implies a pulse rate, *BPM*, as follows:

$$BPM = 60/0.859$$

$$= 70 \text{ bpm}$$

To sketch the pulse, use the form given in Figure 9.3, and let $T = 0.859$ s, $T_D = 0.437$ s, and $|V_S| = 12$ V.

REFERENCES

Citron, P., *et al.* "Cardiac Pacing," Chapter 2 in *Therapeutic Medical Devices, Application and Design*, edited by A. M. Cook and J. G. Webster. Englewood Cliffs, NJ: Prentice-Hall, 1982.

Cordis Corporation. "Omnicor System Pacers, Technical Description." Miami: Cordis Corporation, 1976.

Galioto, F. M., Jr. "Cardiovascular Assist and Monitoring Devices." Chapter 3 in *Biomedical Engineering and Instrumentation*, edited by J. D. Bronzino. Boston: Prindle, Weber & Schmidt, 1986.

Neuman, M. R. "Therapeutic and Prosthetic Devices." Chapter 12 in *Medical Instrumentation, Application and Design*, edited by J. G. Webster. Boston: Houghton Mifflin, 1978.

Malvino, A. P. *Electronic Principles.* 3rd ed. New York: McGraw-Hill, 1984.

McWane, J. W., and Lewis, R. *Electronics and Medical Instrumentation Program.* Department of Health, Education and Welfare, Grant #OEG-0-000973-1873(085), 1973.

EXERCISES

1. A pacemaker pulse output drives a heart tissue at 200 Ω. The pulse waveform is shown in Figure 9.26. The leakage current and circuit drain of the pacemaker are 1 μA while the pulse is off. The battery capacity of the pacemaker is 1 ampere-hour (A-H) at a voltage of 2.5 V.

   (a) Calculate the total energy available from the battery.
   (b) Calculate the energy delivered to the heart by each pulse from the pacemaker.
   (c) Compute the lifetime of the battery in years, provided shelf life will allow it.
   (d) Plot the battery lifetime versus the pulse width T_D from 0.1 to 1 ms. ($T = 1$ s.)
   (e) When $T_D = 0.3$ ms, plot battery lifetime versus the beats per minute, *BPM*.

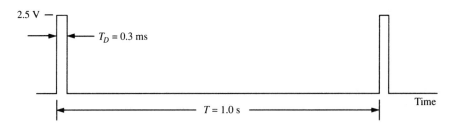

FIGURE 9.26

2. Write a program for Equation (9.2) to compute the battery lifetime of a pacemaker. Use storage registers for A-H, T, V_S, R_H, T_D, and I_D. Check the program by using it to solve Example 9.3 in the text.

3. Beginning with the pacemaker stimulus pulse illustrated in Figure 9.26, make a plot of battery lifetime as a function of pulse duration ranging from 0.1 to 10 ms. The battery parameters are the same as those in Exercise 1.

4. Beginning with the pacemaker stimulus pulse illustrated in Figure 9.26, make a plot of battery lifetime as a function of pulse period T ranging from that corresponding to a pulse rate from 50 to 120 bpm.

5. Beginning with the pacemaker stimulus pulse illustrated in Figure 9.26, make a plot of battery lifetime as a function of leakage current drain I_D from 1 to 100 μA. The battery parameters are the same as in Exercise 1.

6. In the square-wave oscillator in Figure 9.27, calculate the frequency when $R = 2.1$ kΩ, $C = 3$ μF, and $\alpha_1 = 0.5$. α_1 is the fraction of the total wiper arm displacement from the lowest position.

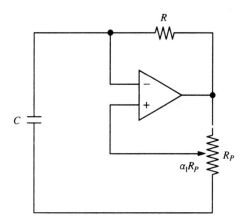

FIGURE 9.27

7. In the square-wave oscillator in Figure 9.27, plot the period of oscillation versus α_1. Let $R = 2.1$ kΩ and $C = 3$ μF.

8. For the square-wave oscillator in Figure 9.27, make a plot of the frequency of oscillation versus α_1. Let $R = 5$ kΩ and $C = 100$ μF.

9. In the circuit described in Exercise 8, compute the value of α_1 that makes the pulse frequency $f = 1.5$ Hz.

10. A square-wave oscillator is given in Figure 9.28. Plot the frequency versus α_2 for this case. $R_1 = 3$ kΩ, $R_2 = 2$ kΩ, $C = 5$ μF, and $R_P = 10$ kΩ.

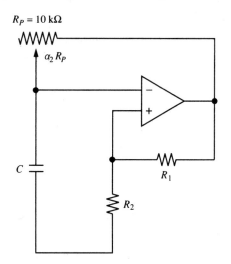

FIGURE 9.28

11. Starting with Equations (9.6) and (9.7), derive Equation (9.8) in the text.

10 Electrosurgical Units and Laser Surgery

The first practical electrosurgical units (ESU) were derived at Harvard University from World War I Navy ship spark-gap transmitters. W. T. Bovie applied the spark output directly to biological tissue, causing it to cut where the tip of the output wire touched the tissue. He developed the device for Harvey Cushing, who used these high-frequency radio currents in neurosurgery in 1925. The use of electrosurgical equipment expanded greatly after 1950, when nonflammable anesthetics were introduced, since ESUs are generally incompatible with the use of flammable anesthetics. Subsequently, the spark-gap Bovie ESU was widely used, but the most recent devices are designed with solid-state circuitry using oscillators with selectable pulse modulation. One obvious advantage the solid-state device has over the spark-gap unit is its smaller size.

10.1 THE BASIC ESU

The basic ESU, illustrated in Figure 10.1, consists of a radio-frequency oscillator operating between 300 kHz and 3 MHz. The cutting electrode has a tapered edge that would be too dull to cut tissue without the RF current produced by the oscillator. When the electrode is held sufficiently far away from the body, no current flows and no cutting action occurs. Voltages on the electrode may range from 1000 to 10,000 volts peak-to-peak (V_{pp}). As the electrode is brought closer to the skin at these voltages, a spark will jump across. The breakdown voltage of air is approximately 30 kV/cm, so if, for example, the electrode voltage is 10,000 V, a spark 0.33 cm in length can be drawn. The existence of sparks in normal ESU application makes

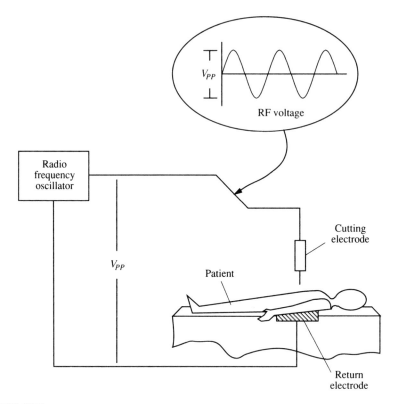

FIGURE 10.1
The essential components of an ESU.

it a fire hazard in the presence of flammable anesthetics or other flammable gases.

When the electrode touches the skin, no spark may be present. When the RF current is applied, it passes through individual cell membranes by capacitive coupling, as explained in Section 2.5. At these high frequencies, large currents flow into the cell, causing it to vaporize, and thereby cause a rupture of the tissue close to the cutting electrode. The current density a short distance from the cutting electrode on the way to the return electrode, as illustrated in Figure 10.1, decreases quickly to harmless levels. As explained in Section 2.5, these currents should not cause muscle contraction or heart fibrillation. The return electrode illustrated in Figure 10.1 must have a large area to minimize the heating effect there and prevent surface burns. One of the hazards with ESU is burns at the return patient-plate electrode because of poor skin contact.

The ESU electrode has several advantages over the traditional stainless steel scalpel. It can often cut faster. Furthermore, the heating effect of

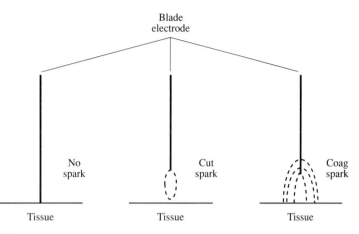

FIGURE 10.2
The skin-electrode contact for various ESU modes.

the cutting currents and sparks has a cauterizing effect on the tissue that inhibits bleeding. Therefore, the ESU can reduce blood loss and minimize the time the patient is in surgery.

Active Electrodes

An active blade-type electrode approximately 1 mm thick and 10 mm wide, used for cutting, is illustrated in Figure 10.2. When the electrode is in the *cutting mode*, a sinusoidal steady-state oscillating current appears at the tip. If the blade is held a short distance from the skin, a sharply directed spark will be drawn to the skin. The voltage along the blade will have the same value everywhere. Therefore, the electric field intensity, in units of volts per meter, will be strongest at the tip, thus producing a well-defined spark and resulting in a cut. The electrode may also be operated in the *coagulation* (or coag) *mode*, produced by a wide spark. The wide spark as shown in Figure 10.2 may be produced by transients on the electrode, which cause a maximum voltage to appear somewhere other than at the tip. The breakdown electric field intensity would then originate from the maximum voltage region on the blade and produce a spraying effect in the spark. The power for the blade would then be spread over a larger region of skin and would tend to cauterize the tissue and coagulate the blood.

Tissue cauterization and coagulation can be facilitated by blunting the tip of the electrode, as illustrated in Figure 10.3. The spark produced by the spherical-tip electrode tends to broaden across the tissue, because there are several equidistant paths from the skin to the electrode surface. The air along all such paths tends to break down simultaneously. The hemostat electrode may be used to lift and clamp, or grasp tissue, especially a bleeding

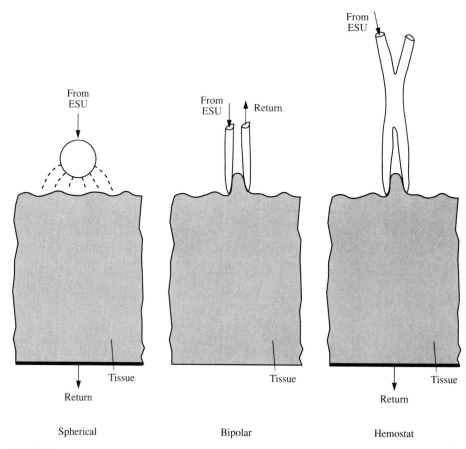

FIGURE 10.3
The spherical, bipolar, and hemostat electrode connections.

vessel. The ESU current then would flow broadly through the grasped tissue, causing a coagulation effect. A bipolar electrode is arranged on the tip of a forceps. Each tip has a separate electrical path, one from the ESU active head and one to the patient return. When in use, these two electrodes contact tissue in close proximity to each other. In this case it is not necessary to have a return, ground-plate electrode. With the bipolar electrode, the current density on both electrodes is equally high. Therefore, each electrode may have both a cutting effect and a coagulation effect.

The Active Electrode Resistance

The active electrode-to-skin resistance, R_E, varies considerably, depending upon how much of the electrode actually contacts the tissue. This variable is changed, or controlled, by the surgeon. It is important to realize that the

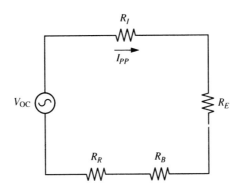

FIGURE 10.4
An ESU electrical equivalent circuit.

amount of power delivered to the tissue for a given ESU instrument voltage depends in turn on this resistance.

An equivalent circuit of the ESU in Figure 10.4 shows its internal resistance, R_I, and R_E, as well as a body resistance, R_B, and return electrode resistance, R_R. The power dissipated by each of these resistances determines the cut, coagulation, warming, or burning effect at each of the sites.

In accordance with the maximum power rule, the maximum power delivered to the patient occurs when R_E equals the sum of the other resistances of the circuit, $R_I + R_B + R_R$.

EXAMPLE 10.1 An ESU illustrated in Figure 10.4 has a peak-to-peak open-circuit voltage $V_{OC} = 1500$ V. If $R_I = 400$ Ω, $R_B = 50$ Ω, and $R_R = 10$ Ω, plot the power absorbed, P_A, at the active electrode as a function of R_E, ranging from 100 to 1000 Ω.

SOLUTION Recall that

$$P_A = \frac{I_{PP}^2}{8} R_E$$

where I_{PP} is the peak-to-peak–value current in the circuit. Also,

$$I_{PP} = \frac{V_{OC}}{R_I + R_B + R_R + R_E}$$

In this case,

$$I_{PP} = \frac{1500}{460 + R_E}$$

Then

$$P_A = \frac{1500^2 R_E}{8(460 + R_E)^2} = \frac{281{,}250 R_E}{(460 + R_E)^2}$$

A plot of P_A appears in Figure 10.5.

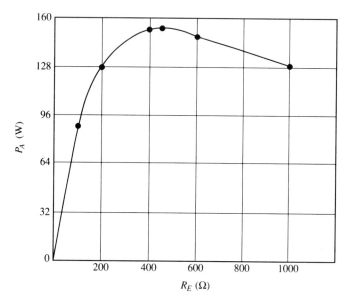

FIGURE 10.5
The power absorbed at an active electrode as a function of electrode resistance.

The Return Electrode

The patient return electrode must be treated carefully in order to avoid the tissue burn hazards associated with it. Any increase in the resistance, R_R, will cause increased power to be dissipated at the skin-electrode interface. In order to minimize R_R, electrode gel should be applied. The return electrode should be placed over a large mass of muscle, such as on the biceps, thigh, or buttock, and the area should preferably be shaved. Adhesive, pregelled electrodes are available, but it is important to be certain the gel has not dried, either in storage, or on the patient during a long operation. Care must also be taken since the contact may inadvertently be changed when the patient is moved.

One method of automatically checking the contact on the return electrode is to monitor its resistance. A change in the resistance can be used to trigger an alarm to warn an attendant.

One method of monitoring the resistance is to separate the return electrode into two parallel areas, as shown in Figure 10.6. The electrodes are then placed in a balanced Wheatstone bridge. Any disturbance in the resistance of the pad will throw the bridge out of balance, causing a voltage V_{OUT} to appear different from the null value. Notice in Figure 10.6 that

$$V_{OUT} = \left(\frac{R_{H1}}{R + R_{H1}} - \frac{R_{H2}}{R + R_{H2}} \right) V_B \tag{10.1}$$

where R is a resistance, R_{H1} and R_{H2} are the resistances of either side of the return electrode, and V_B is a bias voltage. The return electrode should be large enough that the current density is small and does not burn the patient. Normally, a metal-plate electrode taking a conductive jelly to lower the skin resistance is used. The resistance of the electrode is inversely proportional to the surface area. One hazard of such an electrode is that the conductive gel may be unevenly applied, causing hot spots, or the gel may dry, causing the same effect. To avoid this, a capacitively coupled electrode may be used.

The impedance of the capacitive electrode in Figure 10.7 is

$$Z_C = \frac{1}{j2\pi f C_E} \tag{10.2}$$

where

$$C_E = \epsilon_o \epsilon_r \frac{A}{d}$$

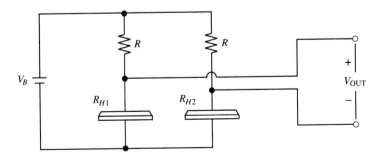

FIGURE 10.6
A return electrode alarm circuit.

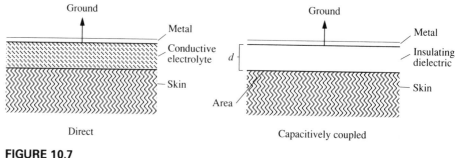

FIGURE 10.7
Types of ESU return electrodes.

and A is the area of the plates, d is the distance between them, and ϵ_o (8.85 pF/m) and ϵ_r are the free space and relative dielectric constants, respectively.

EXAMPLE 10.2   A capacitively coupled return electrode dielectric on an ESU has a thickness $d = 0.0025$ cm. The dielectric constant of the insulator ϵ_r is 3.2. Compute the impedance versus area for the electrode against a person's skin for an ESU operating at 500 kHz.

SOLUTION   Consider the case $A = 120$ cm². Then, using the previous capacitance formula,

$$C_E = \frac{(120 \text{ cm}^2)(1 \text{ m})(3.2)(8.8 \text{ pF/m})}{(0.0025 \text{ cm})(100 \text{ cm})} = 0.013 \ \mu F$$

This capacitance in Equation (10.2) gives

$$|Z_C| = 1/[2\pi(500)(10^3)(0.013)(10^{-6})] = 25$$

Similar calculation yields the following table:

Area (cm²)	Electrode impedance (vars)
120	25
60	50
12	250

The increased electrode impedance, along with the increased current density due to the smaller electrode area, increases the power loss and, therefore, increases the heat on the patient.

A Block Diagram

A generic solid-state ESU block diagram is given in Figure 10.8, along with example waveforms available at the output electrode for the cut, coag, and blend modes of operation. In this circuit the power output of the cut waveform may be up to 400 W into a 500-Ω load. Open-circuit voltages may range from 1000 to 10,000 V peak-to-peak. In Figure 10.8 the coag pulse train is a digital pulse that modulates the RF output according to selected duty cycles as follows:

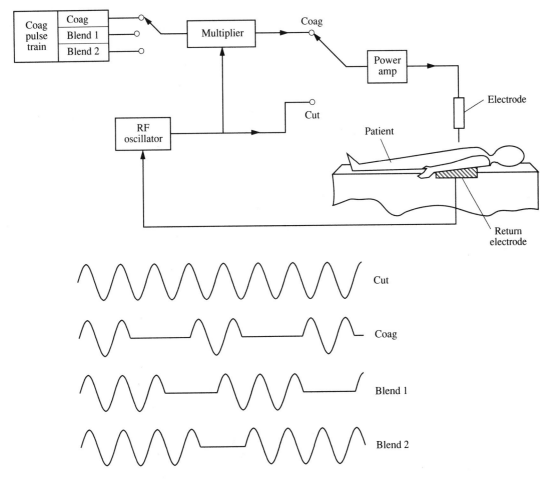

FIGURE 10.8
An ESU with cut, coagulation, and blend modes, and the waveforms of these modes.

Pulse train	Duty cycle (%)	Power (W)
Cut	100	400
Coag	33	132
Blend 1	50	200
Blend 2	75	300

The waveforms are also illustrated for the selected settings. The cut setting is used to cause vaporization of the cell. The coag setting, on the other hand, heats the tissue, causing relatively deep dehydration and tissue cauterization. Blend 1 and 2 controls are used by the surgeon along with the power amplifier gain control to create the degree and speed of coagulation desired. The power in the blend settings is selected in fixed, repeatable steps by adjusting the duty cycle of the applied RF waveform. In order to measure the power output of an ESU, as well as its leakage currents, an ESU analyzer like that illustrated in Figure 10.9 is used.

In summary, the ESU is a high-power device used on patients when they are the most vulnerable and defenseless—during surgery. Safety in its use is therefore of the highest priority. Several safety hints are listed in Box 1.

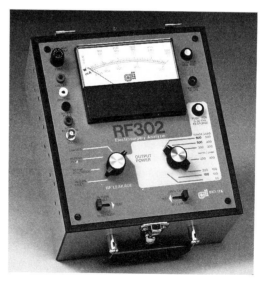

FIGURE 10.9
An electrosurgery analyzer. (Courtesy of Bio-Tek Instruments, Inc.)

Box 1

ESU SAFETY HINTS

- Do not use in the presence of combustible materials such as flammable anesthesia agents or flammable disinfection agents.
- Bowel gas contains explosive methane. Use protective measures during electrosurgery involving the bowel or colon.
- Low-frequency leakage currents may be present in the ESU pencil electrode, presenting a microshock hazard.
- Check the patient for alternative return paths for the ESU current to avoid burns. Isolate the ESU circuit.
- Place the dispersive patient electrode as close as possible to the operative site.
- Avoid placing the dispersive electrode over scar tissue, bony prominences, unshaved hairy areas, metal implants, or wet areas.
- Place the dispersive electrode at right angles to a pacemaker to avoid ESU interference.
- Rigid-metal dispersive electrodes should only be used on the buttocks, where the weight of the body will maintain good contact.
- Adhesive disposable electrodes should not be used where the weight of the body would put uneven pressure on the electrode, causing hot spots and possible burns.
- Be alert to electromagnetic radio frequency interference from the ESU upon monitoring equipment in the vicinity.

10.2 SINUSOIDAL OSCILLATORS

The ESU requires the use of sinusoidal radio frequency signals. The general form of a sinusoidal oscillator consists of the isolated blocks shown in Figure 10.10, where K is an amplifier of gain K, and β is a feedback element.

The gain of this circuit, $A_V = V_{OUT}/V_1$, is given by the following analysis:

$$V_{OUT} = KV_X = K(V_1 + \beta V_{OUT})$$

Solving for A_V gives

$$A_V = \frac{V_{OUT}}{V_1} = \frac{K}{1 - K\beta} \tag{10.3}$$

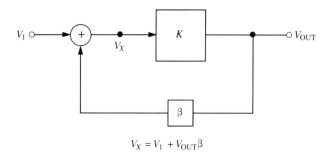

$$V_X = V_1 + V_{OUT}\beta$$

FIGURE 10.10
The basic sinusoidal oscillator.

Notice in Equation (10.3) that when

$$K\beta = 1 \tag{10.4}$$

the gain A_V becomes infinite. This means that the smallest bit of random noise produces an output voltage when the loop gain $K\beta = 1$.

Such an output is self-sustaining because this loop gain equals 1. The circuit therefore oscillates. In this sinusoidal oscillator both K and β may be functions of frequency. When they are, the frequency of oscillation is found by solving Equation (10.4) when the gain expressions for K and β are known in terms of frequency and the circuit element values. When this condition holds for only one frequency, the circuit becomes a pure sinusoidal oscillator.

The example oscillator circuit in Figure 10.11 utilizes operational amplifiers and is analyzed as follows. The rule for ideal diff amps is $V_1 = V_2$. Also, by voltage division, we have for the K side

$$\beta = \frac{V_2}{V_{OUT}} \qquad K = \frac{V_{OUT}}{V_2}$$

and then

$$V_2 = \frac{R_2}{R_1 + R_2} V_{OUT} \tag{10.5}$$

Again, by voltage division for β we have

$$\beta = \frac{V_1}{V_{OUT}}$$

Then

$$V_1 = \cfrac{\cfrac{\dfrac{R}{j\omega C} V_{\text{OUT}}}{R + \dfrac{1}{j\omega C}}}{R + \dfrac{1}{j\omega C} + \cfrac{\dfrac{R}{j\omega C}}{R + \dfrac{1}{j\omega C}}}$$

Simplifying this gives

$$V_1 = \cfrac{\dfrac{R}{j\omega C} V_{\text{OUT}}}{\left(R + \dfrac{1}{j\omega C}\right)^2 + \dfrac{R}{j\omega C}}$$

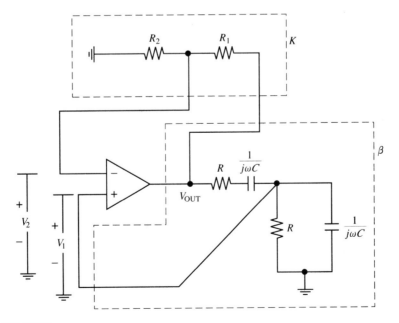

FIGURE 10.11
A sinusoidal oscillator circuit.

Expanding the square yields

$$V_1 = \frac{\dfrac{R}{j\omega C} V_{\text{OUT}}}{R^2 - \left(\dfrac{1}{\omega C}\right)^2 + \dfrac{3R}{j\omega C}} \qquad (10.6)$$

Because K, from Equation (10.5), is a real number, the oscillator condition $K\beta = 1$ implies that β must be real as well. To make that happen in Equation (10.6), let

$$\omega C = \frac{1}{R} \qquad (10.7)$$

Substituting this into Equation (10.6) gives

$$\frac{V_1}{V_{\text{OUT}}} = \frac{1}{3}$$

Because $V_2 = V_1$ at the input to the diff amp, Equation (10.5) then gives

$$\frac{R_2}{R_1 + R_2} = \frac{1}{3} \qquad (10.8)$$

The conclusion we draw from this analysis is that the oscillator radian frequency $\omega = 2\pi f$ is computed from Equation (10.7), and the choice of R_1 and R_2 is made to satisfy Equation (10.8) in the ideal case. Conversely, Equations (10.7) and (10.8) may be taken as the design equations for the sinusoidal oscillator in Figure 10.11 from which we can compute the component values that produce oscillations at a desired frequency.

EXAMPLE 10.3 Design an oscillator using the circuit in Figure 10.11 to have a resonant frequency of 500 kHz.

SOLUTION The resistors R and C are chosen to satisfy Equation (10.7). Arbitrarily let $R = 10 \text{ k}\Omega$. Then

$$C = \frac{1}{2\pi f R} = \frac{1}{2\pi (5)(10^5)(10^4)}$$

or

$$C = 31.8 \text{ pF}$$

The condition in Equation (10.8) is also satisfied if $R_1 = 20$ kΩ and $R_2 = 10$ kΩ.

10.3 AN ESU POWER AMPLIFIER

In order to supply energy of about 400 W to an electrosurgical electrode, a reasonably efficient power amplifier is required. Any waste heat may be dissipated in an aluminum or copper heat sink, sometimes force-cooled with a fan. The problem of dissipating the waste heat in ESU amplifiers is sufficiently difficult that the duration of continuous cutting allowed is limited by the manufacturer's specifications. If the heat is not dissipated from the power transistor chip, junction temperatures in excess of 250 °C occur and the device may fail.

An example power amplifier is given in Figure 10.12. The first stage driver amplifier supplies the base of the power transistor with a peak-to-peak voltage V_{BPP}. An ideal representation of the transistor voltage-current characteristic is given in Figure 10.13.

The operation of the amplifier is described as follows. When V_B is zero, the transistor is turned off, and V_{CE} nearly equals V_{BB}. As V_B increases above the forward base to emitter voltage (0.7 V in silicon), the transistor begins to conduct. When V_B reaches its peak voltage, V_{BPP}, V_{CE} will

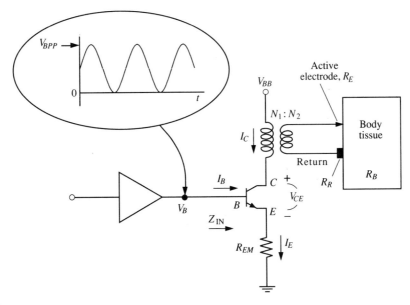

FIGURE 10.12
An ESU power amplifier.

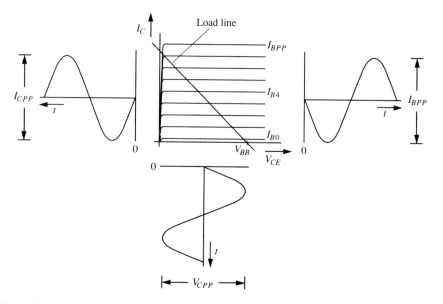

FIGURE 10.13
Power transistor voltage-current characteristics.

be nearly zero, and the current I_C will equal its peak value I_{CPP}. I_{CPP} induces the peak-to-peak voltage into the active electrode through the $N_1 : N_2$ turns ratio of the transformer. A detailed ideal analysis follows to determine the requirements on the components and to compute the amplifier power gain.

When the transistor is fully on, $I_C = I_{CPP}$, and $V_{CE} = 0$. Then, from Figure 10.12,

$$V_{BB} = I_{CPP} (R_{EQ} + R_{EM})$$

where V_{BB} is the bias voltage, R_{EM} is the emitter bias resistance, and

$$R_{EQ} = \left(\frac{N_1}{N_2} \right)^2 R_L \qquad (10.9)$$

where $R_L = R_E + R_B + R_R$ is the total load resistance on the ESU, called the body-electrode resistance. In the transistor with current gain β,

$$I_{CPP} = \beta I_{BPP}$$

Thus,

$$R_{EQ} + R_{EM} = \frac{V_{BB}}{\beta I_{BPP}} \qquad (10.10)$$

This gives a means of choosing proper resistor values for obtaining a full-swing output for a given available current from the previous stage, I_{BPP}. Usually, however, the voltage output maximum capability of the previous stage V_{BP} is given. It is then necessary to calculate the input impedance Z_{IN} from Figure 10.12. Kirchhoff's voltage law around the base loop gives

$$V_B = V_{BE} + \beta I_B R_{EM}$$

When $V_B = V_{BPP}$ and $V_{BPP} \gg V_{BE}$ ($V_{BE} = 0.7$ V in silicon), we can usually approximate

$$V_{BPP} \approx I_{BPP} \beta R_{EM}$$

and

$$R_{EM} \approx \frac{V_{BPP}}{\beta I_{BPP}} \tag{10.11}$$

Thus, using this equation, one can find the R_{EM} for a given β on the transistor, required to give a full-swing output when V_B is at its peak value, V_{BPP}. Equations (10.9), (10.10), and (10.11) are design equations for the amplifier in Figure 10.12.

EXAMPLE 10.4   In the power amplifier of Figure 10.12, find the values of R_{EM} and the turns ratio $N_1:N_2$ required to have the amplifier go through a full-swing output for maximum sinusoidal voltage V_{BPP}. Let $V_{BPP} = 20$ V and the transistor current gain $\beta = 20$. The ideal op amp has the output impedance of zero and a peak saturation current of 0.5 A. The battery voltage is 200 V, and the body-electrode impedance, R_L, is 500 Ω.

SOLUTION   Since $I_{BPP} = 0.5$ A, the required values of R_{EM} and the input impedance of the transformer R_{EQ} are given by Equation (10.10) as

$$R_{EM} + R_{EQ} = 200/[0.5(20)] = 20 \ \Omega$$

Then to find R_{EM} we have, from Equation (10.11),

$$R_{EM} = \frac{20}{20(0.5)} = 2 \ \Omega$$

Then the previous equation yields

$$R_{EQ} = 20 - 2 = 18 \ \Omega$$

Equation (10.9) gives the turns ratio as

$$\frac{N_1}{N_2} = \sqrt{\frac{18}{500}} = 0.1897$$

EXAMPLE 10.5   An ESU amplifier in Figure 10.12 delivers 30 W into a 5000-Ω body-electrode resistance, R_L. The turns ratio in the transformer $(N_1:N_2) = 0.0666$. The battery voltage $V_{BB} = 200$ V, the transistor current gain $\beta = 70$, and $R_{EM} = 2\ \Omega$. Compute the values of V_{BPP} and I_{BPP} required from the first stage.

SOLUTION   From Equation (10.9),

$$R_{EQ} = (0.06667)^2 5000 = 22\ \Omega$$

The power into the transformer is given by

$$\frac{I_{CPP}^2}{8}\, R_{EQ} = 30$$

Therefore

$$I_{CPP} = 3.3\ A$$

Then for a $\beta = 70$, we get

$$I_{BPP} = \frac{3.3}{70} = 47\ mA$$

The corresponding value of V_{BPP} is then computed from Equation (10.11) as

$$V_{BPP} = (70)(47 \times 10^{-3})(2) = 6.6\ V$$

10.4 TROUBLESHOOTING AN ESU

Troubleshooting an ESU often begins with a symptom written on a work request, which can sometimes be a rather vague instruction such as "ESU is broken. Please fix it." A logical first step to better define the symptom would be to interview the operator, if possible. An alternative is to test the ESU with an *electrosurgical analyzer*. This test equipment can be used to measure the output power in all modes of ESU operation. It can also be used to measure the RF leakage to ground, as well as low-frequency currents. It is especially important for the troubleshooter to detect 60-$\sim$ leakage currents, because they can cause microshock.

The service manual accompanying the ESU often provides helpful troubleshooting guides. Module-level troubleshooting can be done by following block schematics, or diagrams, provided in the manual.

For example, a block diagram of the Valleylab Model SSE4 ESU, shown in Figure 10.14, can be used as a troubleshooting aid. There are two

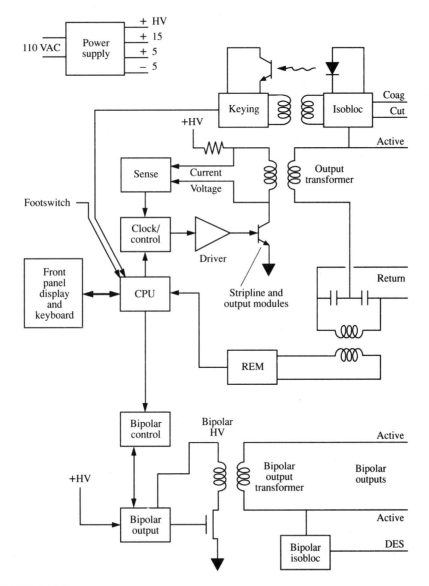

FIGURE 10.14
A model SSE4 block diagram. (Courtesy of Valleylab, Inc.)

outputs to the ESU electrodes in the figure: The bipolar outputs are on the lower right side of the schematic; the monopolar active output and the patient return are located just above the center. The keying switches on the electrodes feed into the upper right corner of the schematic. Optical coupling isolates the electrodes, as do transformers on both the monopolar and bipolar electrodes. The patient is completely isolated from unwanted signals generated within the unit. Keying of all ESU functions is controlled by the central processing unit (CPU) of the microprocessor. (See Chapter 13 on microprocessors.)

The service manual for the SSE4 gives a troubleshooting guide in the form of common symptoms, and suggested remedies, stated in terms of the

---

Troubleshooting Tip

Turn the power off before removing or inserting any circuit board. Otherwise, transients induced may damage the board.

---

block schematic modules. These modules are keyed to circuit boards that the manufacturer recommends should be stocked in the hospital as replacement parts. An outline of some symptoms and possible remedies follows:

Symptom: There is no RF output from the monopolar ESU electrode.
Possible causes: High-voltage power supply. Fuse blown. Surgical pencil open-circuited.

Symptom: There is RF output in all modes except one.
Possible causes: If the bipolar mode is at fault, the bipolar control module should be checked. If a monopolar mode has failed, the clock/control module should be checked.

Symptom: The power output in the monopolar modes is more than 30% below normal.
Possible cause: Some components in the power amplifier stripline and output modules may have failed.

Symptom: The display is dead.
Possible cause: The low-voltage power supplies may be faulty.

More detailed troubleshooting guides are provided in the service manual, keyed to the unit module schematics. There a symptom is described and a relevant troubleshooting tree is given. The troubleshooting tree lists steps that should be taken in sequence until the fault is located and corrected.

10.5 LASER SURGICAL DEVICES

Laser light differs from ordinary light in that it is *coherent*, which means that all of its light waves are in phase. Laser light is also *monochromatic*, which means that all of the light waves are of the same frequency. The effect of these two properties is that the light can be very sharply focused, much more sharply than sunlight can be focused with a magnifying glass to burn paper. In fact, laser light can be focused to the size of a living cell. In laser surgery, all of the energy of the beam can be focused on the cell, causing it to vaporize, and thereby cutting the tissue. This explains the first major advantage of the laser for surgery—namely, it is more precise than either the knife (surgical scalpel) or the ESU electrode. Furthermore, the laser beam can be directed down narrow passages, such as are encountered in eye and brain surgery, too small for ESU electrodes or surgical scalpels. These advantages are balanced by the fact that laser surgical units are more expensive, larger, and sometimes awkward to manipulate.

The CO_2 Laser

The laser light is generated in the gas laser tube depicted in Figure 10.15. The tube contains a mixture of carbon dioxide, nitrogen, and helium gases at a low pressure maintained by the vacuum pump. In the flow-type laser shown, the gas is continuously changed because the laser process destroys CO_2 molecules that must be replaced and it is supplied by the storage bottle. A d.c. voltage is applied to the gas. As with most gases, if the voltage is high enough, the gas will break down, or ionize, and cause a current stream of ions. The stream of ions causes laser action by colliding with the atoms of the gas, causing them to rise to an excited state. An atom in an *excited state* has some electrons that have moved from lower energy orbits to higher energy orbits, which are unstable. When the atom returns to its stable state, it emits a photon of laser light, at an energy level and frequency specific to the gas. This photon eventually collides with another excited atom and stimulates it to emit a photon of light in phase with it, thus adding to it. The laser light beams traveling along the axis of the tube are reflected by the mirrors at either end, reinforcing the light along the axis and causing it to build in intensity. One of the mirrors in the tube is partially transmitting, thereby allowing the beam to exit the tube and travel along the optical guidance system. Such a system, called the *beam manipulator*, may consist of hollow tubes articulated by elbows containing lenses and mirrors that direct the laser light around the corners down the center of the tube. The output of the tube is focused by an output lens system.

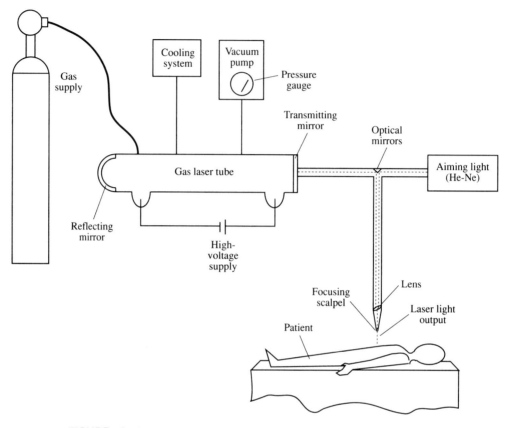

FIGURE 10.15
A CO_2 laser block diagram.

The focal point of the output beam must be adjusted to fall on the tissue to be cut. The size of the focal point, called the *spot diameter*, determines the energy density applied to the tissue for a given beam power. The surgeon adjusts the spot diameter with the output lens system. To *cut*, the beam is adjusted for a small spot diameter; to *coagulate*, a larger spot diameter is chosen.

The size of the spot must be adjusted before the laser is turned on, in the case of the CO_2 laser, because the light is infrared and thus invisible to the eye. In any case an unfocused beam would cause tissue damage if it were run at high power. Therefore, low-power focusing light, called *aiming light*, is run through the output lens system to calibrate the focal spot before the high-energy laser light is applied. A low-power helium-neon (He-Ne) laser is often used as an aiming light because it produces visible, red light.

The CO_2 laser emits light at power levels ranging from 20 to 100 W.

The Argon Laser Surgical Unit

Like CO_2, argon is a gas. The argon laser therefore works on basically the same principle as the CO_2 laser. The most distinctive difference is in the wavelength of the laser light emitted. CO_2 emits light primarily at a wavelength of 10.6 μm, in the invisible, infrared range, whereas argon emits laser light at 0.488 μm, blue light, and 0.515 μm, green light.

The wavelength of laser light gives rise to *selective absorption* of the light energy by tissue. CO_2 laser light is absorbed by water, which makes up the bulk of tissue and cells, and so it is effective at cutting tissue. Argon, however, passes through water without being absorbed, but is absorbed by dark tissue such as hemoglobin or tissue containing melanin. Thus argon laser light is not so effective in cutting, and is used instead to coagulate tissue. It is used, for example, in retinal reattachment, because the light beam passes through the vitreous humor and is selectively absorbed by the detached retina, which is thereby rebonded.

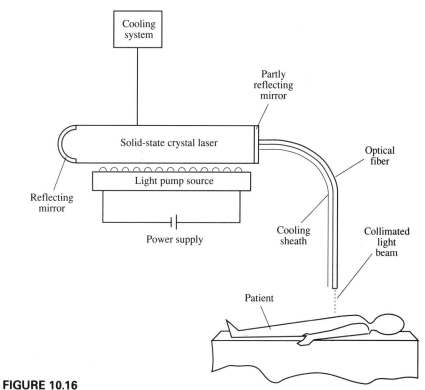

FIGURE 10.16
An Nd:YAG laser block diagram.

The argon laser operates at power levels from 0.01 to 20 W, which is adequate for the coagulation and bonding task.

The Nd:YAG Laser

A common crystal laser for medical applications uses an artificial crystal neodymium-doped yttrium aluminum garnet (Nd:YAG). Nd:YAG produces laser light at a wavelength of 1.06 μm. To generate laser light, the crystal is placed between two reflecting mirrors, as in Figure 10.16 (page 335). An electrical source produces noncoherent light, containing 1.06-μm rays, which is directed toward the Nd:YAG. This light stimulates laser action, as described for the CO_2 laser, and is referred to as a *light pump*. The Nd:YAG laser light can be coupled to the patient through optical fibers somewhat more efficiently than the longer-wavelength CO_2 laser. Optical fiber cooling is achieved by passing air along the fiber's length. The Nd:YAG laser lies between the CO_2 laser and argon laser in its effectiveness at cutting tissue. Because of its visible wavelength, it is nearly as effective as the CO_2 laser in cutting heavily pigmented tissues. Like the CO_2

Box 2

LASER SAFETY TIPS

- Position the laser beam with a low-power aiming light before applying full power.
- Calibrate the aiming lights to ensure accuracy.
- Keep reflective surfaces, which may misdirect the laser beam, away from the surgical field.
- Cover plastic or rubber tubing with adhesive metal foil to avoid burning by the laser beam.
- Do not use a laser with flammable anesthetics or in an oxygen concentration above 40%.
- Use suction to remove laser smoke from the surgical field.
- Do not allow the laser beam to contact OR personnel.
- Wear eyeglasses with filters to prevent a reflected laser beam from entering the eyes.
- Eliminate flammable drapes, and cover the windows with opaque material.
- Place wet sponges around the surgical field to prevent tissue damage if the beam is accidentally misdirected.

laser, the Nd:YAG laser can deliver up to 100 W of light energy. This power is produced at about 15% efficiency. Therefore a cooling system is required to dissipate the waste heat.

Since the laser beam can cause damage at considerable distances from the surgical field, it is necessary to observe safety precautions when using it. Some safety tips are listed in Box 2.

REFERENCES

Absten, G. T., and Joffee, S. N. *Lasers in Medicine.* 2nd ed. London: Chapman and Hall, 1989.

Auth, D. C. "Laser Scalpel." In *Encyclopedia of Medical Devices and Instrumentation*, Vol. 3, edited by J. G. Webster. New York: John Wiley & Sons, 1988.

Bard Staff. *System 5000 Power Plus Technical Manual.* Englewood, CO: Bard Electro-Medical Systems, Inc.

Carr, J. J., and Brown, J. M. "Electrosurgery Generators." Chapter 18 in *Introduction to Biomedical Equipment Technology.* New York: John Wiley & Sons, 1981.

Floyd, T. L. *Electronic Devices.* Columbus, OH: Merrill Publishing, 1984.

Gerhard, G. C. "Electrosurgical Unit." In *Encyclopedia of Medical Devices and Instrumentation*, Vol. 2, edited by J. G. Webster. New York: John Wiley & Sons, 1988.

Jacobson, B., and Webster, J. G. *Medicine and Clinical Engineering.* Englewood Cliffs, NJ: Prentice-Hall, 1977.

Pearce, J. A. *Electrosurgery.* New York: John Wiley & Sons, 1986.

Surgilase Staff. *Laser Surgery Basic Training Manual.* Providence, RI: Surgilase, Inc., 1984.

Valleylab Staff. *SSE4 Service Manual*, Part #A945100042A. Boulder, CO: Valleylab Inc., 1983.

EXERCISES

1. An ESU has an internal impedance of 350 Ω. It drives a pencil electrode of variable impedance. The open-circuit voltage in the pure-cut mode is 2000 V peak-to-peak. Make a plot of the power delivered to the electrode versus its impedance. Assume the patient-plate electrode impedance is negligible.

2. A double-section pad patient-return electrode measures 5 Ω resistance in each section when properly applied. During an operation one of the pad sections loses contact over 10% of its surface. In Figure 10.17, compute the change in output voltage V_{OUT} resulting from this loss of contact.

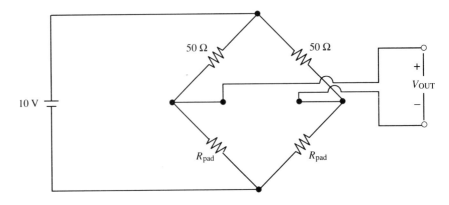

FIGURE 10.17

3. A certain ESU produces the following open-circuit voltages in the pencil electrode:

Mode	Open-circuit voltage, peak-to-peak	Duty cycle (%)
Cut	2500	100
Blend 1	3000	75
Blend 2	3000	50
Blend 3	2500	25

In each case compute the average power delivered to the load of 500 Ω. The internal impedance of the ESU is also 500 Ω.

4. The cable of an ESU pencil electrode becomes wrapped around a surgeon's hand such that 5 cm^2 of cable is separated from the hand by $\frac{1}{16}$ in. of rubber insulation. The relative dielectric constant is 2.5 in the insulation. The surgeon's finger also inadvertently comes in contact with the patient-return plate, producing a 500-Ω resistance at the point of contact. Estimate the power absorbed at the finger contact when the ESU open-circuit voltage is 3000 V peak-to-peak, the internal resistance of the ESU is 500 Ω, and the frequency is 500 kHz. Do you think this would give the surgeon a burn?

5. The sinusoidal oscillator in Figure 10.11 has $R_1 = 2$ MΩ and $C = 0.02$ μF.

   (a) Compute the value of R and R_2 such that the circuit oscillates at 700 kHz.
   (b) Compute the resonant frequency if $R = 200$ Ω and $C = 0.002$ μF.

6. The ideal diff amp in Figure 10.12 drives a power transistor having a current gain $\beta = 40$. This amplifier puts out a voltage $V_{BPP} = 10$ V and when properly loaded delivers 1 mA, I_{BPP}.

   (a) Find an R_{EM} that gives a full-swing output such that $V_{CE} \approx V_{BB}$ in the power amplifier of Figure 10.12.

(b) Calculate the value of R_{EQ} when the battery voltage $V_{BB} = 100$ V.
(c) Calculate the power efficiency of this amplifier.

7. An ESU produces 9000 V peak-to-peak at the tip of a pencil electrode. What is the maximum length of the arc that it will produce?

8. An ESU delivers 250 W of power in the pure-cut mode. What will be the delivered power in the blend mode of Exercise 3 if the voltage level is the same but the duty cycle is 25%?

9. An ESU delivers 350 W of power at an efficiency of 45%. How much power must be dissipated in a heat sink when the unit is in operation?

10. The electrosurgical unit amplifier in Figure 10.18 has $V_{BPP} = 10$ V and $I_{BPP} = 0.5$ mA, given in peak-to-peak values. $V_{BB} = 200$ V and $\beta = 70$. The body-electrode resistance is 500 Ω.
    (a) Find I_C, the collector current.
    (b) Compute the power loss in the resistor R_{EM}.
    (c) If the peak-to-peak value of $V_{CE} = V_{BB}$, compute the power loss in the transistor.
    (d) The turns ratio of the ideal transformer is 3.29:1. Compute the power delivered to the body tissue.
    (e) Find the net efficiency defined by

$$\eta = P_{\text{OUT}}/(P_{\text{OUT}} + P_{\text{LOSS}})$$

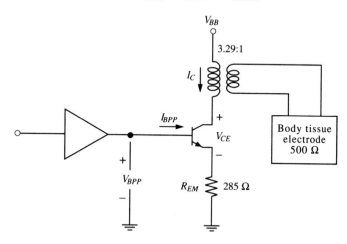

FIGURE 10.18

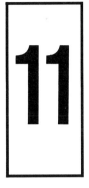

Catheters and Blood Pressure Monitoring

11.1 CIRCULATION SYSTEM MEASUREMENTS

Blood pressure is one of the most critical of the vital signs, because it indicates whether the blood is circulating to the body tissues. Low blood pressure may indicate severe bleeding or heart failure. The techniques of blood pressure measurement range from palpation of the pulse on the radial artery of the wrist to direct measurements by means of catheters inserted into veins, arteries, and vital organs such as the heart or lung.

The primary source of the blood pressure is the heart, although some secondary pumping action occurs as a result of motion of skeletal muscles such as those in the leg.

Pumping Action of the Heart

The electrical depolarization of the heart, as described in Section 2.3, causes first the atrium muscle and then the ventricle to contract. These two cavities of the heart are connected by one-way, self-acting valves, as illustrated in Figure 11.1.

The pumping cycle may be traced in this figure as follows. After the *P*-wave on the ECG in Figure 11.2(a), the atrium contracts and the ventricle remains at rest. This forces blood through the tricuspid valve from the right atrium (RA) into the right ventricle (RV) and through the mitral valve from the left atrium (LA) into the left ventricle (LV). During this action, the pulmonary and aortic valves are kept closed by the high pressure in the

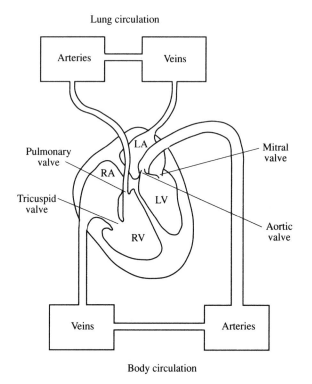

FIGURE 11.1
The circulation system.

pulmonary artery and the aorta. The ventricles therefore fill with venous blood. Following the *QRS* complex of the ECG, the ventricles contract while the atria are at rest. This contraction is strong enough to force blood through the pulmonary valve to the pulmonary artery and into the lungs. At the same time, the blood is forced through the aortic valve into the systemic arteries, as indicated in Figure 11.2. The sound associated with the opening of the aortic valve is the first heart sound. This action causes the blood pressure to rise to its peak value in the arteries, called *systole* in Figure 11.2. During the *T*-wave of the ECG, the ventricles begin to relax, and the pressure in them falls below the aortic pressure level. The higher pressure in the aorta forces the aortic valve closed. This closure is so rapid that it causes a sound detectable with a stethoscope, called the second heart sound. It also causes a characteristic notch in the pressure pulse called the *dicrotic notch*. The ventricles then rest, and the aortic pressure falls to its minimum value, called *diastole*. The cardiac cycle then repeats at a normal heart rate of approximately 75 beats per minute. Figure 11.3 illustrates a noninvasive pressure monitor.

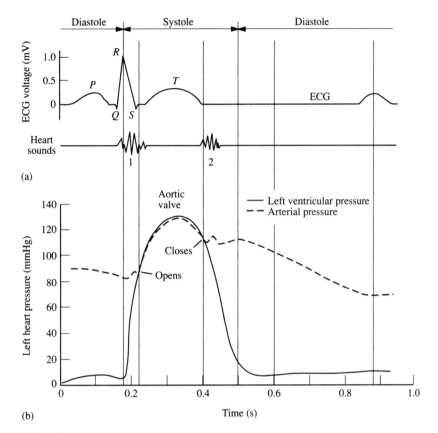

FIGURE 11.2
Correlation between ECG, heart sounds, and blood pressure.

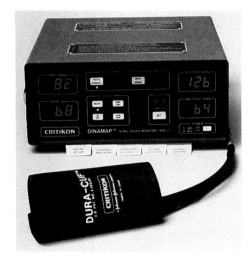

FIGURE 11.3
An automated blood pressure transducer
and monitor. (Courtesy of Critikon, Inc.)

Arterial Pressure Measurement

Arterial pressure is usually measured noninvasively, since this technique is accurate, painless, and convenient to use. The measurement is made with a sphygmomanometer, illustrated in use in Figure 11.4. A pressure cuff is wrapped around the upper arm. The cuff pressure is increased until the pressure on the brachial artery exceeds the systolic arterial pressure, SYST. This stops blood flow in the artery. A stethoscope is then placed on the skin above the brachial artery. No sounds are heard. As the cuff pressure is released, the pressure on the artery falls below SYST, allowing blood to flow through a constriction in the artery. The turbulence of the blood flow makes a pulsing noise known as *Korotkoff's sounds*. The pressure at which these sounds begin is noted as SYST. The cuff pressure is further released, and Korotkoff's sounds continue until the brachial artery opens completely and the turbulence stops. The silence returns when the cuff is at the diastolic pressure, DIAS. Blood pressure is measured automatically in the pressure monitor shown in Figure 11.5.

Physicians need to know the arterial systolic (SYST) and diastolic (DIAS) pressure in order to assess the health of the patient. It is also important to know the mean arterial pressure (MEAN). The average pressure is the arithmetic mean, AVE, given by

$$AVE = \frac{SYST + DIAS}{2}$$

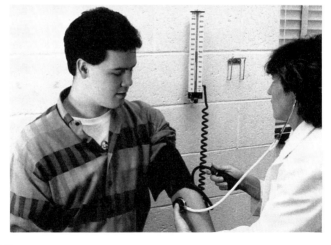

FIGURE 11.4
A sphygmomanometer being used to measure blood pressure.

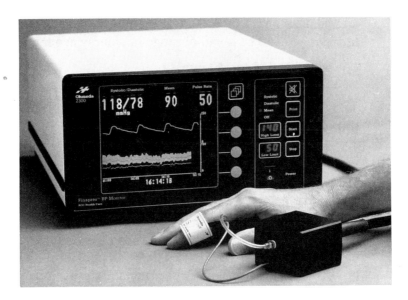

FIGURE 11.5
A blood pressure monitor using a finger-mounted transducer. (Permission granted by Ohmeda, a division of the BOC Group, Inc.)

This average pressure has only limited use for diagnostic purposes, because it does not reflect the duration of the pulse systole. The functional mean, MEAN, is computed by dividing the area under the pressure, p, curve by its duration. A mathematical expression for this calculation is

$$\text{MEAN} = \frac{1}{T} \int_0^T p \, dt \tag{11.1}$$

where t is the time and T is the period of the pressure wave. In a normal individual the atrial pressure integrated by Equation (11.1) yields

$$\text{MEAN} = \frac{1}{3} (\text{SYST} - \text{DIAS}) + \text{DIAS} \tag{11.2}$$

This equation implies that the mean pressure is computed from the systolic and diastolic pressures when the pressure pulse is normal. To compute the MEAN when the pulse is abnormal, it is necessary to know p as a function of time. MEAN is then computed with signal processing circuitry or a microprocessor circuit, using Equation (11.1). To obtain the pressure as a function of time directly, invasive measurement methods are used. A typical arterial pressure is SYST = 120 mmHg and DIAS = 80 mmHg, as illustrated in Figure 11.2. The nominal range in values encountered is as follows:

SYST   115 to 140 mmHg
DIAS   60 to 90 mmHg
MEAN 80 to 105 mmHg

Invasive Blood Pressure Measurement

In order to diagnose the health of the heart, it may be necessary to measure the blood pressure directly. This may be done by inserting a sterile, saline-filled catheter into the blood stream. The pressure at the tip of the catheter is then transmitted through the catheter fluid to an external pressure transducer. The physician may choose to enter the catheter into the carotid, femoral, or brachial arteries, as illustrated in Figure 11.6. Alternatively, he or she may choose to enter the femoral, brachial, subclavian, or internal jugular veins. By either method the physician then has access to the central venous pressure (*CVP*), the pressure in the veins leading to the heart. The catheter may be inserted into the right atrium of the heart to measure the right atrial pressure (*RAP*). Further insertion of the catheter through the tricuspid valve will put the tip of the catheter into the right ventricle (RV). In order to understand how the pressure is transmitted from the tip of the catheter to the pressure transducer, it is necessary to review hydrodynamics. The hemodynamics of blood in vessels and the hydrodynamics of fluids in catheters follow the same rules.

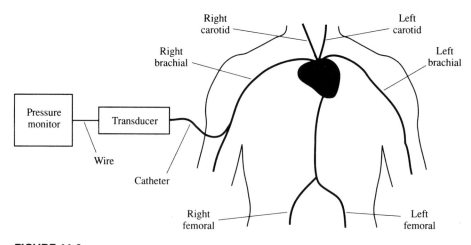

FIGURE 11.6
A pressure monitor connected to a catheter inserted into a blood vessel.

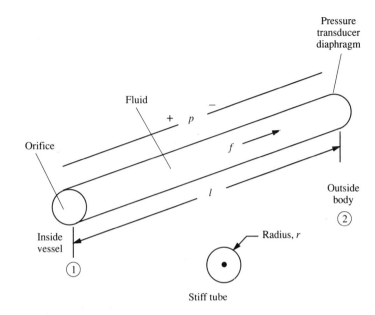

FIGURE 11.7
A catheter modeled as a straight, stiff tube.

Fluid Resistance

The flow of fluid in a catheter, f, in Figure 11.7 is proportional to the pressure difference p that causes it:

$$p = R_C f \qquad (11.3)$$

where R_C is the resistance of the tube. The MKS units of pressure are newtons per square meter, and f has units of mass per unit time, kilograms per second. The MKS units of the resistance are then newton-kilograms per meter to the fifth power (Ns/m^5). In Equation (11.3)

$$p = p_1 - p_2$$

where p_1 and p_2 are the gauge pressures at two specific points. *Gauge pressure* is the pressure relative to atmospheric pressure.

Equation (11.3) is analogous to Ohm's law. The pressure difference p corresponds to voltage, and the flow f corresponds to current. It is important to notice that when f is zero in Equation (11.3), p is also zero. This means that when $f = 0$, $p_1 = p_2$. In other words, when the flow in a closed tube is zero, the pressure at the input equals the pressure at the output. The resistance the tube presents to a flowing fluid is primarily due to the friction between the fluid and the inside surface of the tube. The resistance is proportional to the length of the tube, *l*, and the viscosity, η, of the fluid. The relative amount of fluid that comes in contact with the surface area of the tube is inversely proportional to the square of the radius of the tube. Furthermore, the fluid volume per unit length is inversely proportional to the square of the radius. Therefore, the resistance goes as the inverse of the fourth power of the radius. That is,

$$R_C = \frac{8\eta l}{\pi r^4} \tag{11.4}$$

Instrumentation for Direct Pressure Measurement

Direct measurement of pressure in a blood vessel is made with a catheter having an orifice at the end placed in the vessel and a pressure transducer at the end outside the body, as shown in Figure 11.7. To transmit the pressure with fidelity, the catheter should be as short as is practical, stiff, and noncompliant (*compliance* is the tendency of the catheter to bulge under pressure). It should also have as large a diameter as possible that will allow it to be threaded through the vein. These parameters must, however, be traded off. A noncompliant catheter is difficult to make turn corners in the blood vessels, and a large-diameter catheter is more likely to disturb blood flow and create embolisms. To prevent clotting, the catheter may be continuously infused with an anticoagulant solution. Medication is infused at a slow rate with an intraflow flush valve, illustrated in Figure 11.8. The in-

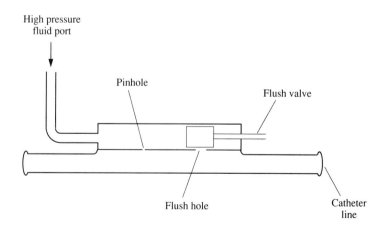

FIGURE 11.8
Intraflow flush valve assembly.

fusing fluid is put under relatively high pressure by squeezing its container with an elastic bag filled with air. The infusing fluid is then driven through the pinhole at a slow rate. When it is time to flush the catheter and cause the fluid to flow rapidly, the flush valve on the intraflow device is pulled to expose the large hole. The high-pressure fluid then flows into the catheter. This action may be used to eliminate any bubbles in the catheter. Since bubbles are compliant, they distort the pressure wave transmitted along the catheter.

Pressure Transducer Calibration

The calibration procedure is illustrated for the system in Figure 11.9. In order to eliminate a constant error due to hydrostatic pressure differences, the

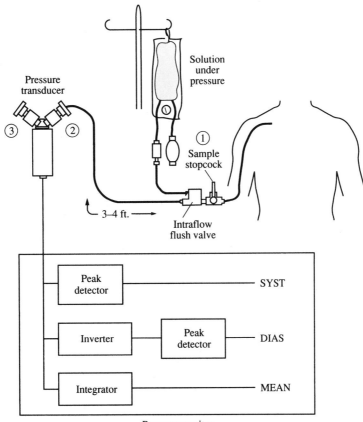

FIGURE 11.9
A block diagram of an illustrative monitoring system with associated transducer, catheter, and tubing.

pressure transducer is placed at the same height as the catheter tip. An internal and external catheter are used. To flush the external catheter free of bubbles, stopcock 1 is closed and stopcocks 2 and 3 are opened. The solution under pressure is infused into the external catheter by opening the flush valve of the intraflow device. Excess fluid and the bubbles will exit through stopcock 3.

The pressure transducer can be calibrated by connecting a mercury manometer to stopcock 2 and opening it while closing stopcock 3. The height of the mercury column (in mmHg) should equal the reading on the monitor connected to the pressure transducer.

In Figure 11.9 the electrical signal output from the pressure transducer goes to a pressure monitor. A peak detector circuit measures the peak, or systolic value, of the pressure wave. In another channel, the wave is inverted before it is passed through a peak detector. In this manner the minimum value of the pressure wave is measured. The display therefore equals the diastolic pressure DIAS. To compute the mean pressure for the pressure wave, it is necessary to integrate it according to Equation (11.1). A third channel in the monitor uses integrator circuitry to produce a voltage proportional to the mean pressure displayed as MEAN. Figure 11.10 illustrates a blood pressure monitor displaying an ECG and blood pressure (BP) pulse. An associated disposable pressure transducer is shown in Figure 11.11.

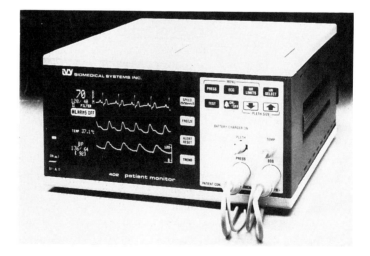

FIGURE 11.10
A patient monitor for blood pressure, ECG, and temperature. (Courtesy of Biomedical Systems, Inc.)

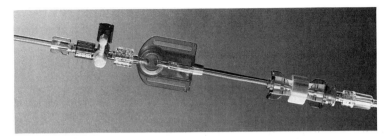

FIGURE 11.11
A disposable pressure transducer. (Courtesy of Baxter Healthcare Corporation. © 1987 Baxter Travenol Laboratories, Edwards Critical Care Division)

Pressure Measurements in the Heart

Physicians sometimes need to know the pressure in the heart and in the large veins feeding it. A catheter may be used to make such measurements. The catheter may be threaded into the brachial vein so that the diaphragm in the tip reaches the superior vena cava. There the central venous pressure (*CVP*) is measured. The position of the catheter is determined by means of an x-ray fluoroscope and by monitoring the blood pressure pulse. The tip of the catheter is usually made of a radio-opaque material that gives clear x-ray images. The catheter may be further inserted into the right atrium, as shown in Figure 11.12(a), to record the right atrial pressure *RAP*. The characteristic, *RAP*, should appear on the monitor as shown in Figure 11.13. Further insertion of the catheter will drive it through the tricuspid valve into the right ventricle, where it measures the right ventricle pressure (*RVP*). The distinctive jump in pressure will serve as an indicator that the right ventricle has been entered. There is some hazard associated with this maneuver, since the tissue could be perforated or arrhythmias could be introduced into the heart.

In seriously ill patients, the physician may need to know the pressure in the pulmonary artery (*PAP*). It was not usually possible to thread the catheter into this space without assistance, until 1970, when Swan and Ganz invented a balloon-guided catheter for this purpose. A balloon-tipped catheter is shown in Figure 11.14. A separate lumen in the catheter passes air to the balloon from a syringe. When the balloon is inflated, the blood flowing by it creates a force that drags the catheter forward. (See Figure 11.12b.) A hazard in the procedure is that if the balloon breaks, an air bubble will get into the bloodstream and may cause harmful side effects. Furthermore, if the balloon material breaks loose, it may lodge in the system and create clotting.

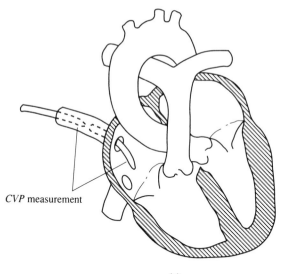

(a)

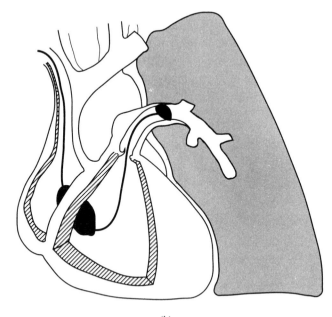

(b)

FIGURE 11.12
(a) A balloon-tipped catheter insertion into a heart atrium. (b) The inflated balloon pulls the catheter into the lung. (From *Guide to Physiological Pressure Monitoring AN739*, Hewlett-Packard Company. Reproduced by permission)

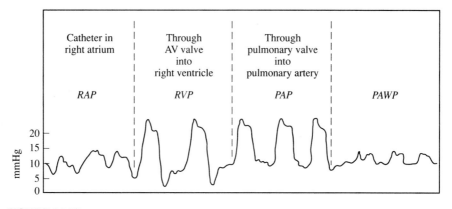

FIGURE 11.13
Pressure waveform changes as a catheter is inserted through the heart into the lung. (From *Guide to Physiological Pressure Monitoring AN739*, Hewlett-Packard Company. Reproduced by permission)

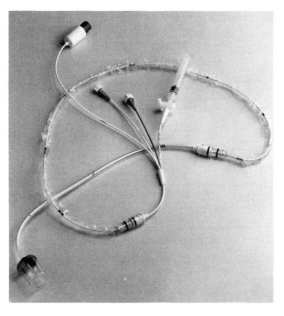

FIGURE 11.14
A catheter tipped with an inflatable balloon. (Courtesy of Arrow International, Inc.)

After the balloon passes through the pulmonary valve of the heart into the pulmonary artery, it is deflated, and the pulmonary artery pressure *PAP* is measured.

With the catheter in the pulmonary artery, it is possible to measure the pressure in the left atrium, which is done by stopping the blood flow in the artery momentarily by inflating the balloon. To do this, the balloon is wedged against the sides of the artery. The pressure measured by the diaphragm is called the pulmonary artery wedge pressure, *PAWP*. Beyond the inflated balloon, there exists a stagnant pool of blood reaching to the left atrium of the heart. Since the flow *f* is zero, Equation (11.3) applies, and the pressure at both ends of this pool of blood is equal. Therefore, *PAWP* equals the left atrium pressure, *LAP*. This pressure may be monitored only for short periods of time because stagnant blood tends to clot. Also, it is important to recognize artifacts in the wedge pressure, such as the effect of muscle contraction due to respiration, illustrated in Figure 11.15. The low rate of respiration compared with the heartbeat is easily recognizable in the figure.

A Swan-Ganz® catheter for measuring blood pressures in the heart is shown in Figure 11.16. This catheter has an inflatable balloon near the tip for guiding the catheter and for measuring *PAWP*. It also has a lumen for

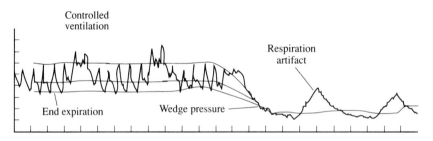

FIGURE 11.15
The respiration artifact in a wedge pressure measurement. (Courtesy of Hewlett-Packard Company)

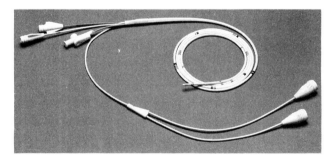

FIGURE 11.16
A five-lumen catheter showing insertion depth markings. The Swan-Ganz® flow-directed catheter. (Courtesy of Baxter Healthcare Corporation. ©1987 Baxter Travenol Laboratories, Edwards Critical Care Division)

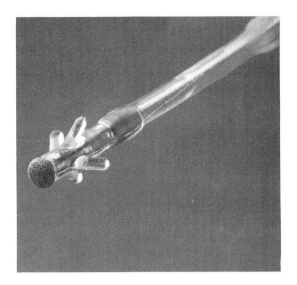

FIGURE 11.17
A catheter with tines for lodging surface electrodes into muscle. The Capsure® lead.
(Courtesy of Medtronic, Inc. Reprinted by permission. ©1987 Medtronic, Inc.)

injecting cold sterile saline into the bloodstream. A thermistor downstream in the catheter records the temperature changes in the blood after the saline is injected. It passes the resulting electrical signal back through a catheter lumen containing a wire connected to a monitor. From this data, it is possible to compute the flow rate of the blood in the blood vessel containing the catheter. A catheter for sensing organ muscle potentials carries lead wires within it. An example appears in Figure 11.17.

11.2 CATHETER MEASUREMENTS

The catheter considered here is a fluid-filled tube designed to be passed into the cavities of the body, such as the gastrointestinal tract, the urinary canal, or the nasal passage, and invasively into the veins and arteries. In a particularly important application, it is used to transmit pressure from a body cavity such as a heart ventricle or cerebral ventricle to an external pressure transducer for measurement and monitoring.

An important analysis problem occurs in the fluid-filled catheter, as shown in Figure 11.7. The catheter is a compliant tube of radius r and length l. If a pressure difference exists between the orifice and the diaphragm, the fluid inside the catheter will tend to move. In addition, the sides of the tube will tend to bulge. The greater the tube's compliance, the larger the bulge due to applied pressure.

An analysis of this catheter will show how the pressure difference across the catheter is analogous to voltage. Furthermore, the rules of voltage circuit analysis apply in sinusoidal steady-state analysis of a catheter containing fluid.

The Equivalent Circuit of a Catheter

In the section of catheter shown in Figure 11.18, the pressure, p, in newtons per square meter (N/m^2), is a function of time, and it causes a fluid flow f in units of cubic meters per second (m^3/s). The length, l, is in meters, and the tube wall consists of a stiff material that may have a very low compliance.

In the following section, we will show that there exists an exact electrical equivalent circuit to a catheter that will allow us to compute the actual pressure inside a ventricle containing a catheter from the measured data outside the body. To establish this analogy, we need a mathematical definition of compliance and inertance.

Fluid Inertance

The flow of a fluid consists of a movement of mass and therefore has inertia. The measure of inertia in a fluid catheter is called inertance, L_C. Inertance is governed by Newton's law: force is equal to mass times acceleration (or the first derivative of velocity). For pressure and flow, this law is expressed as

$$p = L_C \frac{df}{dt} \tag{11.5}$$

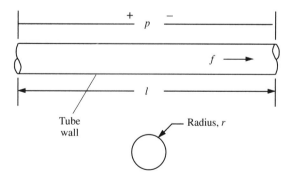

FIGURE 11.18
Catheter variables illustrated.

where L_C is a constant. The relationship between p and f is given in Figure 11.18. The units for L_C are newtons per square meter per cubic meter per second squared (Ns^2/m^5). The inertance, L_C, of the catheter fluid is analogous to the inductance in an electrical circuit, which is a measure of the inertia of current.

Compliance

A pressure difference between points 1 and 2 in Figure 11.19 will cause the compliant wall to expand, and the fluid will flow into or out of the space created, as illustrated in the figure. The compliance is defined in terms of this pressure and the volume of expansion, *vol*, as

$$C_C = \frac{vol}{p} \tag{11.6}$$

This makes intuitive sense, since larger pressure will cause a larger volume of expansion. Also, it is clear that the volume of expansion from time t_0 to t is given by

$$vol = \int_{t_0}^{t} f \, dt$$

Thus the formula for compliance is obtained by combining these two equations:

$$p = \frac{1}{C_C} \int_{t_0}^{t} f \, dt \tag{11.7}$$

The units for compliance from Equation (11.6) are therefore cubic meters per newton per square meter (m^5/N).

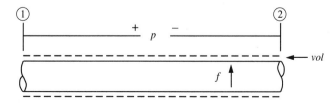

FIGURE 11.19
Volume expansion due to compliance.

The Fluid-Electrical Analogy

If Equations (11.3), (11.5), and (11.7), which define resistance R_C, inertance L_C, and compliance C_C, are arranged in Table 11.1 along with similar formulas for electrical components R, L, and C and the variables current and voltage, an exact analogy is apparent.

Because the same mathematical rules that describe the relationship of pressure to flow describe the relationship of voltage to current, all of the results of electrical circuit theory so far established apply to the fluid catheter. That is, pressure, p, plays the role of voltage, and flow, f, plays the role of current. Furthermore, Kirchhoff's laws hold, and phasor analysis is valid.

A comparison of the phasor analysis formulas is given in Table 11.2, where P is the magnitude and phase of the pressure and F is the magnitude and phase of the flow, both being complex numbers. ω is the radian frequency.

The laws of phasor analysis developed so far apply for the catheter. They give the relationships between the elements of the equivalent circuit, R_C, L_C, C_C, and the variables P and F.

TABLE 11.1
Fluid-Electrical Analogy

Electrical	Fluid
$v = Ri$	$p = R_C f$
$v = L\, di/dt$	$p = L_C\, df/dt$
$v = (1/C) \int i\, dt$	$p = (1/C_C) \int f\, dt$

TABLE 11.2
Phasor Domain Formulas

Electrical	Fluid
$V = RI$	$P = R_C F$
$V = j\omega L I$	$P = j\omega L_C F$
$V = I/(j\omega C)$	$P = F/(j\omega C_C)$

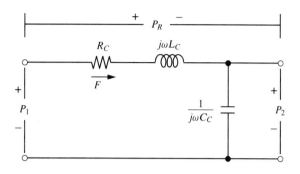

FIGURE 11.20
A catheter equivalent circuit.

The Catheter Equivalent Circuit

Because of the analogy developed earlier, an electrical equivalent circuit can be drawn for Figure 11.18 as given in Figure 11.20. In this equivalent circuit the flow F goes through the resistance R_C and the inertance L_C. Another component of flow goes in a perpendicular direction into the compliance represented by C_C. Using phasor theory, it is possible now to compute the gain function P_2/P_1 for this catheter circuit as a function of frequency. P_1 and P_2 represent the sinusoidal variations with respect to a reference at atmospheric pressure.

The Physical Formulas for Catheter Components

Equation (11.4) shows that the fluid resistance is a physical quantity, strongly dependent upon the catheter radius. Formulas are likewise available for the inertance and compliance.

To compute the inertance, we note from Equation (11.5) and Newton's law that

$$L_C = \frac{m}{A^2} \tag{11.8}$$

where m is the fluid mass, ρ is its density, and A is the cross-sectional area of the catheter. Since the radius of the catheter is r, this formula becomes

$$L_C = \frac{\rho l}{\pi r^2} \tag{11.9}$$

The compliance of a tube, diaphragm, or other object, such as a bubble in fluid, is simply measured by applying the definition in Equation

(11.6). The compliance of a water-filled catheter with a zero-compliance wall is measured to be

$$C_C = 0.53 \times 10^{-15} \, VOL \qquad \text{(in m}^5\text{/N)} \qquad \textbf{(11.10)}$$

where *VOL* is the volume in milliliters (ml).

Frequency Response of a Catheter with a Diaphragm

The catheter shown in Figure 11.7 has a diaphragm on the end that serves as the moving element in a pressure transducer outside of the body. It records the measured pressure P_{MEAS}, which differs from the actual pressure in the ventricle, P_{ACT}. To find the frequency response of the catheter, we calculate its gain, defined as

$$G_P = \frac{P_{\text{MEAS}}}{P_{\text{ACT}}} \qquad \textbf{(11.11)}$$

By design, the diaphragm usually has a higher compliance, C_D, than the wall of the catheter or its fluid, C_C. As shown in Figure 11.21, they add in parallel, as do capacitors in electrical circuits. This circuit in the phasor domain is set up so that the G_P can be computed as a function of frequency.

Applying the voltage division principle, we can compute that for $\omega = 2\pi f$ the gain function becomes

$$G_P = \frac{\dfrac{1}{j2\pi f(C_C + C_D)}}{R_C + j\left(2\pi f L_C - \dfrac{1}{2\pi f(C_D + C_C)}\right)} \qquad \textbf{(11.12)}$$

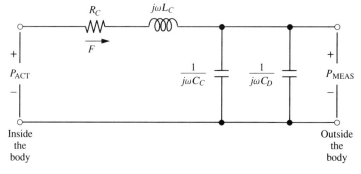

FIGURE 11.21
Equivalent circuit of a catheter with a diaphragm.

EXAMPLE 11.1 Write a computer program that computes G_P for any frequency, f, in Figure 11.21.

SOLUTION Equation (11.12) is programmed according to the flow diagram in Figure 11.22. An example program, Program A-18, appears in Appendix A.

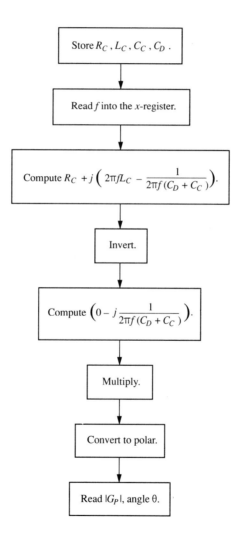

FIGURE 11.22
Flow diagram for calculating Equation (11.12).

EXAMPLE 11.2 A typical medical catheter has a length of 2 m, a radius of 0.46 mm, and walls with zero compliance. It is water-filled, and has a diaphragm in a pressure transducer of compliance 2.04×10^{-15} m^5/N. Compute the components of the equivalent circuit in Figure 11.21, $\eta = 0.001$ Ns/m^2 at 20 °C.

SOLUTION   From Equation (11.4), we have $R_C = (8)(0.001)2/\pi(0.46 \times 10^{-3})^4 = 11.374 \times 10^{10}$ Ns/m^5. From Equation (11.9), and $\rho = 1$ g/cm^3, or 1000 kg/m^3 for water,

$$L_C = (10^3)(2)/\pi\ (0.46 \times 10^{-3})^2 = 3.008 \times 10^9$$

The compliance of the water in the catheter is obtained from Equation (11.10). In this case, the volume $VOL = \pi r^2 l$.

$$VOL = \pi(0.46 \times 10^{-3})^2\ (2) = 1.33 \times 10^{-6}\ \text{m}^3$$

Converting to milliliters,

$$VOL = (1.33 \times 10^{-6}\ \text{m}^3)(10^6\ \text{ml/m}^3) = 1.33\ \text{ml}$$

The compliance for water, from Equation (11.10), is then

$$C_C = (0.53 \times 10^{-15})\ (1.33\ \text{ml})$$
$$= 0.704 \times 10^{-15}\ \text{m}^5/\text{N}$$

EXAMPLE 11.3   Draw an equivalent circuit for the catheter in Example 11.2 and compute the transfer gain, G_P, as a function of frequency including phase and angle. The diaphragm has a compliance $C_D = 2.04 \times 10^{-15}$ m^5/N.

SOLUTION   The equivalent circuit is given in Figure 11.23. Plugging the component values illustrated there into Equation (11.12) yields the result

$$|G_P| = -4.34\ \text{dB, and}\ \theta = -173.8°$$

when f is taken as 90 Hz. A plot of this equation as a function of f for $|G_P|$ appears in Figure 11.24.

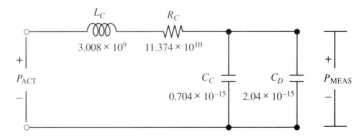

FIGURE 11.23
Equivalent circuit for Example 11.3.

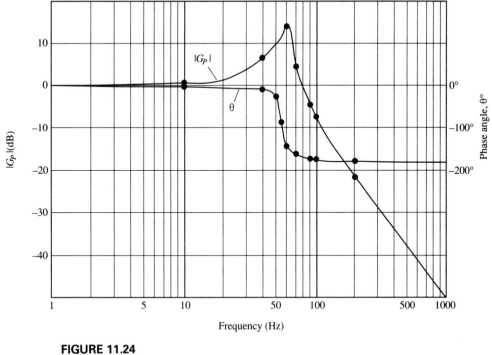

FIGURE 11.24
Frequency response computed in Example 11.3.

Tuning a Catheter

The purpose of the catheter in pressure measurement is to faithfully transmit pressure from a body ventricle to the external pressure transducer. In the previous section, the frequency response of the catheter was described and computed. Here, a means is specified to modify that frequency response. A further objective is to help you understand the effects of physical constraints of certain medical procedures, such as the requirement for a fluid leak in the catheter, or for an extended length of catheter. The frequency response of the catheter is affected by bubbles in the fluid, by a leak of fluid out of the catheter, and by a pinch in the catheter tube. The following analysis allows you to specify these effects.

Pinches, Bubbles, and Leaks in a Catheter

A pinch in a catheter is modeled by a short section of catheter, l_P, with a diminished radius, r_P, as illustrated in Figure 11.25. The pinch introduces a resistance given from Equation (11.4) as

$$R_P = \frac{8\eta l_P}{\pi r_P^4} \tag{11.13}$$

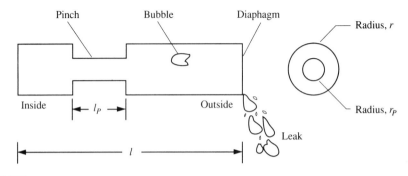

FIGURE 11.25
A catheter with a pinch, bubble, and leak.

Here we assume that the pinch has a cylindrical shape, and that $l_P \ll l$, thus introducing an approximation to the actual case. The pinch also introduces an inertance in the form given by Equation (11.9):

$$L_P = \frac{\rho l_P}{\pi r_P^2} \qquad (11.14)$$

The compliance of the pinch may usually be neglected as a small quantity. Both L_P and R_P are in series with R_C and L_C in the equivalent circuit.

A leak in a catheter is simply created by a hole. The resistance R_H is given by Table 11.2 as the ratio of pressure P_H and flow F_H through the hole,

$$R_H = \frac{P_H}{F_H} \qquad (11.15)$$

where P_H is the pressure difference inside and outside the catheter. Therefore, resistance is modeled in shunt to the diaphragm compliance.

A bubble in the catheter appears in shunt also with the diaphragm, since a bubble adds compliance to the system. This is true because of the analogy made in Table 11.2: since capacitances arranged in parallel add, so do compliances in parallel. A measurement of the compliance of a bubble shows that it changes volume 1 ml per cm of H_2O for each liter of bubble volume, VOL_B. Thus the compliance C_B for the bubble is

$$C_B = VOL_B \qquad \text{(in ml/cm } H_2O)$$

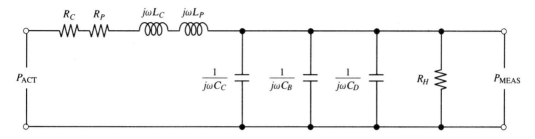

FIGURE 11.26
An equivalent circuit for a catheter accounting for a pinch, a bubble, and a leak.

where VOL_B is the bubble volume in liters. To convert this equation to MKS units, we first note that 1 cm H_2O = 0.000967814 atm, 1 kg/m^2 = 9.67841 × 10^{-5} atm, and 1 ml = 10^{-6} m^3. Therefore

$$C_B = VOL_B(1.02)10^{-8} \qquad \text{(in m}^5\text{/N)} \qquad \textbf{(11.16)}$$

The equivalent circuit in Figure 11.23 can now be modified to account for R_P, L_P, R_H, and C_B, as given in Figure 11.26.

The gain function for Figure 11.26 results from voltage division directly as

$$\frac{P_{\text{MEAS}}}{P_{\text{ACT}}} = \frac{\dfrac{-jR_H}{2\pi f C_{EQ}}}{R_H - \dfrac{j}{2\pi f C_{EQ}}}{R_{EQ} + j2\pi f L_{EQ} - \dfrac{\dfrac{jR_H}{2\pi f C_{EQ}}}{R_H - \dfrac{j}{2\pi f C_{EQ}}}} \qquad \textbf{(11.17)}$$

where $R_{EQ} = R_C + R_P$, and $C_{EQ} = C_B + C_D + C_C$.

In order to calculate this equation as a function of frequency f, Program A-19 is given in Appendix A.

EXAMPLE 11.4 Redo Example 11.3 using Program A-19 for Equation (11.17).

SOLUTION To eliminate the effect of R_H in Program A-19, take a value $R_H = 10^{30}$, essentially a closed hole. Then $L_{EQ} = 3.008 \times 10^9$, $C_{EQ} = 2.744 \times$

10^{-15}, and $R_{EQ} = 11.374 \times 10^{10}$. You may use the program to compute the same curve as that given in Example 11.3.

EXAMPLE 11.5   The catheter in Example 11.2 has a pinch that reduces the radius by one-half, and it has a length $l_P = 1$ cm. Compute the pinch compliance and resistance, then compute the frequency response, G_P.

SOLUTION   The pinch resistance is computed from Equation (11.13) as

$$R_P = \frac{8(0.001)(0.01)}{\pi (0.23 \times 10^{-3})^4} = 9.099 \times 10^9 \text{ Ns/m}^5$$

The pinch inertance is computed from Equation (11.14) as

$$L_P = \frac{(10^3)(0.01)}{\pi (0.23 \times 10^{-3})^2} = 60.2 \times 10^6$$

The frequency response results are illustrated in Figure 11.27.

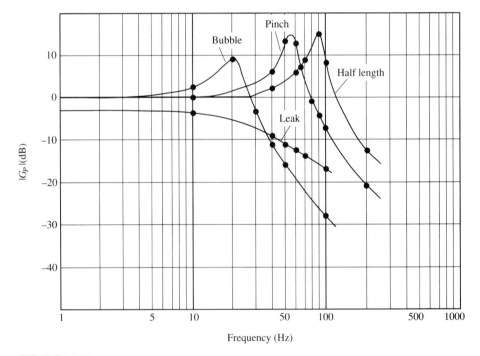

FIGURE 11.27
The effects of a bubble, a pinch, a leak, and length on the frequency response of a catheter.

EXAMPLE 11.6 The catheter in Example 11.5 has a bubble 2×10^{-6} liter in volume. Furthermore, a leak passes at a rate of 0.003 ml/min through a 13.3 N/m^2 pressure. Compute the bubble compliance and the leak resistance. Compute the frequency response $|G_P|$ for the catheter in Example 11.5 adding only the bubble given here. Then repeat the calculation adding only the leak resistance to Example 11.5.

SOLUTION From Equation (11.16) we have $C_B = (2 \times 10^{-6})(10^{-8}) = 2 \times 10^{-14}$ m^5/N. From Equation (11.15) the leak resistance is computed as follows:

$$R_H = \frac{13.3}{0.05 \times 10^{-9}} = 2.66 \times 10^{11} \quad \text{(in Ns/m}^5\text{)}$$

where the flow in MKS units is

$$F = \left(\frac{0.003 \text{ ml}}{\text{min}}\right)\left(\frac{\text{min}}{60 \text{ s}}\right)\left(\frac{1 \text{ cm}^3}{\text{ml}}\right)\left(\frac{\text{m}}{100 \text{ cm}}\right)^3 = 0.05 \times 10^{-9} \text{ m}^3\text{/s}$$

The frequency response is computed from Program A-19 in Appendix A. A graph of the results is given in Figure 11.27.

Practical troubleshooting tips for catheters are given in Box 1.

Box 1

TROUBLESHOOTING TIPS FOR CATHETERS

Symptom: False pressure readings due to low frequency response. A normal pressure waveform is not obtained.

Remedy: Eliminate bubbles in the catheter by gently tapping and flushing it.

Make the length of the catheter smaller.

Tighten all stopcocks and make sure that all connections between catheters, pressure transducers, and other elements are leak-free.

Symptom: Catheter whip. That is, the catheter is being pushed by the heart motion. This causes a pressure artifact that is synchronous with the normal pressure wave.

Remedy: Reposition the catheter until the artifact disappears.

REFERENCES

Cromwell, L., Weibell, F., and Pfeiffer, E. A. *Biomedical Instrumentation and Measurements*. 2nd ed. Englewood Cliffs, NJ: Prentice-Hall, 1980.

Ganz, W., and Swan, H. J. C. "Balloon-Tipped Flow-Directed Catheters." In *Cardiac Catheterization and Angiography*, edited by W. Grossman. Philadelphia: Lea and Febiger, 1974.

Geddes, L. A. *The Direct and Indirect Measurement of Blood Pressure*. Chicago: Year Book, 1970.

Guyton, A. C. *Textbook of Medical Physiology*. 3rd ed. Philadelphia: W. B. Saunders Company, 1966.

Hewlett-Packard Company. "Guide to Physiological Pressure Monitoring, Application Note AN739." Waltham, MA: Hewlett-Packard, 1977.

Peura, R. A. "Blood Pressure and Sound." Chapter 7 in *Medical Instrumentation, Application and Design*, edited by J. G. Webster. Boston: Houghton Mifflin, 1978.

Traister, R. J. *Principles of Biomedical Instrumentation and Monitoring*. Reston, VA: Reston Publishing, 1981.

EXERCISES

1. A fluid-filled catheter is 90 cm long and has a diameter of 1 mm. Compute its resistance to blood flow, and state its units in MKS. The viscosity of blood is $0.0028 \ \text{Ns/m}^2$ at 37 °C.

2. A water-filled catheter is 180 cm long and has a diameter of 1 mm. Compute its inertance and compliance. Assume the catheter tube has zero compliance.

3. Find the resistance of the catheter in Exercise 2.

4. Determine the resonant frequency, f_R, of the catheter in Exercise 2. Verify that the units of f_R are s^{-1}.

5. Draw an equivalent circuit for the catheter in Exercise 2, and plot its gain function versus frequency.

6. A normal patient's blood pressure is 120 over 80 mmHg. Compute the average pressure. Also, compute the mean pressure, MEAN.

7. A saline-filled catheter has a viscosity $\eta = 0.0007 \ \text{Ns/m}^2$ at 36 °C, and a length $l = 1.3$ m. Plot the catheter resistance as a function of its radius in meters.

8. A catheter tube with zero compliance is filled with water.

   (a) Plot the catheter compliance per meter length as a function of its radius.
   (b) Plot the inertance per unit length as a function of the catheter radius in MKS units.

9. A catheter has a length of 1.5 m, and a radius of 0.6 mm. It is filled with saline. The diaphragm compliance is $C_D = 1.5 \times 10^{-15}$ m^5/N. Find the resonant frequency f_R.

10. A standard catheter has a radius $r = 1.1$ mm and is terminated with a diaphragm having a compliance $C_D = 2.5 \times 10^{-15}$ m^5/N. The catheter is filled with saline of $\eta = 0.0007$ Ns/m^2 at 37 °C. The length is 1 m, and the orifice end is to be inserted into a heart ventricle. The equivalent circuit of such a catheter is given in Figure 11.21. The actual pressure, P_{ACT}, appears inside the body, and the measured pressure, P_{MEAS}, is taken outside the body by a pressure transducer attached to the diaphragm. Graph the frequency response, or gain, $P_{\text{MEAS}}/P_{\text{ACT}}$, for this catheter. Use 3-∿ semi-log paper and express the gain in decibels.

11. For the catheter in Exercise 10, graph the frequency response, $P_{\text{MEAS}}/P_{\text{ACT}}$, starting with the values given there. Make a series of plots on the same axis, changing the radius values, taking $r = 0.23$ mm, 0.46 mm, 0.92 mm, and 1.1 mm. Use 3-∿ semi-log paper.

12. For the catheter in Exercise 10, make a series of frequency response plots on the same axis, changing the length values, taking $l = 0.5$ m, 1 m, 2 m, and 4 m. Compute the resonant frequency, f_R, in each case and mark on the plots.

13. In the catheter in Exercise 10, a bubble with a volume of 2×10^{-6} liters is placed in the catheter. Make a series of frequency response curves on the same axis for the ratio $P_{\text{MEAS}}/P_{\text{ACT}}$, for 1, 4, and 8 bubbles.

12 Respiratory Equipment and Pulmonary Function Monitoring

12.1 THERAPEUTIC AND DIAGNOSTIC EQUIPMENT

Respiration is the process by which gas is exchanged across cell membranes in all living systems. At the cellular level, oxygen enters the cell and carbon dioxide is excreted. This process occurs even in dormant systems such as seeds. In human beings, the lung transfers O_2 from the ambient air to the blood and exhausts CO_2 into the atmosphere. The blood in turn carries O_2 to and CO_2 from the cells. To control the rate at which this transfer occurs, an elaborate control system has evolved, as illustrated in Figure 12.1.

In this process, contraction of respiratory muscles such as the diaphragm and intercostal muscles between the ribs expands the thorax, creating a negative pressure in the lung, and drawing in oxygen-rich air. The alveoli exchange O_2 for CO_2 in the blood flowing into the lung. The output blood then stimulates CO_2-sensitive cells called CO_2 receptors in the arteries near the carotid sinus. These cells, along with stretch receptors in the respiratory muscles, send out nerve impulses to the medulla oblongata region of the brain stem. The output from the brain stem is fed back to the respiratory muscles. This controls the breathing rate. Measurements of blood partial pressure of CO_2, called $^PCO_2$, or partial pressure of O_2, called $^PO_2$, show that the respiration rate is controlled by these factors. An increase in $^PCO_2$ increases the breathing rate, as illustrated in Figure 12.2. CO_2 is a waste product of respiration that must be swept away as it builds up in the lung. On the other hand, as $^PO_2$ increases, the breathing rate slows down, as indicated in the figure. In this case, the demand for oxygen-rich fresh air decreases.

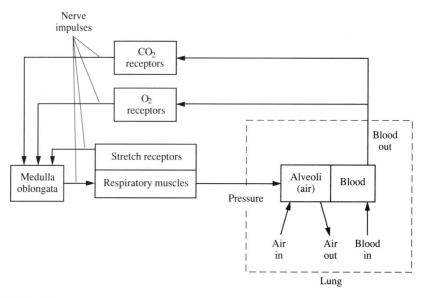

FIGURE 12.1
A simplified block diagram of respiratory control.

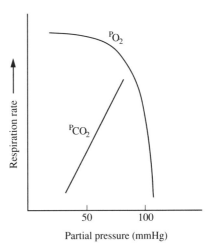

FIGURE 12.2
The effect of blood $^PCO_2$, and $^PO_2$ on the respiration rate. (From B. Jacobson, J. G. Webster, *Medicine and Clinical Engineering*, Englewood Cliffs, NJ: Prentice-Hall, 1977.)

In order to diagnose diseases of the lung such as emphysema or bronchitis, clinicians need to measure air volumes and flow rates. The nominal volumes, illustrated in Figure 12.3, are measured by spirometers and plethysmographs, such as are described further on in this chapter. Commonly measured volumes are defined as follows:

TV Tidal volume: The volume of air exchanged in relaxed breathing, nominally 0.6 liters.

IRV Inspiratory reserve volume: The additional air one can inhale with maximum inspiratory effort above a relaxed inspiration, nominally 3 liters.

ERV Expiratory reserve volume: The additional air one can exhale with maximum effort beyond a relaxed expiration, nominally 1.2 liters.

VC Vital capacity: The total volume of air one can exchange with maximum effort, nominally 5 liters.

RV Residual volume: The air that remains in a normal lung after full expiratory effort, nominally 1 liter.

FRC Functional residual capacity: The amount of air remaining in the lung after a relaxed expiration, nominally 2.2 liters.

TLC Total lung capacity, nominally 6 liters.

Parameters that relate to the airway resistance are defined as follows:

FVC_1 Fractional volume capacity (1 second): The amount of air a subject can force into a spirometer chamber after taking a maximum inspiratory breath, and exhaling with full force for 1 second.

FVC_2 Fractional volume capacity (2 seconds): The same as FVC_1, except it is measured for 2 seconds.

FEF_1 Forced expiratory flow (1 second): The average flow over 1 second.

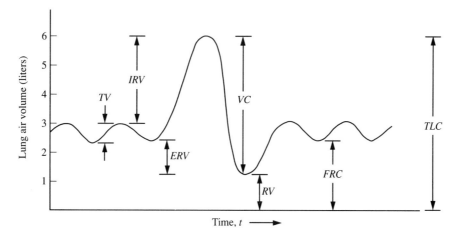

FIGURE 12.3
Lung air volumes important to clinical diagnosis.

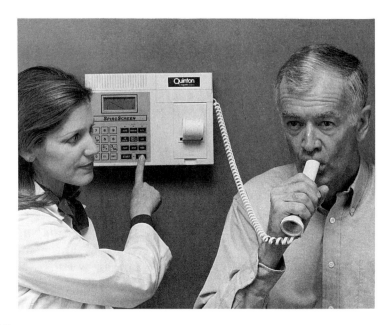

FIGURE 12.4
A patient having his pulmonary functions measured with a spirometer. (Courtesy of Quinton, Inc.)

An instrument for measuring the pulmonary functions is illustrated in Figure 12.4.

12.2 THE VENTILATOR

As part of intensive care, patients often require assistance with breathing. An artificial ventilator may be used to provide oxygen-enriched, medicated air to a patient at a controlled temperature. Ventilation assistance is provided under either of two conditions: (1) breathing initiated by a timing mechanism or (2) patient-initiated breathing. Automatically timed breathing is usually provided for patients who cannot breathe on their own. It provides inspiration and expiration at fixed rates and durations except for periodic sigh; a sigh is a rest period for the patient. Patient-initiated breathing may be given to one who has difficulty breathing due to high airway resistance. The patient's effort to inhale triggers the respirator unit to deliver air at the positive pressure prescribed.

Ventilator Modes of Operation

The following definitions are commonly used to describe respirator/ventilator operation:

CMV   Continuous mandatory ventilation: Once initiated by either the ventilator operator or the patient, the breath is driven to the patient.

CPAP   Continuous positive airway pressure: Breaths are spontaneous, unless the operator intervenes. The spontaneous breaths are determined entirely by patient effort. However, the air/oxygen mixture is set by the ventilator.

SIMV   Synchronized intermittent mandatory ventilation: These breaths are initiated by either the machine, the operator, or the patient. The breaths may be either spontaneous or mandatory. That is, if the patient does not breathe within a preset time period, the ventilator will deliver a breath.

PEEP   Positive end-expiratory pressure: The pressure maintained by the ventilator that the patient must exhale against.

Apena   The patient has stopped breathing.

Sigh   A breath delivered by the ventilator that differs in duration and pressure from a nominal breath.

Nebulizer A device for producing a fine spray of liquid or medication into the patient's air.

To illustrate the types of pneumatic circuits that operate in a ventilator as illustrated in Figure 12.5, we give the following description based on a simplified block diagram (Figure 12.6).

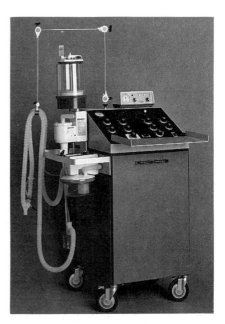

FIGURE 12.5
A pneumatic ventilator, Model MA-1.
(Courtesy Puritan-Bennett Corporation)

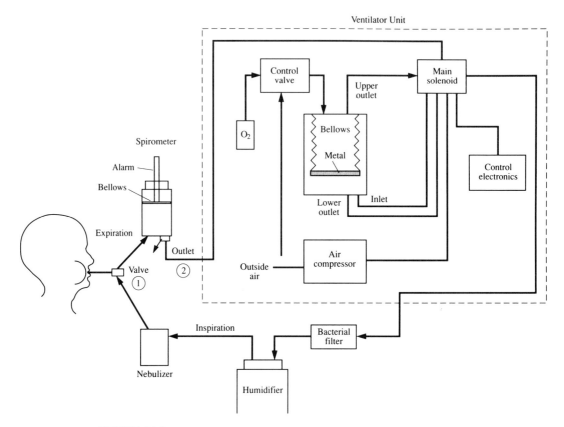

FIGURE 12.6
Airway paths and tubing on a ventilator.

The block diagram shows the external flexible tubing and the ventilator unit. Air from the ventilator during patient inspiration passes through a bacterial filter and humidifier. A nebulizer may spray medication into the air. This air then forces valve 1 up to close off the spirometer and deliver air to the patient. After the inspiration air is turned off by the ventilator, valve 1 drops and the patient exhales into the bellows, which has its outlet valve held closed pneumatically by the ventilator unit. During the subsequent patient inspiration cycle, that valve will open, causing the bellows to fall and empty.

During patient expiration, the direction of the air in the pneumatic system is determined by the main solenoid, which is switched appropriately by the system electronics, shown in the block diagram. Room air is drawn from the air inlet filter by the main compressor and is directed through the main solenoid to hold closed the upper outlet valve of the bellows located inside the unit. Next, the weight of the bellows causes the bottom bellows chamber outlet valve to open, as the main solenoid directs air to close the inlet bellows chamber valve. The weight of the falling bellows draws oxygen-enriched air into it in preparation for the patient-inspiration part of the cycle. The oxygen content of the air flowing into the bellows is controlled by a percentage control valve, which regulates the resistance to room air and oxygen appropriately.

At the end of patient expiration, the system electronics trip the main solenoid, thereby initiating the patient-inspiration part of the cycle.

During patient inspiration, the compressor draws room air through an air filter and then through the main solenoid. It forces the bottom inlet valve of the internal bellows chamber open and forces the bottom bellows chamber outlet valve closed. The high pressure in the bellows chamber compresses the bellows, forcing open the upper outlet valve set free by the main solenoid. This allows the oxygen-enriched air to pass through the main bacteria filter into the external tubes and then to the patient lungs. A sensitivity control monitors the negative pressure necessary to initiate inspiration when the respirator is used in the patient-initiated breathing mode called the *assist mode*. A nebulizer compressor may draw air from the bellows and

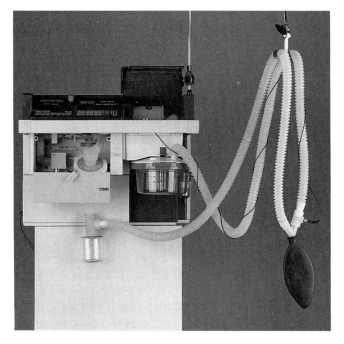

FIGURE 12.7
A positive-pressure ventilator with its tubing connected to a model lung. (Courtesy of Puritan-Bennett Corporation)

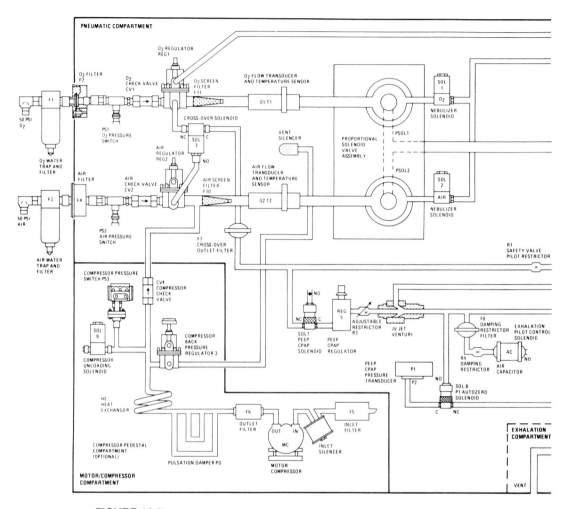

FIGURE 12.8
Block diagram of a Model 7200 ventilator. (Courtesy of Puritan-Bennett Corporation)

force it through an aspirator to mix medication into the patient-inspired air. When inspiration is complete, the main solenoid switches the direction of the pneumatic air to repeat the expiration cycle, and so on.

Figure 12.7 (p. 377) shows a specific respirator. The black bag at the end of the tubing simulates a compliant lung. This respirator may be operated using compressed air from the hospital air supply. In that mode, the ventilator can be removed from its internal compressor, thereby decreasing it in size; turning off the compressor also reduces problems in instru-

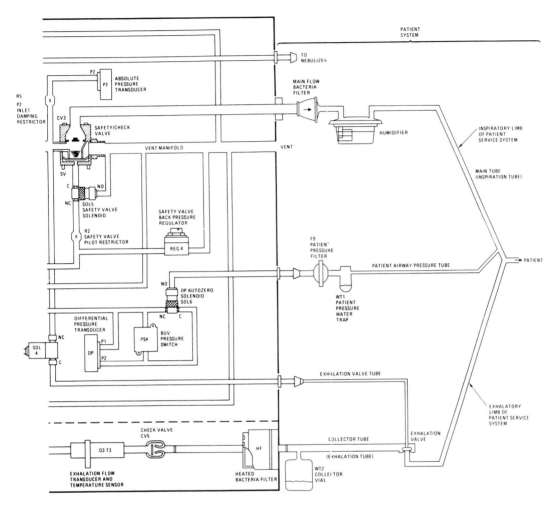

FIGURE 12.8 (continued)

ment noise control. A block diagram of the example ventilator appears in Figure 12.8. It consists of three subsystems: the pneumatic compartment, the exhalation compartment, and the motor/compressor compartment. The motor/compressor is used as an option if hospital air is not available or if the air pressure falls below 35 psi.

To aid patient respiration, hospital air and oxygen enter the pneumatic compartment, where it is filtered. A check valve reduces the pressure to a nominal 10 psi. A proportional solenoid valve assembly allows the air/oxygen mix to be controlled by the system electronics. A check valve, CV3 in the figure, directs air to the patient during the inspiration cycle. During the subsequent expiration phase, the system electronics opens the check valve, CV5, to provide a vent for the patient exhalation air. In this case, the pneumatically operated valves of older ventilators have been replaced by valves controlled with microprocessor-based electronics. A small positive-pressure ventilator is illustrated in Figure 12.9, in both front and back views.

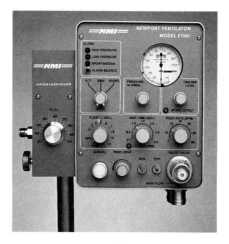

(a)

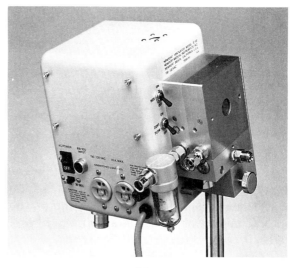

(b)

FIGURE 12.9
A positive-pressure ventilator showing (a) front and (b) back view. (Courtesy of Newport Medical Instruments, Inc.)

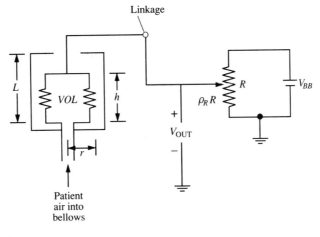

FIGURE 12.10
A spirometer.

12.3 A SPIROMETER

A spirometer consists essentially of a bellows designed to be as light as possible, in order to minimize airway resistance error. In its simplest form, the bellows is mechanically articulated to a biased potentiometer such that the wiper arm voltage is proportional to volume, VOL. The maximum volume, VOL_{max}, of the spirometer in Figure 12.10 is

$$VOL_{max} = L\pi r^2$$

The mechanical linkage may be adjusted such that

$$\rho_R = \frac{V_{OUT}}{V_{BB}} = \frac{VOL}{VOL_{max}}$$

where ρ_R is a proportionality constant giving the fractional position of the wiper arm on R. Therefore

$$VOL = \frac{V_{OUT}}{V_{BB}} VOL_{max} \qquad (12.1)$$

EXAMPLE 12.1 A spirometer has a radius of 18 cm and a maximum height of 10 cm. If $V_{BB} = 10$ V, plot the air volume versus the output voltage, V_{OUT}.

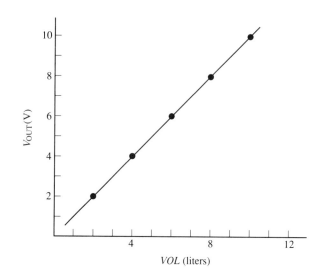

FIGURE 12.11
Spirometer *VOL* versus V_{OUT}.

SOLUTION   The maximum volume $VOL_{max} = 10\pi(18)^2 = 10.2$ liters. So, from Equation (12.1),

$$V_{OUT} = 0.982 \ VOL$$

The result is plotted in Figure 12.11, where *VOL* is expressed in liters.

A spirometer measuring only $4 \times 7 \times 1\frac{1}{2}$ in. is illustrated in Figure 12.12.

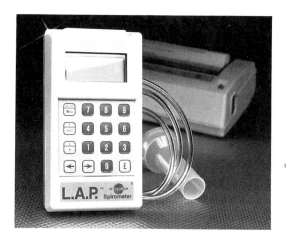

FIGURE 12.12
A portable spirometer with a mouthpiece.
(Courtesy of Timeter Instrument Corporation)

12.4 PNEUMOTACHOGRAPH AIRFLOW MEASUREMENT

Patient airflow may be measured by changes in resistance of a thermistor in the airstream due to the cooling effect of flowing air. But it must be calibrated to compensate for changing ambient temperature. To eliminate this disadvantage, a strain-gauge wire mesh is often used, as shown in Figure 12.13. The airflow in either direction puts a strain on the screen and changes the resistance of its strain gauge. The strain gauge is a component of a Wheatstone bridge as shown in Figure 12.14. Here the change in re-

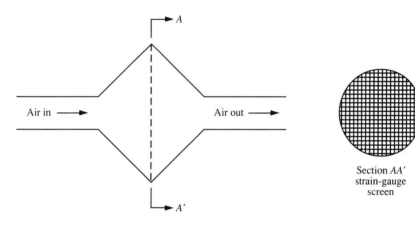

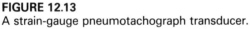

FIGURE 12.13
A strain-gauge pneumotachograph transducer.

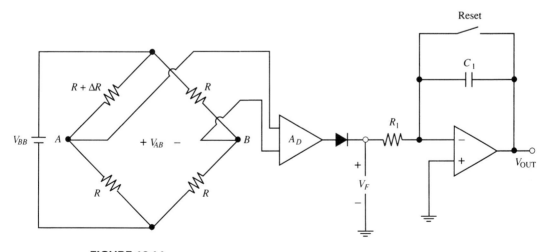

FIGURE 12.14
A circuit for measuring airflow rate and volume.

sistance, ΔR, is proportional to the airflow, F, past the wire mesh in Figure 12.13:

$$F = k\Delta R \qquad (12.2)$$

where k is the pneumotach coefficient in units of liters per second ohm (liter/sΩ). The wire mesh is made part of a Wheatstone bridge having elements R in each branch.

To compute the voltage that is proportional to flow, the Wheatstone bridge is analyzed by voltage division for bias voltage V_{BB}, so that

$$V_{AB} = \left(\frac{R}{R + \Delta R + R} - \frac{R}{2R} \right) V_{BB}$$

And by finding a common denominator,

$$V_{AB} = \left(\frac{-R\Delta R}{4R^2 + 2R\Delta R} \right) V_{BB}$$

The circuit may be designed so that $R \gg \Delta R$, and we have

$$V_{AB} = \frac{-\Delta R}{4R} V_{BB}$$

For a controlled gain differential amplifier, with a gain A_D, we then have

$$V_F = -A_D \left(\frac{\Delta R}{4R} \right) V_{BB} \qquad (12.3)$$

Then from Equation (12.2) into (12.3), we have

$$V_F = \frac{-A_D V_{BB} F}{4kR} \qquad (12.4)$$

The conclusion from this result is that the voltage V_F is proportional to flow when ΔR is small.

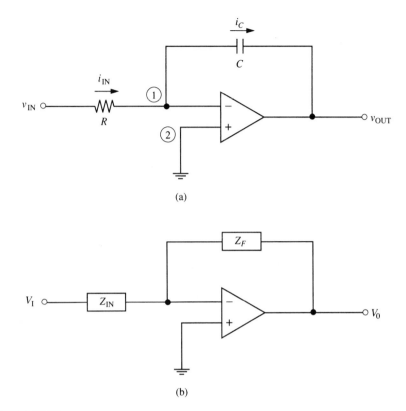

FIGURE 12.15
An integrator circuit (a) in the time domain and (b) in the phasor domain.

The Integrator Circuit

An ideal diff amp can be used to construct a circuit for which the output voltage is proportional to the integral of the input voltage. Such a circuit, shown in Figure 12.15, is called an integrator.

To analyze in the time domain note that node 1 is held at zero volts, thus

$$i_{IN} = \frac{v_{IN}}{R}$$

Also, by the definition of a capacitor,

$$v_{OUT} = -\frac{1}{C} \int_{t_0}^{t} (i_C) \, dt$$

where t is the time and t_0 the initial time. Combining the previous two equations, noting that $i_C = i_{IN}$, gives

$$v_{OUT} = -\frac{1}{RC} \int_{t_0}^{t} (v_{IN})\, dt \qquad (12.5)$$

Thus we conclude that the circuit integrates and inverts the input voltages. Inverting is indicated by the minus sign.

The circuit can also be analyzed in the sinusoidal steady-state phasor domain using Figure 12.15(b). The gain equation yields

$$V_0 = -\frac{Z_F}{Z_{IN}} V_I \qquad (12.6)$$

Then, since $Z_F = 1/j\omega C$ and $Z_{IN} = R$,

$$V_0 = -\frac{V_I}{j\omega RC} \qquad (12.7)$$

Comparing Equation (12.7) with (12.5), we can conclude that integration in the time domain in sinusoidal steady state is equivalent to division by the factor $j\omega$ in the phasor domain.

Pneumotachograph Volume Measurements

A volume exhaled by a patient is measured with the pneumotachograph by first closing and then opening the reset switch in Figure 12.14. This sets the initial charge on the capacitor to zero and fixes V_{OUT} at zero in the figure. The patient is then asked to exhale through the pneumotach mouthpiece. The resulting change in ΔR creates a voltage V_F as a function of time in proportion to flow as given in Equation (12.4).

EXAMPLE 12.2 A patient exhales rapidly at a constant rate of 2 liter/s for 3 s, as shown in Figure 12.16. The diff amp gain is -200 and the pneumotach coefficient is 100 liter/sΩ. Compute and plot the output voltage when the Wheatstone bridge bias is 10 V and the bridge resistances are 10 Ω each.

SOLUTION The voltage V_F is computed as a function of time from Equation (12.4) as

$$V_F = [(200)(10)/4(100)(10)]F = 0.5F \text{ V}$$

F is in liter/s. Therefore, V_F is 1 V for 3 s, as shown in Figure 12.16.

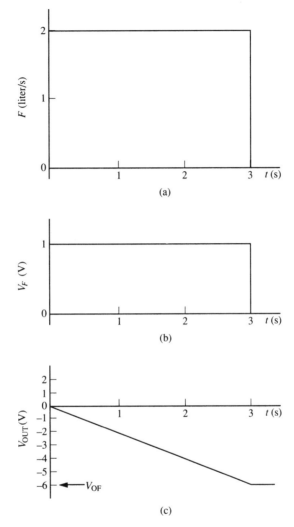

FIGURE 12.16
(a) Flow through the pneumotach. (b) Voltage out of the diff amp. (c) Voltage out of the integrator.

The air volume expired by the patient, beginning at time $t = 0$, when the reset is activated, equals the area under the flow versus time curve, as for example in Figure 12.16(a). Mathematically this area is computed by integration. In the circuit in Figure 12.14, the integrator circuit output voltage, V_{OUT}, is proportional to the volume of air expired from the time $t = 0$ to the time, t, desired. After the patient has stopped exhaling, the voltage V_{OUT} will remain constant in proportion to the total volume of air expired until the reset switch is closed. When the reset switch is set, and then opened at $t = 0$, the output voltage in Figure 12.14 follows from Equation (12.5) as

$$V_{OUT} = -\frac{1}{R_1 C_1} \int_0^t (V_F)\, dt$$

Substituting this into Equation (12.4) gives

$$V_{OUT} = \frac{1}{R_1 C_1} \int_0^t \left(\frac{A_D V_{BB}}{4kR}\, F \right) dt$$

The constant can be removed from under the integral sign:

$$V_{OUT} = \frac{A_D V_{BB}}{4R R_1 C_1 k} \int_0^t (F)\, dt \qquad (12.8)$$

But the total volume, *VOL*, is

$$VOL = \int_0^t (F)\, dt$$

Thus, putting this into Equation (12.8) gives

$$V_{OUT} = \frac{A_D V_{BB} VOL}{4R R_1 C_1 k} \qquad (12.9)$$

This equation means that V_{OUT} is proportional to the total volume of air that has passed through the pneumotach from $t = 0$ up to the time of observation. The flow, F, is a function of time that may increase, decrease, or stay constant, so long as it goes in one direction.

EXAMPLE 12.3   Calculate the volume exhaled by the patient in Example 12.2 as a function of time, and give the total volume of air exhaled. $R_1 = 500$ kΩ and $C_1 = 1$ μF.

SOLUTION   The voltage V_{OUT} in this case is given by

$$V_{OUT} = -\frac{1}{5(10^5)(10^{-6})} \int_0^t (V_F)\, dt = -2 \int_0^t (V_F)\, dt$$

A plot of this voltage is obtained by measuring the area under the curve in Figure 12.16(b) and multiplying by −2, as shown in Figure 12.16(c). The total volume of air exhaled is found from the value of the voltage V_{OUT} after the flow has stopped, V_{OF}, in this case after 3 seconds. Thus the total volume, from Equation (12.9), is

$$VOL = \frac{-6(4)(10)(5)(10^5)(10^{-6})100}{-200(10)}$$

or

$$VOL = 6.0 \text{ liters}$$

This volume of air expended could also be computed by finding the area under the curve in Figure 12.16(a). This value in the example given is 6 liters also, thus verifying Equation (12.9).

12.5 THE PLETHYSMOGRAPH

The pneumotachograph described in the previous section can be used to measure the rate of airflow during respiration and the vital air capacity of the lung VC, defined in Figure 12.3. It cannot, however, measure the total lung capacity, TLC. The reason for this is that the pneumotachograph can only measure the amount of air a person can exchange in respiration, and cannot detect the residual volume of air, RV, left in the lung after a forced exhaling. To measure the TLC, a body plethysmograph may be used. Illustrated in Figure 12.17, the plethysmograph consists of an airtight chamber the patient can enter and sit in.

The principle of operation of the plethysmograph depends directly on the gas law for an ideal gas of volume VOL and pressure P, namely Boyle's law,

$$P(VOL) = k_1 T \qquad (12.10)$$

where k_1 is a constant and T is the absolute temperature (K). In the chamber, the temperature remains constant. The product of $P\ VOL$ is therefore constant. Taking the derivative of the preceding equation yields

$$d(P\ VOL) = \frac{\partial(P\ VOL)}{\partial P}\ dP + \frac{\partial(P\ VOL)}{\partial VOL}\ d\ VOL$$

P_T - thorax pressure (N/m^2)
TLC - thorax volume (m^3)
P_C - chamber pressure (N/m^2)
VOL_C - chamber volume (m^3)

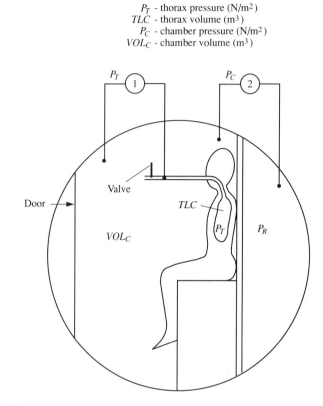

FIGURE 12.17
The body plethysmograph.

Since *P VOL* is constant, $d(P\ VOL) = 0$, so

$$VOL\ dP + P\ dVOL = 0$$

Solving this for an ideal gas at constant temperature gives

$$\frac{dP}{dVOL} = -\frac{P}{VOL} \tag{12.11}$$

This result gives a means of measuring the total lung capacity *TLC*.

Measurement of Total Lung Capacity

To measure *TLC*, the patient enters the chamber shown in Figure 12.17. The door is sealed, and the valve on the mouthpiece is closed. Since the patient cannot breathe with the valve closed, the air pressure in the mouthpiece equals that in the lung, P_T. That is, when the flow of air is zero, the pressure drop from mouthpiece to lung is also zero. With the valve closed, a formula for the thoracic volume is derived as follows.

The gas equation for constant temperature, Equation (12.11), holds inside the lung, sealed with the valve closed, yielding

$$\frac{dTLC}{dP_T} = -\frac{TLC}{P_T} \tag{12.12}$$

That equation also holds in the chamber, so that

$$\frac{dVOL_C}{dP_C} = -\frac{VOL_C}{P_C} \tag{12.13}$$

Here VOL_C is the chamber volume and P_C is the chamber pressure. Because the chamber is closed, any increase in the thoracic volume introduced by breathing motions causes a decrease in the chamber volume of air. That is,

$$dVOL_C = -dTLC$$

Then, putting this into Equations (12.12) and (12.13) yields

$$\frac{TLC}{P_T}\, dP_T = -\frac{VOL_C}{P_C}\, dP_C$$

During the test $P_C = P_T$ approximately, since the changes in pressure induced by breathing motions are small when the patient is resting. Thus we have

$$TLC \approx -VOL_C\, \frac{dP_C}{dP_T} \tag{12.14}$$

This equation gives the means for measuring the lung volume, TLC, by the following steps:

1. Close the mouthpiece valve on the patient sealed in the chamber.
2. Ask the patient to make breathing motions.
3. Read the change in pressure dP_T on meter 1.
4. Read the change in pressure dP_C in the chamber on meter 2.

5. Since the chamber volume VOL_C is a known specification of the plethysmograph, use the result of steps 3 and 4 to compute *TLC*, using Equation (12.14).

EXAMPLE 12.4   A plethysmograph chamber volume is 20×10^4 cm^3. The maximum thorax pressure is 30 psi, and the minimum is 5 psi, when the mouthpiece valve is closed and the patient goes through breathing motions. Simultaneously, the chamber pressure goes from 14.13 psi minimum to 15.0 psi maximum. Use this data to calculate the total lung capacity.

SOLUTION   Write Equation (12.14) in the following form:

$$TLC \approx -VOL_C \frac{P_{C\max} - P_{C\min}}{P_{T\min} - P_{T\max}}$$

$$= -20(10^4) \frac{15 - 14.13}{5 - 30} \qquad (\text{in cm}^3)$$

$$= 6.96 \text{ liters}$$

12.6 TROUBLESHOOTING PNEUMATIC EQUIPMENT

Faults in pneumatic equipment arise from airway obstructions caused by debris, often from patient breathing. Airway leaks are a persistent problem. These types of faults can often be found by visual inspection and by making sure the connections are tight.

A calibration analyzer for making ventilator calibrations and for troubleshooting ventilator problems is shown in Figure 12.18.

Modern microprocessor-based instruments have extensive self-diagnostic test circuits built in. Troubleshooting the Model 7200 ventilator shown as a block diagram in Figure 12.8 should begin with a reading of the power-on self-test (POST). POST is activated automatically each time the ventilator is turned on, even if it is connected to the patient. POST tests such items as the microprocessor and the printed circuit boards.

Additional troubleshooting can be performed by an extended self-test (EST). EST thoroughly tests the ventilator, including the pneumatic and electronic circuits. EST computes the system compliance and checks for airway leaks. The patient must be removed from the ventilator during execution of an EST procedure. A failure diagnosed by EST makes service mandatory before the equipment can be used again. EST produces error codes on the ventilator display that the troubleshooter may interpret by referring to the maintenance manual for the equipment.

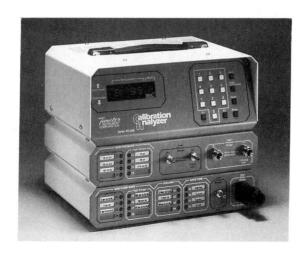

FIGURE 12.18
A calibration analyzer for making ventilator corrections. (Courtesy of Timeter Instrument Corporation)

REFERENCES

Egan, D. F. *Fundamentals of Respiratory Therapy*. St. Louis: C. V. Mosby, 1977.

Hunsinger, D. L., Lisnerski, K. J., Maurizi, J. J., and Phillips, M. L. *Respiratory Technology Procedure and Equipment Manual*. Reston, VA: Reston Publishing, 1980.

Puritan-Bennett. *7200 Series Microprocessor Ventilator Service/Maintenance Manual Rev. E 12-84*. Overland Park, KS: Puritan-Bennett, Inc., 1984.

Reiser, S. J., and Anbar, M. *The Machine at the Bedside*. Cambridge, UK: Cambridge Univ. Press, 1984.

Smith, W. "Ventilators and Respiratory Equipment." Chapter 13 in *Therapeutic Medical Devices*, edited by A. M. Cook and J. G. Webster. Englewood Cliffs, NJ: Prentice-Hall, 1982.

EXERCISES

1. The spirometer in Figure 12.10 has a radius of 5 cm. Plot the volume versus the height, h, of the spirometer from 0 to 10 cm.

2. From the result in Exercise 1, make a plot of volume, VOL, in Figure 12.10 versus voltage V_{OUT} when $V_{BB} = 10$ V.

3. The pneumotachograph illustrated in Figure 12.14 has $R = 1$ kΩ and $V_{BB} = 10$ V. The pneumotach coefficient is 2 liter/sΩ. If the diff amp gain is 10, plot the output voltage versus flow rate in units of liter/s.

4. The pneumotachograph illustrated in Figure 12.14 has $R_1 = 100$ kΩ and $C_1 = 0.1$ μF. Plot the volume of the air passing through versus the output voltage, beginning at $t = 0$. At $t = 0$, the volume $VOL = 0$. Here, $R = 1$ kΩ, $V_{BB} = 10$ V, and the pneumotachograph coefficient $k = 2$ liter/sΩ. The diff amp gain equals 10.

5. A plethysmograph chamber measures 22×10^4 cm^3. The maximum thorax pressure is 30 psi and the minimum pressure is 5 psi when the mouthpiece is closed and the patient goes through breathing motions. Simultaneously, the chamber pressure goes from 14.2 psi minimum to 15.1 psi maximum. Use this data to calculate the total lung capacity.

13

The Central Station Monitor, Microprocessor-Based Equipment, and System-Level Troubleshooting

The vast increase in the use of medical equipment was driven by the invention of the transistor in 1948, and by the subsequent development of solid-state electronics, which made possible the small, dedicated computer. The importance of the computer in medical equipment increased rapidly in the 1970s, in particular with the invention of the computer tomography (CT) scanner, an instrument that would be virtually impossible without dedicated computers. Many types of medical equipment are improved by the incorporation of dedicated computers, even though, in principle, they worked fine without them. This is not the case with CT scanners and magnetic resonance imagers (MRI). For them the dedicated computer has always been an essential element.

The microprocessor, or computer on a chip, is the component that makes inexpensive dedicated computers possible. By 1970 manufacturers could fabricate a thousand transistors on a chip about one square inch in size. This made possible dedicated computers such as the ordinary pocket calculator. At present, a million gates can be fabricated on a chip, which means that relatively powerful computers can be made quite small. These chips are so inexpensive that a computer once costing one or two thousand dollars is now available for about ten dollars. Because of this, they are now widely used in calculators, watches, automobiles, and many types of medical equipment.

Microprocessors are used, for example, to do signal processing on an ECG waveform. That is, they save time by computing heart *P-R* intervals and heart rates and by doing arrhythmia analysis. Holter ECG waveform storage devices are now available to monitor heart patients and to store selected arrhythmia events for later analysis. They are used to save nurses' time in central station monitoring. In pulmonary instrumentation they compute such variables as vital capacity, forced expiratory flow, and peak flow rates. They are used in anesthesia machines to monitor gas flow and blood gas parameters. They are used in electroencephalography to monitor frequency and the power spectrum.

Because microprocessors are so widely used, the engineer and technician working with hospital equipment clearly need to be familiar with them. In this chapter the discussion centers on the microprocessor. In particular, we wish to learn about microprocessors so that we can troubleshoot them in existing circuits. The data available for this task is, fundamentally, the voltage on the pins. Measurement of this data can lead to a decision as to whether the chip needs to be replaced.

13.1 MACHINE LANGUAGE

In order to understand microprocessors it is necessary to know their language. The language of microprocessors is made up of words having only two symbols, 1 and 0. The voltage on each node in the microprocessor has one of these two values, so the voltage is called either the 0 state or the 1 state. State 1 is often defined as 5 V and state 0 as 0 V. In digital logic, 1 and 0 may be given other meanings: 1 can mean true and 0 false, or 1 can mean HI and 0 LO.

The groups of 1s and 0s that make up machine language are called bits, bytes, nibbles, and words. A *bit* is the smallest unit of information and is either a 1 or a 0. To have one bit of information is to know whether the state of one node in the microprocessor is either 0 or 1. A *byte* is defined as 8 bits of information. It consists of a set of eight 1s or 0s. A *nibble* is made up of 4 bits of information, or half a byte. The length of a *word* depends upon the type of microprocessor. In some machines a word is 8 bits, in others 12 or 16 bits.

The words of a microprocessor are binary numbers. The *binary number system* is made up of the two numbers 0 and 1. Therefore it is referred to as a base two number system. The decimal number system, used in ordinary arithmetic, is a base ten system. The binary number system is more convenient for computers because each node has two states, 0 and 1.

The binary numbers using 4 bits are listed in order from lowest to highest as follows:

Binary number				Decimal equivalent
a_3	a_2	a_1	a_0	
0	0	0	0	0
0	0	0	1	1
0	0	1	0	2
0	0	1	1	3
0	1	0	0	4
0	1	0	1	5
0	1	1	0	6
0	1	1	1	7
1	0	0	0	8
1	0	0	1	9
1	0	1	0	10
1	0	1	1	11
1	1	0	0	12
1	1	0	1	13
1	1	1	0	14
1	1	1	1	15

To determine how many units are counted by a binary number, A_2, we convert it to a decimal number, A_{10}, by the formula

$$A_{10} = a_n \times 2^n + \ldots + a_1 \times 2^1 + a_0 \times 2^0 \qquad (13.1)$$

where a is either 1 or 0, and n is an integer.

EXAMPLE 13.1 Convert the binary number $A_2 = 1011_2$ to its decimal equivalent.

SOLUTION Applying Equation (13.1) to this case, we have

$$A_{10} = 1 \times 2^3 + 0 \times 2^2 + 1 \times 2^1 + 1 \times 2^0$$

Performing the indicated operations yields

$$A_{10} = 1 \times 8 + 0 \times 4 + 1 \times 2 + 1 \times 1$$
$$= 11_{10}$$

Here we include the base numbers. Usually, when the base is clear by context, it is dropped in the notation. The fact that 1011_2 is equivalent to 11_{10} may also be deduced by reference to the table above.

13.2 MICROPROCESSOR BLOCK DIAGRAM

The microprocessor is most clearly introduced if we consider a specific unit and start with the simplest case. Our discussion is based on the INTEL 8080A microprocessor. Other microprocessors will have a different programming language, and will even use slightly different generic names. For example, the heart of the microprocessor is called the *central processing unit* (*CPU*) by INTEL, whereas Motorola prefers to call it a microprocessor unit (MPU). The microprocessor is the most complex single-chip electronic component to date. The process of understanding each new chip is rather complicated, but after understanding one chip, it will be an easier matter to learn other chip types, because similarities will become evident.

A simple, practical microprocessor unit is shown in Figure 13.1. It consists of two major chips: the CPU and the memory. These chips, along with an input unit and an output unit, make up a minimal microprocessor. These units are connected by cables of wires called *buses*, consisting of groups of perhaps 8, 16, or more wires, depending upon the size of the machine. The buses shown in the figure are called the data bus, the address bus, and the control bus. The *data bus* carries digital words between all of the chips in the microprocessor. The *address bus* carries words from the CPU to the memory in order to connect desired memory locations to the data bus. The *control bus* carries words from the CPU to the other chips of the microprocessor in order to control the timing of their operations.

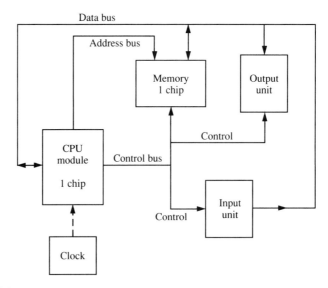

FIGURE 13.1
A block diagram of a simple microprocessor.

The *input unit* in the figure typically consists of a keyboard of numbers and letters called alphanumerics. An operator may enter data into the microprocessor by punching the keys on the input unit. Each word of information will appear at any point in time as a binary number on the data bus. An 8-bit binary number, for example, would require an 8-wire data bus. Such a data signal may be applied to either the output unit, the memory, or the CPU. The double arrow on the data bus means that the data may travel in either direction on the bus.

The CPU is the most complex chip. It is, in fact, a complete computer on a chip, containing a small internal memory, an arithmetic logic unit (ALU), and control circuits. The CPU does logical processing using the digital logic elements: AND, OR, and inverter functions. It does arithmetic by addition, multiplication, division, and subtraction. It also makes decisions by comparison of options. If the memory were larger, the CPU, with the input unit, output unit, and data bus, would constitute a microprocessor. However, for practical applications, a separate memory chip is required.

The memory chip consists of 8-bit *registers*, which are eight nodes on the chip, each of which holds either a 1 or 0 state. Each register constitutes a memory location. A *memory location* is a fixed physical region on the chip surface, perhaps as small as $10 \mu m \times 100 \mu m$, where eight flip-flop digital circuits are etched, each of which can hold a 1 or 0 voltage state. An 8-bit signal on the address bus will turn on the appropriate gates in the memory chip so that the memory location corresponding to the number on the address bus will be connected to the data bus through a path consisting of those gates. That is, each memory location has an 8-bit address that may be presented as an 8-bit binary number on the address bus by the CPU. The direction of flow of the address is from the CPU to the memory chip, as indicated by the arrow on the address bus in Figure 13.1.

The bus from the CPU carries signals that cause the memory circuits to operate in proper time sequence. It also delivers command signals to the input and output units. The output unit in a simple form may be formed by eight terminal posts, each carrying a voltage corresponding to either a 1 or 0 state, thereby providing an 8-bit signal output. A light may then be connected to each post, turning either ON or OFF corresponding to the state of each bit. The row of eight lights may then be visually observed and read as an 8-bit binary number.

The CPU

The central processing unit contains an arithmetic logic unit (ALU), a timing and control module, and eleven internal registers. The ALU, illustrated in the CPU diagram (Figure 13.2), is the most complex region of the chip. Here the routines necessary to perform the arithmetic operations and the

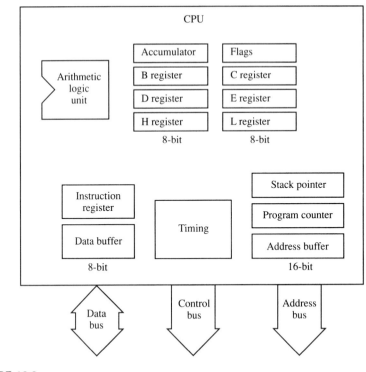

FIGURE 13.2
A CPU block diagram.

logic functions are located. These routines can be accessed by way of either the accumulator or the instruction register. Another way of saying this is that the ALU contains internal programs that may be called up by a binary number in the instruction register. Then a number in the accumulator is operated on—for example, multiplied, if the operation the program calls for is a multiplication routine.

The registers are symbolized by a box with eight slots, each representing the location of one of the eight bits; as, for example,

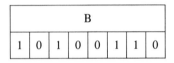

Here the register B is shown to contain the binary number 10100110.

The *accumulator* is an 8-bit register that holds the data from the data bus, which is to be operated upon by the ALU or other processing routines. The result of these operations is placed in the accumulator, and the original data is wiped out. The accumulator may be thought of as the entry and exit port of the CPU. For example, in the HP-15C calculator, the accumulator serves as the *x*-register.

The *flag register* contains five bits, each of which will change the processing procedure in accordance with data or program instructions. The flags indicate the readiness state of the input units, the sign of the data, and whether or not limits are exceeded or thresholds are reached. The flags then change the processing accordingly.

The 8-bit registers B, C, D, E, H, and L comprise a small, six-location memory fabricated in the CPU chip. This memory is usually used for temporary storage for numbers to be operated on at some point in time. Instruction commands can be used to move data from one of these registers to the other or into the accumulator.

The *program counter* consists of two 8-bit registers, one called LO and the other HI. The program counter contains a binary number that is the memory address of the next instruction to be executed after the current operation is completed. It may also be the address of data stored in memory. The 16-bit program counter register holds the maximal number

$$1\ 1\ 1\ 1\ 1\ 1\ 1\ 1\ 1\ 1\ 1\ 1\ 1\ 1\ 1\ 1_2 = 65{,}535_{10}$$

This means it can address 65,535 (usually rounded off to 64K) memory locations through a 16-wire address bus. In the case of the 8080A microprocessor, only 10 bits of the possible 16 bits in the program counter are used, and the memory size is therefore limited to 1023, rounded off to 1K, locations.

The *stack pointer* is a specialized address register giving the address to a group of memory locations called a stack. More specifically, it is a 16-bit register giving the address to the location at the top of the stack. When a number is placed on top of the stack, it *pushes* the existing number there into another location in the stack. Conversely, when a number is drawn out of the stack, it is replaced by another number popped from another location within the stack. In the HP-15C calculator, the *x*-, *y*-, *z*-, *t*-registers are a stack that operates in this fashion.

The instruction register, an 8-bit register, holds the binary number corresponding to a program instruction taken from the memory. In a sense it is the address of the proper subroutine within the CPU to execute the instruction.

The timing circuit in the CPU (Figure 13.2) receives the clock pulse and distributes the control signals to the memory, the input unit, and the output unit.

The Memory Chip

Microprocessors usually have separate memory chips. This is necessary because space is limited on the CPU chip, and because separate chip memories allow for expandability. There are two general types of memory chip, *ROM* (read only memory) and *RAM* (random access memory). The contents of the ROM are permanent (that is, they are not destroyed when the power is shut off), and in normal usage they can only be read, not changed or replaced. The RAM is sometimes called a read/write memory. Random access means that any location can be addressed at will, and one can either read or use the contents of that address. Furthermore, the contents of that location can be changed.

A variation of these memory types is the *PROM* (programmable read only memory). PROM chips can be programmed on a special device separate from the microprocessor but cannot be changed otherwise during microprocessor operation. A further variation, *EPROM*, is an erasable, programmable read only memory that can be either erased or programmed with a special device separate from the microprocessor. This programming device is not usually part of the equipment using the microprocessor and would be considered fabrication, or maintenance, hardware.

To understand how memories work, refer to Figure 13.3. The memory chip has some pins that connect to the address bus and other pins connecting to the data bus. The function of the address bus voltages is to activate the proper gates so that a conducting path is made through the chip to the data bus pins. That is, the address voltage connects the memory lo-

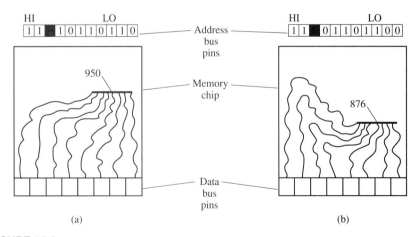

(a)   (b)

FIGURE 13.3
Addressing memory locations.

cation at that address to the data bus. For example, Figure 13.3(a) illustrates that the address $1110110110 = 950_{10}$ connects the 950th memory location to the data bus pins. In a second example, Figure 13.3(b), the 876th location is shown to be connected to the data bus, when the address pins have the states given by the binary number $1101101100 = 876_{10}$.

Input/Output Units

The input unit of a microprocessor dedicated to medical equipment is often an arrangement of manually operated switches. These may be the power switch, gain and sensitivity controls, numbers, and letters. An example input unit is illustrated in Figure 13.4. These inputs have meaning to the user as mathematical or alphabetical symbols. For microprocessor use, it is essential to convert them to machine language binary numbers.

A commonly used code for converting keyboard symbols to machine language is called the American Standard Code for Information Interchange, or ASCII code, given in Table 13.1. For operation of a printer, the code symbols in the table are extended to include the lowercase numbers, and the printer operations LF (line feed) and CR (carriage return):

CR 0001101
LF 0001010

The input unit is designed so that keying the letter A, as given in the table, results in the data bus receiving the number 1000001 from the input unit. Likewise, the letter Q would put the machine language 1010001 on the data bus.

A digital output unit would do the opposite: it would display the letter A when 1000001 appeared on the data bus connected to it. It would display the number 3 when 0110011 appeared on the data bus.

A simple output unit may simply be a set of eight terminal pins. The set of voltage states on the terminals may be interpreted as a binary num-

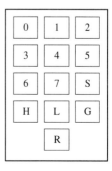

FIGURE 13.4
An input unit of a microprocessor.

TABLE 13.1
The Binary ASCII Code

Character	Binary	Character	Binary
@	1000000	space	0100000
A	1000001	!	0100001
B	1000010	"	0100010
C	1000011	#	0100011
D	1000100	$	0100100
E	1000101	%	0100101
F	1000110	&	0100110
G	1000111	'	0100111
H	1001000	(	0101000
I	1001001	)	0101001
J	1001010	*	0101010
K	1001011	+	0101011
L	1001100	,	0101100
M	1001101	−	0101101
N	1001110	.	0101110
O	1001111	/	0101111
P	1010000	0	0110000
Q	1010001	1	0110001
R	1010010	2	0110010
S	1010011	3	0110011
T	1010100	4	0110100
U	1010101	5	0110101
V	1010110	6	0110110
W	1010111	7	0110111
X	1011000	8	0111000
Y	1011001	9	0111001
Z	1011010	:	0111010
[	1011011	;	0111011
\	1011100	<	0111100
]	1011101	=	0111101
^	1011110	>	0111110
←	1011111	?	0111111

ber. Then voltages may be used to turn on LED lamps so that the result can be read. On the other hand, these voltages may be used to drive switches and relays. And certainly they could be fed through a digital-to-analog (D/A) converter to drive conventional meter movements or to create a trace on an oscilloscope screen.

13.3 A MICROPROCESSOR-BASED MONITOR

Many modern patient-care instruments, such as we discussed in the previous chapters, use microprocessors for control functions and for signal processing. The analog circuitry such as diff amps and drivers discussed previously is still used, especially for amplifying signal levels and for transforming physiological parameters such as pressure, flow, and temperature into voltage high enough to be processed by microprocessors.

To illustrate the role of microprocessors, and to point out some relevant troubleshooting techniques, we will describe the block diagram of the Hewlett-Packard model 78534 monitor. This instrument is designed to monitor patient ECG, heart rate (*HR*), pressure, temperature (*T*), and respiration rate. The monitor may also be used as a component of a *central monitoring station*. The central monitoring station is a unit that makes it possible for one nurse to watch over the physiological parameters of many patients at one time.

The signal flow in the 78534 monitor block diagram (Figure 13.5) begins in the upper left-hand corner. At the front panel inputs there are receptacles for the patient transducers. The pressure transducer plugged into one of these ports requires an excitation voltage. It may have a sensitivity of either 5 or 40 microvolts per volt of excitation per millimeter of mercury (μV/V/mmHg). It requires a balanced bridge circuit, as discussed in Chapter 4, along with amplifiers to raise the voltage to approximately 1 V for signal processing. The ECG transducers are usually surface electrodes on the limbs, labeled RA, LA, LL, RL, and C, as described in Chapter 6. The temperature transducers utilize thermistors as described in Chapter 4. Respiration is measured by monitoring the resistance between the RA and LL electrodes. Expansion and contraction of the chest during breathing changes the torso resistance considerably during the breathing cycle. This resistance is measured by means of bridge circuits, as discussed in Chapter 4.

Each of the blocks in Figure 13.5 represents a separately removable circuit board of the monitor. This makes it convenient to do board-level troubleshooting in the hospital environment. Figure 13.6 illustrates a proper technique for extracting circuit boards.

In Figure 13.5 the protect board (A20) provides coupling of the ECG, pressure, and temperature signals to the monitor. It has components that protect the monitor from overvoltage such as defibrillator pulses or power-line surges. The signals are routed from board A20 to either the ECG board (A17), or the pressure, respiration, and temperature (P.R.T.) board (A18), as appropriate. Board A17 contains ECG circuits similar to those discussed

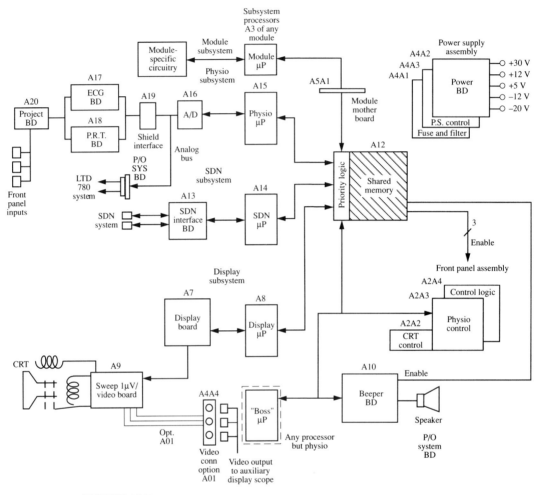

FIGURE 13.5
The model 78534 block diagram. (Courtesy of Hewlett-Packard Company)

in Chapter 6. The common-mode and input circuits are optically isolated from signal processing circuits to protect the patient from leakage currents and microshock hazards. Likewise, the P.R.T. board contains linear bridge circuits for detecting changes in pressure and temperature transducer parameters. Various filters are included to suppress noise and to eliminate plumbing resonances in the catheter and pressure transducer assemblies.

The outputs of these two boards, through a shielded interface, go, in a sense, from the floating world to the grounded world. The *floating world* is the isolated circuitry connected to the patient. The *grounded world* is the

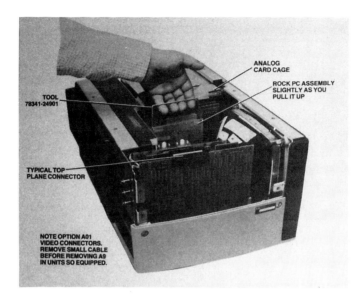

FIGURE 13.6
PC board extraction technique. (Courtesy of Hewlett-Packard Company)

nonisolated circuitry of the signal processing units. The analog bus seen between boards makes the patient data available to various types of recording devices, if the data is to be recorded.

The data is sampled by a control signal from the physio microprocessor board (A15) in a timed sequence, so that the ECG, pressure, respiration, and temperature data are kept separate. The ECG is sampled every 2 ms. Also, every 32 ms the pressure and respiration waves are sampled four times. The temperature is sampled every 64 ms. Other data sampled includes the power supply voltages and the ECG and pressure alarms.

These sampled signals are applied to an analog-to-digital (A/D) converter. A simple A/D converter consists of a resistor tapped at several places, as shown in Figure 13.7. In that example, the higher the voltage V_{ANAL} level, the more channels have 1-state outputs from the threshold detectors TD. In this case, V_{ANAL} is digitized into eight separate levels. For example, if V_{ANAL} equals the threshold voltage of the circuit V_T, only the top channel in the figure will have a 1-state output. However, if V_{ANAL} is eight times this value, all channels will have a 1-state output. In practical A/D converters this idea can be extended so that V_{ANAL} is separated into 512 levels for greater accuracy. Each level is coded into an 8-bit binary number for transmission along an 8-wire bus.

After passing through the A/D converter in Figure 13.5, the sampled, digitized data is ready to be processed in a microprocessor, called the physio μP board A15. Physically, the three microprocessor boards A15, A14, and A8 are the same, having the same circuits, although the components attached to each board's connecting cables are different. This is convenient

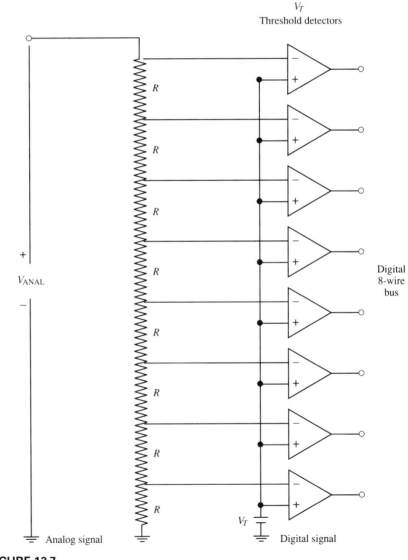

FIGURE 13.7
The A/D converter concept.

for design, maintenance, and troubleshooting. If a failure is suspected, the boards can be interchanged. If the interchange affects the symptoms of the failure, one of the boards would be suspected of being faulty. By the process of elimination, the faulty board can be identified and replaced, or sometimes repaired on site.

The physio μP board in Figure 13.5 transfers the sampled physiological data to the shared memory (A12) and stores it in a RAM. Take, for example, the ECG data, which exists in the shared memory as a wave record. This data is transferred to the display μP, board A8. A8 encodes the waveform into four-brightness-level picture elements, called pixels. The pixels appear as dots of light on the cathode-ray tube (CRT).

The microprocessor computes the *R-R* interval of the ECG to determine arrhythmias and pulse rate (*PR*). It also computes the respiration rate (*RR*). Furthermore, it warns of heart stoppage, called *asystole*, when it occurs.

An example display from the 78534 monitor in Figure 13.8 shows an example ECG wave from lead II accompanied by alphanumeric labels. In

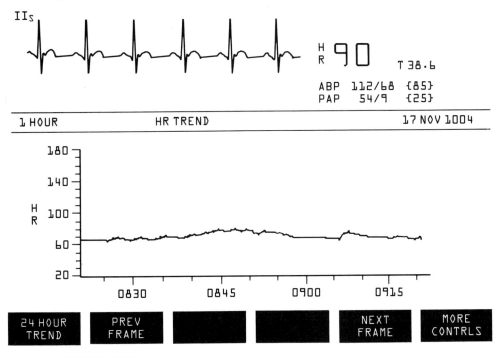

FIGURE 13.8
An example model 78534 display. (Courtesy of Hewlett-Packard Company)

this case the heart rate HR is 90 bpm, T is 38.6 °C, arterial blood pressure (ABP) is 112/68, and the mean pressure, in parentheses, is 85 mmHg. The pulmonary arterial pressure (PAP), obtained with an intervenous catheter, reads 54/9 on the display, with a mean pressure, indicated in parentheses, of 25 mmHg. The memory capability of the monitor is used in this case to record heart rate trends over a one-hour period. This display is mapped on the display board, labeled A7 in Figure 13.5. It can then be called up on the CRT through a video board for visual observation by the operator. The block diagram in Figure 13.5 also shows power supply boards and a provision for additional module capability.

Further detailed information, excepting microprocessor programs, is available in the manufacturer's service manual. The actual microprocessor software would have to be obtained from the manufacturer.

It is possible to transfer the data prepared for display to a remote location. In order to transfer the display data over external cables, the data must be modified. In the figure, boards A13 and A14 comprise the serial distribution network (SDN). The SDN performs the modifications. The operation of these boards will be explained in the next section in connection with central station monitoring.

Central Station Monitoring

Central station monitoring is done by delivering data from several bedside monitors to a single location. A monitor at that central location presents the data in a form convenient for observation by a single nurse. The central monitor illustrated in Figure 13.9 shows ECGs from six bedside monitors displayed simultaneously on a single screen. In this case, one nurse can continuously watch all patients. Otherwise the nurse would have to go to each bedside and could miss a critical event. In another way of displaying the data, shown in Figure 13.10, the remote-location monitors are arranged side by side so that one observer can scan them all. The advent of microprocessors and dedicated computers has greatly expanded the amount of information that can be presented at the central location. In the case of the 78534 monitor (Figure 13.5), the microprocessor in the SDN delivers digital patient data to a central location through a dedicated computer, system communication controller (SCC). In the SDN illustrated in Figure 13.11, the SCC coordinates the data within and among several intensive care units (ICU) and critical care units (CCU) and their satellites. The SCC allows each monitor to deliver its information every 32 ms. The SCC will rebroadcast this information to a patient information center or to another monitor within the system. In the case illustrated in Figure 13.11, 14 patient moni-

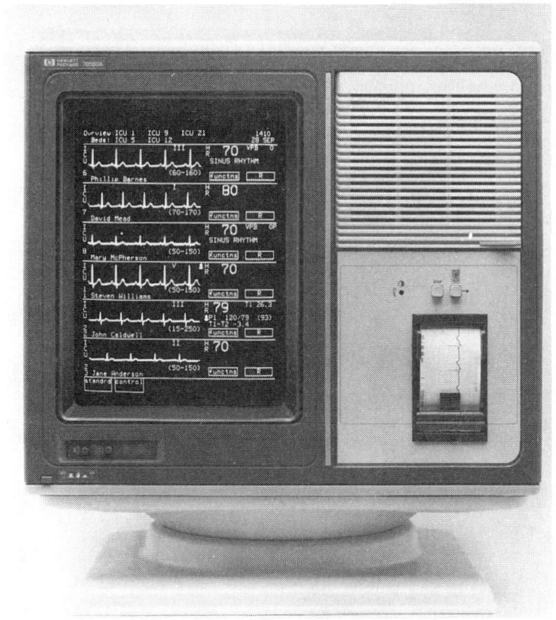

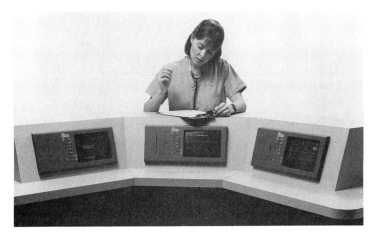

FIGURE 13.9
A central station monitor displaying ECGs from several different patients simultaneously.
(Courtesy of Hewlett-Packard Company)

FIGURE 13.10
A surveillance system for several bedside monitors located at a central nurses' station.
(Courtesy of Corometrics Medical Systems, Inc.)

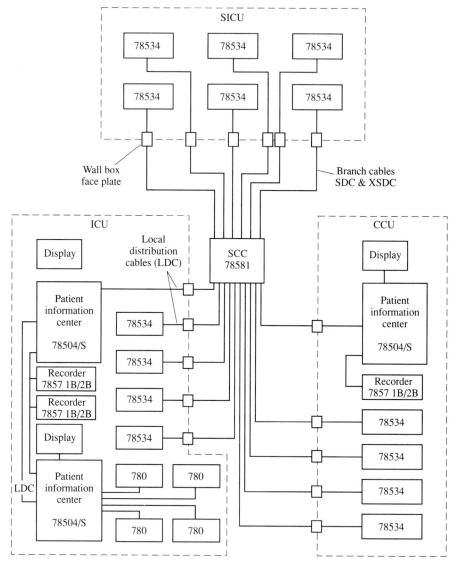

FIGURE 13.11
A typical SDN configuration. (Courtesy of Hewlett-Packard Company)

tors are coordinated by the SCC. In this way, patient alarms can be delivered to several different patient-care areas. In the evening while patients are sleeping, or when there is a small patient load, one nurse can monitor the entire system, while in peak periods, several nurses can be on watch. The result is an increase in the quality of patient care, and by fewer nurses, which can mean lower labor costs.

Troubleshooting Microprocessor-Based Equipment

In troubleshooting equipment, you have to find the one small part that has caused the fault. Since instruments often have millions of parts, you must use a systematic approach to finding the faulty part. One logical procedure, discussed in Chapter 3, is to begin at the system level. At that level you would distinguish between a problem with the central monitoring system and a problem caused by operator error. This simply involves going over the operating procedure to ensure that the equipment was being operated correctly. An interview with the operator is often helpful in making this determination. A particularly common operator-error problem involves the patient transducer attachments and the patient leads. These components should always be checked, if possible, as this can often lead to a quick fix.

If the hardware is at fault, you would next identify the module causing the problem. For example, in the central monitoring system in Figure 13.11, you would need to determine whether the problem is in the SCC, a 78534 monitor, or some other component of the system. Since there are several monitors in this system, it may be helpful to interchange monitors to distinguish between a SCC problem and a 78534 problem. If it is determined that there is a fault in the 78534 monitor, troubleshooting would involve first checking system connections. The cables in any system are very vulnerable to failure. They get abuse from pulling, rough handling, and normal wear. Also, they usually have spring contacts subject to fatigue and surfaces that can corrode and get dirty. Careful visual inspection of the cables for frayed ends or signs of wear is an important technique. Moving and pulling the cable to see if it affects the problem will often identify a fault.

A next logical step is to open the instrument case. Again, visual inspection is important. Look for smoke. Look for signs of burning or overheating. Touch the parts (avoiding electrical shock, of course). It is always a rule of thumb that if an electronic part, with the exception of vacuum tubes, is too hot to touch, it may be overheated.

A next step is to focus on more minute parts, such as a circuit board. A guide to logical deduction at this level is the module block diagram. The 78534 block diagram in Figure 13.5, for example, is drawn to show the relationship between the boards in the monitor. The physical location of each board in the monitor, seen with the outside cover removed, is given in Figure 13.12. There are often test points at convenient locations on the boards, so that you can check for proper supply voltages and do signal tracing. The

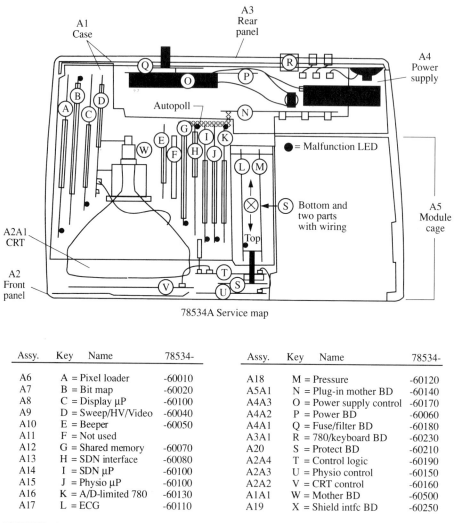

78534A Service map

Assy.	Key Name	78534-
A6	A = Pixel loader	-60010
A7	B = Bit map	-60020
A8	C = Display μP	-60100
A9	D = Sweep/HV/Video	-60040
A10	E = Beeper	-60050
A11	F = Not used	
A12	G = Shared memory	-60070
A13	H = SDN interface	-60080
A14	I = SDN μP	-60100
A15	J = Physio μP	-60100
A16	K = A/D-limited 780	-60130
A17	L = ECG	-60110

Assy.	Key Name	78534-
A18	M = Pressure	-60120
A5A1	N = Plug-in mother BD	-60140
A4A3	O = Power supply control	-60170
A4A2	P = Power BD	-60060
A4A1	Q = Fuse/filter BD	-60180
A3A1	R = 780/keyboard BD	-60230
A20	S = Protect BD	-60210
A2A4	T = Control logic	-60190
A2A3	U = Physio control	-60150
A2A2	V = CRT control	-60160
A1A1	W = Mother BD	-60500
A19	X = Shield intfc BD	-60250

FIGURE 13.12
An aid to locating circuit boards and unit modules. (Courtesy of Hewlett-Packard Company)

maintenance manual supplies expected signal measurements at the test points. It is also useful to compare a failed instrument with one that is working properly by comparing test-point waveforms. A list of trouble-shooting tips is given in Box 1 to provide you with examples of the kinds of troubles that would lead you to identify specific boards as being faulty.

Box 1

ILLUSTRATIVE TROUBLESHOOTING TIPS

(Figure 13.5)

Isolate lead problems:
>   If one channel of the ECG fails, check the lead on that channel.
>   If all ECG channels fail, but the P.R.T. channels work, the ECG board may be bad.
>   If pressure works, but respiration does not, check the respiration connecting leads.
>   If the local module works but does not broadcast on the central monitoring station, interchange the display μP board and the SDN μP to test for a microprocessor problem.

Check bus cables:
>   Reverse the buses at both ends if physically possible. If the trouble is affected, the cable is probably at fault.

A board changing convenience:
>   The physio μP, SDN μP, and display μP boards have identical circuits on them and can be interchanged.

Self-Test

The advent of microprocessors has greatly expanded the capability of instrument self-testing. In an instrument that has a self-testing feature, an error message will appear on the display unit that either identifies the problem or helps you identify the problem. For example, self-testing may be used to troubleshoot the 78534 monitor.

The 78534 monitor has three self-test levels: background self-test, manually initiated self-test, and extended self-test. The *background self-test* occurs automatically to inform an unsuspecting user of an equipment problem. In a potentially hazardous situation, this may be a visual or audio alarm. The *manually initiated self-test* is made by a user depressing a test button to check out the instrument before use. The *extended self-test* is more elaborate and is usually done by a specialist. It is made with simulated data, such as an ECG simulator, applied to the input of the instrument under test. In all cases, error codes are written on the output display to indicate faults.

Error codes consist of four alphanumeric symbols. The service engineer may consult an error code table to get more details. Some of the error codes are very specific, pointing out a component such as "ECG lead I." Another code reads "ECG alarm slider value too high." Such problems can be checked immediately by the operator. Other error codes are not so specific. They may reveal errors on the board level, indicating that a particular circuit board should be changed. Switching the board will get the equipment on line, so that component-level testing can be done without jeopardizing the equipment operation. You should realize that error codes are not infallible and may not identify the problem sufficiently to get the equipment back into use. Considering the complexity of modern medical equipment, making accurate self-testing algorithms is a challenging design task.

Component-level testing of boards may be done either by a technician in the shop on a spare unit, or by the manufacturer. The choice of whether to do component-level troubleshooting on site should be made on the basis of cost. If the faulty component can be located in a short time, it pays to fix it on site. However, the cost of shipping a board to the manufacturer is often small compared to the cost of time spent in troubleshooting. The manufacturer can often do the repair more economically, since it will have specialists who repair the boards more frequently than users and who have specialized test equipment to troubleshoot the boards. A further consideration is that with some equipment, particularly large-scale equipment like the CT scanner, the downtime created by a component failure can cost as much as $1000 per hour. In this case, the cost in time to ship the board out for repair, or even to order a new one, may be high compared to the time it takes the in-house technician to fix it on site.

A Logical Approach to Troubleshooting

Your fundamental assets for troubleshooting equipment are your knowledge and your analytical ability. These assets are augmented by the equipment service manual, which contains equipment specifications, operation instructions, equipment theory, maintenance procedures, troubleshooting charts, and diagnostic aids. Other assets include the knowledge about the equipment and the experience of the equipment operator, your co-workers, the operating technician, and the manufacturer's service representative. For specific equipment, the equipment records reveal weaknesses, previous problems, and failures. This data is often recorded on a shop computer for easy access and convenient data processing. A broader database is often available from the manufacturer.

A step-by-step approach to utilizing these assets is given in Chapter 3, Figure 3.15. The flowchart in the figure suggests when to interview the operator, access data records, perform equipment diagnostic checks, measure circuit data, use the manufacturer's resources, or turn to the equipment manual. These are only suggestions.

Factors to consider when deciding whether to implement a particular step include cost and convenience. For example, you may not be able to look through equipment records because the hardware happens to be off the site where the records are while being repaired. It is sometimes necessary to adapt procedures to utilize equipment and parts available. Almost any procedure that gets the equipment back into operation safely, accurately, reliably, and economically is valid.

REFERENCES

Bronzino, J. D. *Computer Applications for Patient Care.* Boston: Addison-Wesley, 1982.

Javitt, J. *Computers in Medicine: Applications and Possibilities.* Philadelphia: W. B. Saunders, 1986.

Hewlett-Packard Company. *Monitor Model 78534 Service Manual.* Waltham, MA: Hewlett-Packard, 1988.

Roney, P. R. *Introductory Experiments in Digital Electronics and 8080A Microcomputer Programing and Interfacing*, Vol. 5 and 6. Indianapolis: W. W. Sams & Co., 1987.

Tompkins, W. J., and Webster, J. G. *Design of Microcomputer-Based Medical Instrumentation.* Englewood Cliffs, NJ: Prentice-Hall, 1981.

Triebel, W. A., and Singh, A. *16-Bit Microprocessors.* Englewood Cliffs, NJ: Prentice-Hall, 1985.

EXERCISES

1. Name three inventions that made it possible to build microprocessors.

2. Identify three types of signal processing that can be accomplished on an ECG waveform with a microprocessor.

3. Name three medical instruments that use microprocessing in signal conditioning.

4. Give the definitions of the following terms:
   Bit
   Byte
   Nibble

5. Convert the following binary numbers into decimal form:
   101101
   100111
   001111

6. Write the following numbers in binary coded decimal (BCD) notation. To do this, form each digit as a 3-bit binary number:
   21
   736
   542
   28

7. Convert the following BCD numbers from binary to octal (base eight) form. Each octal digit is to be given by 3 bits of the binary number:
   101001101
   110100111

8. Define the following terms and acronyms associated with a microprocessor:
   Data bus
   CPU
   Address bus
   Control bus
   RAM
   ROM
   PROM

9. Explain the difference between RAM and ROM.

10. Explain how a binary number on the address bus of a memory chip affects it.

11. Match the following components of a CPU chip if possible.
    a. ALU
    b. Accumulator
    c. H-register
    d. B-register
    e. L-register
    f. Instruction register
    g. Stack pointer
    h. Program counter

    __ contains the address of instruction codes
    __ contains the most significant bit (MSB) of the address
    __ is the most frequently used internal memory register
    __ contains routines to carry out program instructions
    __ is the address register for a group of memory locations
    __ contains the least significant bit (LSB) of the address
    __ is a temporary storage register within the CPU
    __ directs which arithmetic logic unit is to be used
    __ controls everything in the CPU

12. Name four physiological parameters of medical diagnostic significance that can be monitored with the unit shown in Figure 13.5.

13. Which of the physiological parameters recorded by the monitor in Figure 13.5 is measured by recording the thorax resistance?

14. Identify three circuit boards in Figure 13.5 that make up the "floating world" in the monitor.

15. What fact about circuit boards A8, A14, and A15 greatly assists in trouble-shooting them?

16. A symptom of a trouble in the 78534 monitor is that no display works properly. Of the following, what is most likely at fault?
    (a) ECG board A17
    (b) Front panel inputs
    (c) A/D board A16
    (d) P.R.T. board A18

17. A symptom of a trouble in the 78534 monitor is that the temperature display is faulty and one ECG display is faulty, but all other ECG displays work fine. What is the most likely fault?
    (a) ECG board A17
    (b) P.R.T. board A16
    (c) Protect board A20
    (d) Front panel inputs

18. The 78534 is part of a central station monitor. No display on the monitor connected to the patient is working. However, the patient's data is measured and appears on the other monitors in the system. Which circuit board has most likely failed?
    (a) Physio μP, A15
    (b) SDN μP, A14
    (c) Display μP, A6
    (d) Shared memory, A12

19. In the A/D converter in Figure 13.7, the applied voltage $V_{ANAL} = 3.75$ V. How many threshold detectors will indicate an excess of 1 V on the input?

PART III
Specialized Medical Equipment

14. Clinical Laboratory Equipment

15. Medical X-Ray Equipment

16. Ultrasonic Equipment

14

Clinical Laboratory Equipment

Most hospitals have a laboratory area separate from patient areas that is used solely for chemical analyses and measurements of body fluids and tissues. Typically, analysis is done on blood and urine and on body tissue. These measurements are made to aid physicians in the diagnosis of disease states and to help them monitor the effects of therapy. For example, when oxygen therapy is given to a patient it is necessary to frequently monitor the partial pressure of oxygen and carbon dioxide in the patient's blood. Accuracy of measurement is critical in the laboratory. And because the chemical parameters are sensitive to environmental factors such as temperature, light, and humidity, equipment calibration must constantly be monitored. The chemical solutions are often active, and cause aging and wearing effects that may impair accuracy. These effects are most clearly evident in the chemical electrode.

14.1 CHEMICAL ELECTRODES

Chemical electrodes produce a potential that depends on the ionic concentration of fluids under test. As discussed in Chapter 2, these potentials are determined by the Goldman equation (Equation 2.4) or the Nernst equation (Equation 2.5). These equations show that these potentials are directly proportional to temperature. Ions that are of particular interest in body fluid analysis include calcium, potassium, sodium, lithium, and the chlorides.

Chemical electrodes range in complexity from a simple solid in contact with the solution under test to multiple-element structures. A chloride membrane electrode, for example, consists of a silver chloride membrane on the tip of a glass tube. A wire from one side of the membrane connects to a high-impedance voltmeter. The membrane potential is a function of the chloride content of perspiration on the skin in contact with the electrode.

The pH Electrode

The pH of normal blood must be maintained within a narrow range in human beings. Therefore, electrodes for accurate and convenient measurement of pH are essential. Furthermore, the pH electrode is a component from which more complex electrodes may be constructed.

The Goldman equation, Equation (2.4), shows that electrolyte membrane potentials are proportional to the logarithm of the ion concentration. In a solution containing the hydrogen ion, a membrane separating two solutions has a potential proportional to the hydrogen $[H^+]$ ion concentration. For example, at 25 °C,

$$V_m = -60 \log [H^+] + C \qquad \text{(in mV)}$$

where C is a constant. Usually, pH meters are calibrated so that the effect of this constant is cancelled. The pH is a measure of the hydrogen ion concentration and is defined as

$$pH = -\log[H^+]$$

Therefore,

$$V_m = 60 \text{ pH} + C$$

In a pH meter, illustrated in Figure 14.1, the constant C is compensated for by calibration so that the meter scale is proportional to pH. V_m is also proportional to the absolute temperature, T, and ranges from zero to several tenths of a volt. The pH electrode consists of a reference terminal and an active terminal. The reference terminal uses a metal, in this case silver-silver chloride (Ag-AgCl), in a potassium chloride electrolyte. A salt bridge consisting of a fiber wick saturated with KCl is inert to the solution under test. However, it maintains the KCl at the potential of the solution and keeps the reference terminal potentials essentially the same regardless of the solution under test. The active terminal is sealed with common glass except for a tip made of pH-sensitive glass. The pH-sensitive glass consists of a hydrated gelatinous glass layer. Its membrane potential is proportional to the log $[H^+]$ and therefore is proportional to the pH of the solution under test. The pH-sensitive glass very slowly dissolves in solution, taking as long

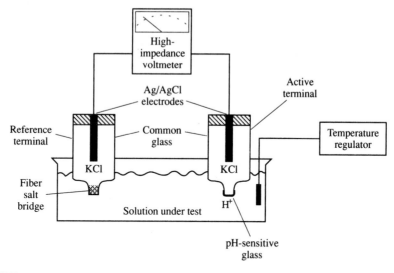

FIGURE 14.1
A pH meter.

as several years to become ineffective. In general, all boundary potentials in the electrode except those across the pH-sensitive glass are independent of the solution, so long as the temperature remains constant. The temperature is held constant in a pH meter by thermal compensation circuits that control the temperature of the sample chamber, as shown in Figure 14.1.

The care of pH electrodes includes cleaning to avoid contamination by the sample solution. They must be replaced periodically because they are a wearing element. To compensate for unknown variables, the meter is calibrated with a solution of known pH when used for tests in the clinical setting.

Troubleshooting Tip

pH electrodes are wearing elements that may fail because of aging.

The pH electrode is also a building block of other chemical electrodes. In particular, it is a component of blood gas analyzer electrodes.

14.2 A BLOOD GAS ANALYZER

A major function of blood is to carry oxygen to the cells and carbon dioxide to the lungs for expiration. These gases mix with the blood to form a partial pressure in the blood.

A blood gas analyzer is used to measure the partial pressure of oxygen, PO_2, the partial pressure of carbon dioxide, PCO_2, and the blood pH. The fundamental measurement from which the others are derived is the pH measurement. In normal blood this must be maintained between 7.34 and 7.44, slightly basic. pH readings from 0 to 7 are acidic, and readings from 7 to 14 are basic. Since pH measurements are very dependent on temperature, that parameter is carefully regulated to normal body temperature, 37 °C. A pH electrode, as illustrated in Figure 14.1, may be used in a blood gas analyzer. Again, because errors in measurement can cause a dangerous misdiagnosis of disease, careful calibration procedures are followed.

The PCO_2 Electrode

The pH electrode is used as a component of a PCO_2 electrode to measure the partial pressure of CO_2 by the arrangement shown in Figure 14.2. Blood or another fluid to be measured enters a sample chamber and comes in contact with a teflon or silicon rubber membrane. This membrane separates the fluid from a sodium solution but is permeable to the CO_2 in the solution. The CO_2 combines with water so as to produce free hydrogen ions in the sodium solution. This changes the solution pH in proportion to the partial pressure of CO_2 in the blood.

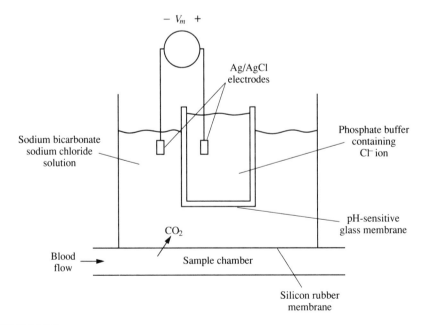

FIGURE 14.2
A cell for measuring PCO_2.

A chemical reaction in the electrode is

$$H_2O + CO_2 \rightleftharpoons H_2CO_3 \rightarrow H^+ + HCO_3^-$$

Notice here that the CO_2 is proportional to the hydrogen ion, H^+. The pH meter then measures pH-sensitive membrane voltage, V_m, which in turn is proportional to the pH. The voltmeter is calibrated in units of $^PCO_2$. The electrode is maintained at body temperature with temperature-regulating circuits. The input impedance of the electrode ranges from 50 to 1000 MΩ; therefore a high-input-impedance voltmeter is required. One form of the $^PCO_2$ electrode is called a Severinghaus electrode, named for its developer.

The $^PO_2$ Electrode

The $^PO_2$ electrode known as a Clark electrode, in honor of its inventor, is an oxygen sensor for blood. It consists of two chambers separated by a polypropylene membrane that is permeable to oxygen. The blood sample is injected into the lower sample chamber, as illustrated in Figure 14.3. The upper chamber contains the electrode. The O_2 in the blood permeates the

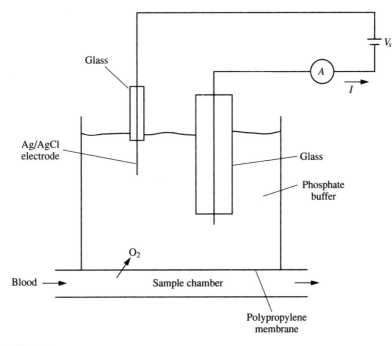

FIGURE 14.3
The Clark electrode for $^PO_2$.

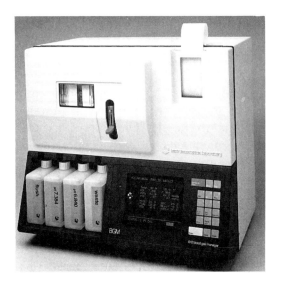

FIGURE 14.4
A blood gas analyzer with an electronic display and hard-copy printout. (Courtesy of Instrumentation Laboratory, Fisher Medical Division)

polypropylene membrane and reacts chemically with a phosphate buffer contained in the upper chamber. The buffer maintains the solution pH at a constant level. The O_2 combines with water in the buffer, producing electrons in proportion to the number of oxygen molecules according to the formula

$$O_2 + 2H_2O + 4e^- \rightarrow 4OH^-$$

The electron current I is measured by the ammeter A in Figure 14.3. The electron current is proportional to the $^PO_2$. The electrons on the left side of the equation that drive the reaction are provided by a source voltage, V_s, that polarizes the electrode and has a value between 0.4 and 0.8 V. The need for this polarizing voltage gives rise to the name *polarographic* electrode for the Clark electrode. The meter scale is then calibrated in units of partial pressure of oxygen ($^PO_2$) in the blood.

This electrode depends on current flow rather than membrane potential, as was the case with the pH-electrode-based devices. As with the other electrodes, procedures for calibration for environmental effects, electrode aging, corrosion, and contamination must be developed and followed.

A blood gas analyzer that measures blood serum pH, $^PCO_2$, and $^PO_2$ is illustrated in Figure 14.4. The sample is drawn into the instrument

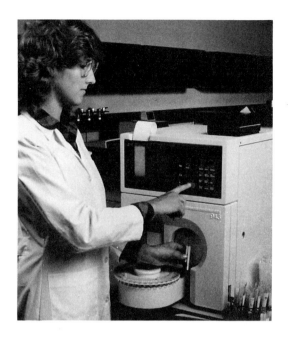

FIGURE 14.5
A laboratory technician analyzing samples. (Courtesy of Instrumentation Laboratory, Fisher Medical Division)

through a capillary. The measured quantities appear on a front panel display and are printed on paper to provide hard copy. In order to calibrate the instrument, two known solutions of pH 7.384 and 6.840 are used. After each sample, a flushing solution cleans the tubing and sample chambers and ejects the waste into the container shown. The laboratory technician in Figure 14.5 is injecting samples for automatic chemical analysis.

Noninvasive Blood Gas Monitoring

The blood gas analyzer described in the previous section makes measurements on blood samples drawn from a patient and carried to the instrumentation. The process has the disadvantages of discomfort to the patient in drawing the blood and a time delay in obtaining the data. Real-time, immediately available measurement of $^PO_2$ and $^PCO_2$, as well as oxyhemoglobin saturation SaO_2, can be achieved by use of noninvasive transducers applied directly to the surface of the skin. Such monitoring instrumentation is especially valuable in the OR, where immediate knowledge of the patient's oxygen and carbon dioxide is of critical importance.

It has long been known that both O_2 and CO_2 diffuse through the skin, as well as through the alveoli of the lung. Although the diffusion is minimal, it can be increased significantly by heating the skin. Therefore, to measure the $^PO_2$, the Clark electrode in Figure 14.3 can be modified by placing it in a heating coil that heats the skin. The polypropylene membrane is placed against the skin, and O_2 passes through it into the electrode, where it can be measured as described earlier.

In a similar manner the $^PCO_2$ electrode may also be modified. Its silicon rubber membrane is then placed against the patient's skin so that real-time $^PCO_2$ measurement can be made.

The $^PO_2$ can also be measured optically by using the fact that oxygenated blood tends to be red, and low-oxygen blood tends to be blue. About 98% of oxygen in the blood combines with hemoglobin (Hb) to form oxyhemoglobin (HbO_2). The ratio of HbO_2 to Hb in the blood is called the percentage oxyhemoglobin saturation (SaO_2). SaO_2 also is related in a known manner to $^PO_2$ for given values of blood pH and temperature. To measure SaO_2 optically, two light-emitting diodes are used side by side to illuminate the tissue, such as a finger tip. One light is red and the other is near infrared. The absorption of the red light is very dependent on the SaO_2, and the infrared light is independent of this value. Therefore the ratio of the light intensity as detected on corresponding photodetector diodes can be used to drive an output display calibrated to give the SaO_2 value. A finger transducer for monitoring blood gas is shown in Figure 14.6. In addition to measuring the SaO_2, the instrument shown in Figure 14.7 measures the end tidal CO_2 ($ETCO_2$). This instrument is called a pulse oximeter, end tidal (POET).

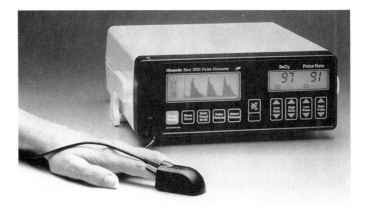

FIGURE 14.6
The saturated blood oxygen (SaO_2) and pulse rate are measured noninvasively through a finger. (Courtesy of Ohmeda)

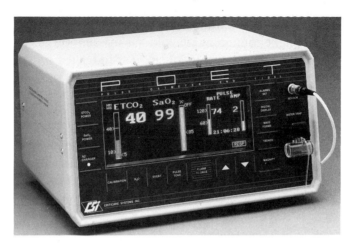

FIGURE 14.7
A device for monitoring O_2 and CO_2. (Courtesy of Criticare Systems, Inc.)

14.3 PHOTOMETERS AND COLORIMETERS

The chemical content of biological substances can be determined by measuring how they either absorb or emit visible light. The colorimeter uses light absorption to determine blood proteins and iron levels. In order to enhance the color of these substances in blood serum, it is necessary to mix it with reagents. Measurements of light emitted by ions, such as sodium or potassium in serum or urine, excited by heat are made with a flame photometer.

A colorimeter consists of a light source broken into its spectrum of colors by a prism or diffraction grating. The individual colors are then passed through the sample. The amount of each color absorbed is measured to determine the type and concentration of substances in the sample. Since these measurements are highly temperature dependent, control of this parameter is necessary.

Diffraction Gratings

Colorimeters and spectrophotometers, which are used to measure the light transmitted and absorbed as it passes through a sample, typically use diffraction gratings to break the light source into individual colors, as defined by their frequencies and wavelengths.

A diffraction grating consists of slits, or openings, on an opaque plate, as illustrated in Figure 14.8. The slits are spaced D meters apart. For each color there is an angle, ϕ, with respect to the plane of the grating, in the direction of which path lengths from adjacent slits differ by integer numbers of wavelengths. Therefore the color experiences constructive interference along that path, which makes it visible to an observer. In Figure 14.8, white light containing all colors is incident on the left side of the plate. An observer moving around a circle as indicated on the right side of the plate would see violet, yellow, or red depending on his or her position. A flame photometer may be constructed with photodetectors at each of those positions. They are interconnected to the potassium, sodium, and lithium channels of the flame photometer.

To find the directional angle ϕ, observe that the difference in path length to an observation point from adjacent slits in Figure 14.8 may be defined as $M\lambda$, where M is an integer $1, 2, 3, \ldots$, etc.

It is left as an exercise (Exercise 7) to show that

$$M\lambda = D \cos \phi \qquad\qquad (14.1)$$

for values of λ for which there is constructive interference at the observation point. In other words, the angle ϕ at which an observer sees the color having a wavelength λ may be computed from Equation (14.1).

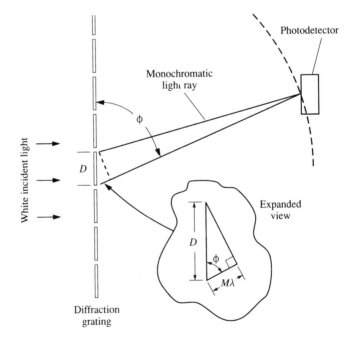

FIGURE 14.8
A diffraction grating showing an incident beam of white light, and a ray of monochromatic light emerging.

In order to cause light of different wavelengths to take a path through the sample under test to the photodetector, it is possible to rotate the diffraction grating on its axis, while holding the detector in one position. By measuring the detector output versus its angle of rotation, it is then possible to record the sample absorption versus light wavelength, or color. This data then leads to the identity of these substances and their concentration.

Flame Photometers

A flame photometer is used to analyze urine or blood in order to determine the concentration of potassium (K), sodium (Na), and lithium (Li). Sodium and potassium are present in normal urine. Lithium is used as a calibrating substance, unless it appears in the serum or urine because of medication.

The first use of flame as a spectroscopic source is attributed to Bunsen and Kirchhoff in 1860. Automated flame photometers came into use after 1945.

A flame photometer operates on the same principle as that used for chemical analysis with a Bunsen burner. A liquid sample, as shown in Figure 14.9, is aspirated into the flame by the gas and air mixture. Depending upon the chemical content of the sample, the flame has different colors resulting from high-temperature thermal collisions that force atoms into excited states. For medical analysis, the commonly analyzed ions, and the respective colors they make in the flame as the excited atoms return to the ground state, are as follows:

Element	Color	Wavelength (Å)
Potassium, K	violet	4047
Sodium, Na	yellow	5890
Lithium, Li	red	6708

The actual intensity of the color is quite variable because of changes in the flow rate of the gas that draws the sample into the flame. Electronic circuitry is used to compensate for the variations.

The light from the flame in the flame photometer is filtered, then directed along individual channels for the three major substances, Li, Na, and K. The simplest filter consists of colored glass. Violet glass, for example, passes violet color in the flame but rejects the other colors. It may be considered an optical filter. Glass filters generally cause relatively high attenuation of the light and tend to get hot. Flame photometers typically use diffraction gratings to filter the light, as described earlier.

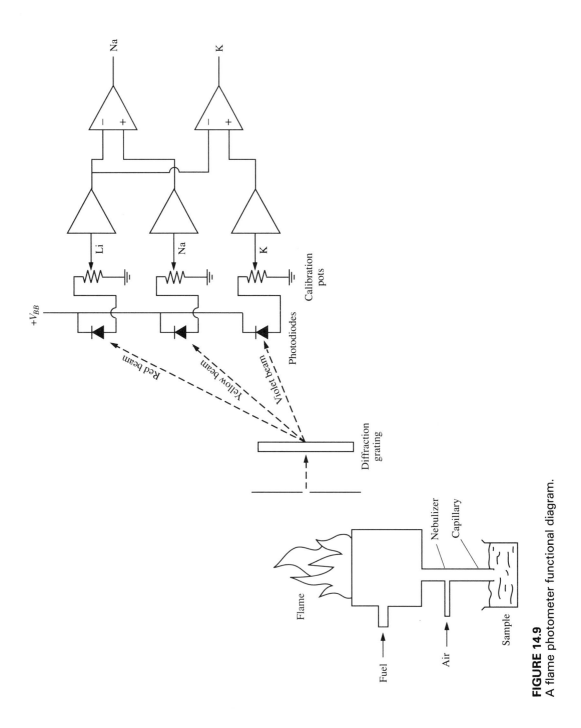

FIGURE 14.9
A flame photometer functional diagram.

The flame photometer illustrated in Figure 14.9 has a separate photodetector for each channel. The photodetector is a reverse-biased diode for which current increases as intensity of light incident upon it increases. Calibration potentiometers in each channel are used to calibrate the instrument with known, standard solutions.

The output of the Na and K channel is compared with that of the Li channel. In normal use the sample to be tested in this instrument should not contain an unknown amount of Li. Rather, a known, standard amount of Li is added to the sample. The output Na and K concentrations are calibrated in terms of differences with the known Li, called a *stock standard*. This procedure compensates for variations in the flame that are common to all channels.

EXAMPLE 14.2 In a flame photometer, the flame and aspirator have to be calibrated with lithium. The example calibration circuit in Figure 14.10 is adjusted such that the voltage V_{OUT} is zero when a known concentration of lithium is aspirated into the flame. In this case, the lithium causes a photodetector output of +2 V. Calculate the fraction needed to make $V_{OUT} = 0$, where the resistance of the potentiometer from the wiper arm down is αR_{OUT}.

SOLUTION Since V_{OUT} must be zero, we can calculate $I = 2/50\,\text{A} = 0.04\,\text{A}$. Because $V_{OUT} = 0$, the current through the 10-kΩ resistor is zero, so $I_1 = I = 0.04\,\text{A}$. The voltage $V_1 = -I(100) = -4\,\text{V}$. Then Kirchhoff's current law (KCL) at node 2 gives

$$\frac{V_2 - (-4)}{10} + \frac{V_2 - (-10)}{\alpha(100)} + \frac{V_2 - 10}{(1 - \alpha)(100)} = 0 \qquad \textbf{(14.2)}$$

and KCL at node 1 gives

$$\frac{-4 - V_2}{10} + (-0.04) + \frac{-4}{200} = 0$$

Solving this equation for V_2 gives $V_2 = -4.6\,\text{V}$. This value in Equation (14.2) gives

$$\frac{-4.6 + 4}{10} + \frac{-4.6 + 10}{100\alpha} + \frac{-4.6 - 10}{100(1 - \alpha)} = 0$$

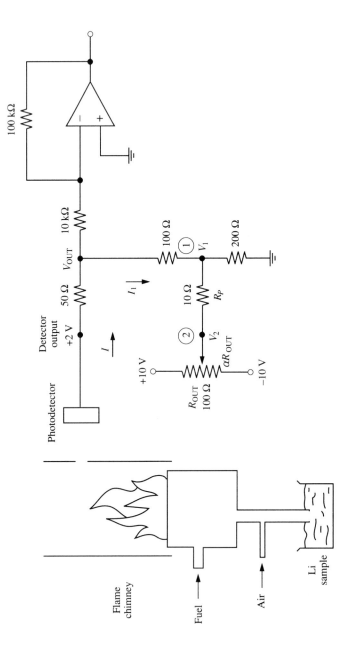

FIGURE 14.10
A simplified flame photometer calibration circuit.

Solving this for α we have

$$0.06\alpha^2 - 0.260\alpha + 0.054 = 0$$

$$\alpha = \frac{+0.260 \pm \sqrt{0.260^2 - 4(0.06)(0.054)}}{2(0.06)}$$

$$= 0.2183 \text{ or } 4.1$$

Since the solution 4.1 is greater than 1, it cannot be the correct value, so $\alpha = 0.2183$. If you repeat this exercise for the case that the resistor between the pot and V_1 is increased to 100 Ω, you will find that no value less than 1 exists. This means the circuit cannot be balanced. A faulty resistor that changed its value to 100 Ω could cause such a trouble.

14.4 BLOOD CELL COUNTER

Knowledge about the number of particles in blood is important data from which a physician can diagnose disease. These particles are commonly known as red blood cells (RBC), white blood cells (WBC), and platelets (PLT). They can be distinguished from each other by virtue of their size and density, as Table 14.1 shows. Because of these distinguishing features it is possible to use a microscope to count the particles or to use electronic circuitry to do the task automatically. Notice in the table that the RBCs are more numerous but smaller than the WBCs. Table 14.1 shows that most of the particles in blood are RBCs. To determine relative proportion of blood volume made up by cell particles, known as the *hematocrit* (*ht*), a centrifuge is used (the centrifuge is sometimes called a hematocrit also). The blood sample is placed on a test tube, which is spun so that the cells are packed on the bottom under centrifugal force. The *ht* value equals the height of the packed cells divided by the height of the blood in the tube. This is typically 45%.

TABLE 14.1
Blood Particles

Type	Density (millions/μl)	Individual size (μm)
RBC	4.26–6.2	6.8 to 7.5
PLT	0.15–0.40	2 to 4
WBC	0.004–0.011	6 to 18

The function of the red blood cell is to carry hemoglobin to the cells of the body. It is important to know the mean volume of each red blood cell (*MCV*) in liters. *MCV* is defined as

$$MCV = \frac{ht}{RBC} \quad \text{(in liters/cell)}$$

where *RBC* represents the density of red blood cells in cells per liter. A measure of hemoglobin is made by destroying the red blood cells with an acid and releasing the red color hemoglobin into solution 1 in a process called *lysing*. The hemoglobin is then separated and weighed. A measure of the mean cell hemoglobin (*MCH*) is then computed by the definition

$$MCH = \frac{\text{hemoglobin (g/liter)}}{RBC \ (\text{liter}^{-1})}$$

The units of *MCH* are grams per cell. The concentration of hemoglobin in the blood is then given by the mean cell hemoglobin concentration (*MCHC*) in grams per liter:

$$MCHC = \frac{\text{hemoglobin (g/liter)}}{ht}$$

A circuit for electronic measurement of the number of cell particles in the blood is shown in Figure 14.11. The transducer consists of an orifice through which the sample is drawn by a vacuum. Since the blood cells have high-resistance membranes, the cells in the orifice increase its resistance R_{OUT}. That is,

$$R_{OUT} = R + \Delta R \qquad \qquad \textbf{(14.3)}$$

where ΔR is the change in resistance due to a cell in the orifice and the value of the orifice resistance clear of cells is R. ΔR produced by each white blood cell is larger than that of a red blood cell or a platelet because its size is greater. The Wheatstone bridge in Figure 14.11 produces a voltage V_{OUT} due to changes in R_{OUT} as follows:

$$V_{OUT} = \left(\frac{R_{OUT}}{R_{OUT} + R} - \frac{1}{2} \right) V_{BB} = \left(\frac{R_{OUT} - R}{2(R_{OUT} + R)} \right) V_{BB} \qquad \textbf{(14.4)}$$

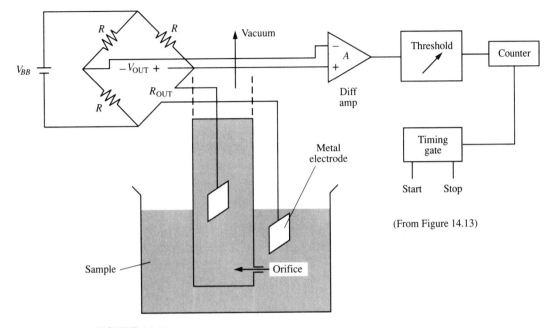

FIGURE 14.11
A circuit for electronic measurement of blood cell count.

where V_{BB} is the bias voltage on the bridge. Inserting Equation (14.3) into (14.4) gives

$$V_{\text{OUT}} = \frac{\Delta R}{4R + 2\Delta R} V_{BB}$$

$$\approx \frac{\Delta R}{4R} V_{BB} \qquad\qquad (14.5)$$

where $\Delta R \ll R$. Therefore V_{OUT} is proportional to ΔR, which is in turn proportional to the size of the blood cell in the orifice. In Figure 14.11, V_{OUT} is amplified by a differential amplifier of gain A. An oscilloscope trace of the output is illustrated in Figure 14.12. Notice that the highest peaks are fewest in number. These are due to the WBCs, which are correspondingly largest in size and fewest in number according to Table 14.1. The RBCs are represented by the peaks between threshold T_2 and T_1. They are much greater in number than the WBCs but make less resistance change in the orifice. In the operation of the instrument, the threshold is first set to zero and the counter will read N_0, the total number of particles per liter,

$$WBC + RBC + PLT = N_0 \qquad\qquad (14.6)$$

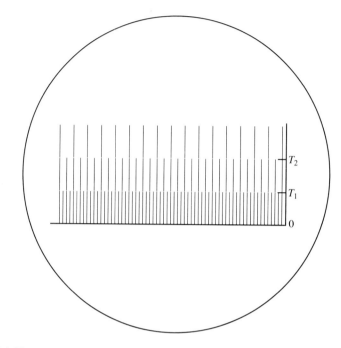

FIGURE 14.12
A blood cell counter display.

where WBC is the number of white blood cells per liter, RBC the number of red blood cells per liter, and PLT the number of platelets per liter. The threshold is then set to T_1 and the counter will read those signals that exceed the threshold and give the number N_1:

$$RBC + WBC = N_1 \qquad\qquad\qquad (14.7)$$

Then the threshold is set to T_2 and the counter will read just WBC. The RBC is then computed from Equation (14.7) and the PLT from Equation (14.6).

EXAMPLE 14.3 In Figure 14.11, the orifice resistance, when there are no blood cells of any type in it, is 1 kΩ. A single RBC in the orifice increases its resistance to 1.01 kΩ. What will be the output voltage V_{OUT} each time an RBC passes into the orifice? The bias voltage $V_{BB} = 10$ V.

SOLUTION The orifice resistance $R = 1$ kΩ. From Equation (14.3) we have $\Delta R = 1.01$ k$\Omega - 1$ k$\Omega = 10.0 \ \Omega$. Then from Equation (14.5),

$$V_{\text{OUT}} = \frac{10(10)}{4(1000)} = 25 \text{ mV}$$

EXAMPLE 14.4 A blood cell counter threshold is set to zero, and the output display reads 5.3100×10^{12} liter^{-1}. The threshold is then set to T_1 in Figure 14.12, and the output reading becomes 5.18×10^{12} liter^{-1}. The threshold is then set to T_2 and the output reading becomes $0.18 \times 10^{+12}$ liter^{-1}. Find *RBC*, *WBC*, and *PLT* in units of cells per liter.

SOLUTION The T_2 threshold reading is $WBC = 0.18 \times 10^{12}$. At threshold T_1 yields

$$RBC + WBC = 5.18 \times 10^{12}$$

Therefore $RBC = 5.18 \times 10^{12} - 0.18 \times 10^{12} = 5.0 \times 10^{12}$ cells per liter. Equation (14.6) then is used to find the platelets:

$$PLT = 5.31 \times 10^{12} - 5.0 \times 10^{12} - 0.18 \times 10^{12}$$

$$= 0.13 \times 10^{12} \text{ cells per liter}$$

The counter must be started and stopped over well-timed periods. A vacuum fluid arrangement for doing this timing is shown in Figure 14.13. To operate the mechanism, valves V and F are both initially opened. This draws a flushing solution through glass tubing into the waste to get rid of any bubbles. Valves F and V are then closed. A sample of dilute blood is then placed in the beaker and valve V is opened. The vacuum thus created will cause the sample to enter the orifice. Simultaneously the mercury will

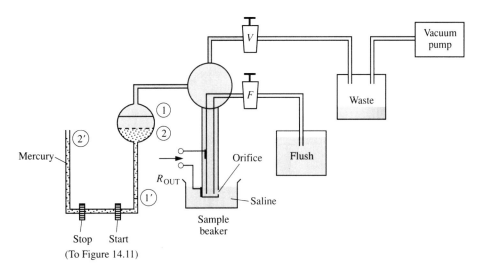

FIGURE 14.13
Glass tubing for a blood cell counter using a mercury timer.

be drawn up into the bulb so that it is confined between the levels 1 and 1'. Valve V is then closed, cutting off the vacuum pump from the sample and mercury. The mercury surface then moves from the levels 1 and 1' to become confined between the levels marked 2 and 2' in the figure as it seeks its own level because of the atmospheric pressure at both ends.

As the mercury surface travels from position 1-1' to position 2-2', it activates first the start switch to begin the counter. When it arrives at the stop switch the counter stops. As the mercury falls it also draws a fixed volume of the sample through the orifice. The counter therefore reads the number of particles per unit volume. This mechanism controls the rate of flow through the orifice so the digital display can be calibrated in units of cells per microliter.

Optical Methods of Cell Counting

The cell counts *RBC*, *WBC*, *PLT*, and *MCV* may also be determined by measuring the light scattered from each cell particle as it passes through an aperture, as illustrated in Figure 14.14. The blood is heavily diluted to reduce the number of particles counted to one at a time. A sheath fluid is directed around the blood stream to confine it to the center of the aperture. The cell is illuminated by a light source such as a laser. The angle of scattered light is different for different-size cells. The scattering angles of platelets and red blood cells are sufficiently separate that these two types of cells can be distinguished by directing the scattered light to different detectors. To separate white blood cells from red blood cells, it is necessary to destroy

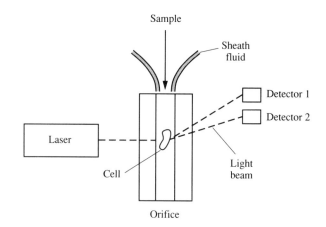

FIGURE 14.14
Optical cell counting.

the red blood cells with a lysing agent. This also frees the hemoglobin so that it can be measured. Instrumentation based on this principle presents a display of *RBC*, *WBC*, *PLT*, *ht*, *MCV*, *MCH*, and *MCHC*.

REFERENCES

Bender, G. T. *Principles of Chemical Instrumentation.* Philadelphia: W. B. Saunders, 1987.

Eggert, A. A. *Electronics and Instrumentation for the Clinical Laboratory.* New York: John Wiley & Sons, 1983.

Instrumentation Laboratory Staff. *IL 143/243 Service Manual.* Lexington, MA: Instrumentation Laboratory, Inc., 1973.

Norman, R. A. *Principles of Bioinstrumentation.* New York: John Wiley & Sons, 1988.

Sutphin, S. E. *Advanced Medical Instrumentation and Equipment.* Englewood Cliffs, NJ: Prentice-Hall, 1987.

EXERCISES

1. A pH electrode and its standard reference are immersed in a buffer of pH 5.25. The attached voltmeter measures a cell potential of 0.203 V. A solution of unknown pH replaces the buffer solution. The voltmeter now reads 0.39 V. Calculate the pH of the unknown solution.

2. Sodium measurements are made with a glass electrode and a calomel electrode reference, both immersed in a 0.15 molar sodium nitrate solution. A voltmeter measures a cell potential at 0.21 V. The sodium nitrate is now replaced with an unknown concentration of the substance. The voltmeter reads 0.25 V. Compute the concentration of sodium nitrate in the unknown.

3. The pH of a serum solution is 7.4 at 25 °C. What is the pH at 37 °C, normal body temperature?

4. In Figure 14.11, the resistance of the orifice is 1 kΩ when there are no blood cells of any type in it. A single RBC in the orifice increases its resistance to 1.02 kΩ. What will be the output voltage V_{OUT} each time an RBC passes into the orifice? The bias voltage $V_{BB} = 15$ V.

5. A blood cell counter threshold is set to zero, and the output display reads 6.32×10^{12} per liter. The threshold is then set to T_1 in Figure 14.12 and the output reading becomes 6.15×10^{12} per liter. The threshold is then set to T_2 and the output reading becomes 0.015×10^{12} per liter. Find the count of the RBC, WBC, and PLT.

6. Modify Example 14.2 such that the 10-Ω resistor is changed to $R_P = 100 \ \Omega$. All other conditions in the problem remain the same. Compute the value of α in the pot that balances the circuit and makes $V_{OUT} = 0$.

7. Adjacent slits in a diffraction grating are shown in Figure 14.8. Constructive interference occurs for those angles ϕ with the plane of the diffraction grating that make the path lengths an integer multiple M of the wavelength of the light, λ, incident on the grating. Show that constructive interference occurs when $M\lambda = D \cos \phi$, where $M = 1, 2, 3 \ldots$.

8. A diffraction grating has 600 grooves per millimeter. At what angle with the plane, ϕ, will the light be deflected from sodium in a flame of a flame photometer?

9. For the diffraction grating in Exercise 8, find the ϕ angles at which potassium light emerges.

10. Repeat Exercise 9 for lithium.

11. A blood gas analyzer measures the RBC count in a sample of blood at 5×10^{12} per liter. The mean cell volume (MCV) is 80 femtoliters (fl) (1 fl $= 10^{-15}$ liters). Find the percentage of the blood volume made up of RBCs. This quantity is called the hematocrit, ht.

12. Find the number of grams of hemoglobin per cell when a liter of blood in Exercise 11 contains 150 g of hemoglobin.

15

Medical X-Ray Equipment

15.1 X-RAYS

The discovery of x-rays by Roentgen in 1895 was a total surprise to him and everyone else at the time. He was not searching for a way to see into the body without surgery. Rather, he was investigating the cathode rays of a vacuum tube diode when he noticed changes being caused in photographic material, not directly involved with his experiments. His curiosity and his willingness to act on impulse and be diverted from the task at hand drove him to investigate further.

Within a period of only days he subsequently discovered that x-rays

- cause barium platinocyanide to exhibit fluorescence.
- affect photographic emulsions.
- discharge electrified objects.
- make certain materials transparent.
- can be collimated into pinholes.
- are created by a high-energy cathode-ray tube.
- are more efficiently produced by heavy elements.

Within two weeks of their discovery, x-rays were being used in medical diagnosis, and they have been indispensable ever since. When we consider that it took two centuries to develop the internal combustion engine, the lightning speed with which such a revolutionary technique as x-ray diagnosis appeared is nothing less than amazing.

What Roentgen did not discover, however, and what it took scientists about 50 years to fully appreciate is that x-rays can be dangerous when not properly used, and may cause cancer.

Over the years x-ray equipment has been continually improved. Major engineering objectives have been to

- improve the quality of the image.
- heighten the contrast between different tissues.
- improve size resolution.
- minimize the dose of x-rays used on the patient.

The X-Ray Tube

The x-ray tube is simply a glass-enclosed vacuum tube diode consisting of a cathode that thermally emits electrons and an anode that attracts these electrons. A functional diagram of an x-ray tube is given in Figure 15.1, which shows a filament-heated cathode, an anode, and a glass vacuum enclosure. The filament source voltage V_F causes a current I_F to flow through the filament coil, heating the cathode metal. Electrons in the cathode are boiled off the metal into the vacuum. In an x-ray the anode voltage V_A is high enough that these electrons are swept across to the anode and form the beam current, I_B. V_A on the tube is very high, on the order of 100 kV. This high voltage impels the electron to a very high velocity. Approximately 1% of the electrons upon entering the anode collide with atoms and produce x-rays. The x-rays then pass through the tube into space.

To understand how x-rays are produced it is necessary to first consider the beam current. Electrons are boiled off the heated cathode because thermal agitation gives them enough energy to escape from the bonding forces into tube vacuum. The value of that energy, called the work function, E_W,

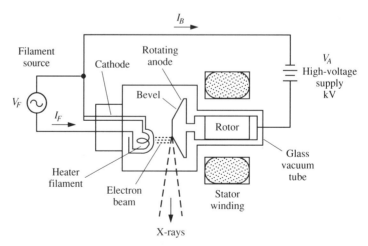

FIGURE 15.1
An x-ray tube with a rotating anode.

TABLE 15.1
X-Ray Tube Cathode Material Coefficients and Work Functions

Cathode	$C_0 \left(\dfrac{\text{A}}{\text{m}^2\text{K}^2} \right)$	E_W (eV)
Tungsten	60×10^4	4.52
Thoriated tungsten	3×10^4	2.63
Oxide coated	0.01×10^4	1

differs among metals. (See Table 15.1.) The value of the current in amperes due to thermal agitation, I_B, is derived from quantum mechanical considerations as

$$I_B = C_0 A_C T^2 e^{-11600 E_W/T} \tag{15.1}$$

where A_C is the cathode area in meters squared, and C_0 is the cathode material coefficient. Values of C_0 for several materials used in cathodes are listed in Table 15.1.

Box 1

FOR FURTHER INFORMATION

When V_A is low enough that a space charge forms around the cathode in the vacuum tube, the beam current is derived on the basis of electron physics as follows:

$$I_{BE} = 2.33(10^{-6}) \frac{V_A^{3/2}}{d^2} A_C \quad \text{(in amperes)}$$

where d is the distance in meters from the cathode to the anode, and A_C is the cathode area in square meters. In a properly designed x-ray tube, d is small enough that $I_B < I_{BE}$ for all medical x-ray tube anode voltages. Therefore I_B limits the current in the tube; that is, I_B represents the upper limit for the tube current. The current, I_{BE}, follows the preceding equation, known as the Langmuir-Childs law, and describes the current in typical power supply diodes (see Seely, Chapter 1), where V_A is low enough that a space charge forms around the tube.

Equation (15.1) calculates the beam current only under the assumption that the anode voltage V_A is large enough to sweep all electrons boiled off the cathode across the vacuum. This is usually the case in x-ray tubes. The current computed by Equation (15.1) is limited by the temperature, T, and is called the thermally limited current. If V_A is not high enough, however, a space charge of electrons will form around the cathode, and they will simply fall back into it. In that case Equation (15.1) does not compute the correct value of beam current. Rather, the current would be determined by the anode voltage and is called the electronic current, I_{BE}. Of course, when the x-ray tube voltage V_A is turned off, such a space charge is formed around the cathode. Further information about the electronic current is given in Box 1 on the preceding page.

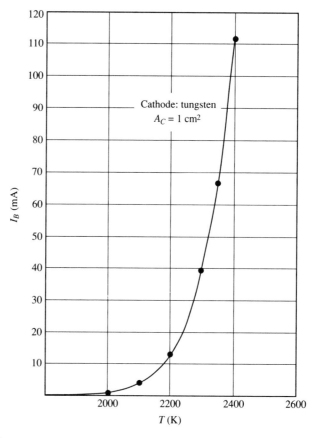

FIGURE 15.2
The thermally limited beam current versus cathode temperature of a tungsten cathode.

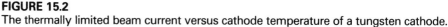

EXAMPLE 15.1 An x-ray tube has no space charge around the cathode. The cathode is tungsten, and it has a surface area of 1 cm². Plot the beam current versus temperature.

SOLUTION Using the values for tungsten from Table 15.1 in Equation (15.1) gives

$$I_B = (60 \times 10^4) A_C T^2 e^{-11600(4.52)/T}$$

The area is then $A_C = (1 \text{ cm}^2)(1 \text{ m}/100 \text{ cm})^2 = 10^{-4} \text{ m}^2$. Therefore,

$$I_B = 60 T^2 e^{-52432/T} \qquad \text{(in A)}$$

A plot of I_B is given in Figure 15.2.

Figure 15.2 shows that the beam current can be controlled with the temperature of the cathode. In x-ray tubes, this method is used. This is done by keeping the anode voltage high enough to prevent a space charge buildup around the cathode. To control the cathode temperature, the operator normally varies the filament voltage. This allows the operator to change the beam current while holding the anode voltage constant.

The Nature of X-Rays

An x-ray is produced by an electron beam when one of the electrons collides with an atom in the anode. The collision causes one of the orbiting electrons of the atom to shift to a higher energy orbit. It then falls back to its rest state and emits a photon of x-ray. This is known as *characteristic radiation*. The energy shifts, K_α and K_β, illustrated in Figure 15.3, represent different orbital shifts in the atom. Characteristic radiation is used to study the atomic structure of materials and is not typically used in medical x-ray applications. A second type of collision, scattering of the incident electron, produces a spectrum of x-ray radiation, called *bremsstrahlung radiation*. This radiation is caused by changes in the velocity of the beam electron that reduce its kinetic energy by a factor equal to the energy in the x-ray.

Bremsstrahlung radiation contains most of the x-ray energy. For this reason it is most important in medical applications, which are based on energy absorption rather than on the measurement of particular wavelengths, as in crystallographic studies using x-rays.

The effect of the anode voltage on the radiated photon energy is shown in Figure 15.4. Increased anode voltage at a constant beam current produces

Relative intensity

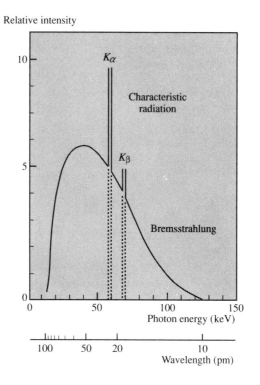

FIGURE 15.3
X-ray spectrum emitted by a tungsten anode at 130 kV. From B. Jacobson and J. G. Webster, *Medicine and Clinical Engineering*, Prentice-Hall. ©1977. p. 406. (Reprinted by permission of Prentice-Hall)

high-energy electrons in the beam. In fact, the energy of the electron, E_E, when it strikes the anode is given by

$$E_E = eV_A \qquad (15.2)$$

where e is the electronic charge on an electron [$e = 1.602 \times 10^{-19}$ coulomb (C)]. E_E is measured in units of electron-volts (eV). An *electron-volt* is defined as the energy acquired by an electron as it is accelerated through one volt. When the electron collides with an atom in the anode, it produces a photon of x-ray having an energy, in accordance with quantum mechanics, given by

$$E_P = hf \qquad (15.3)$$

where h is Planck's constant ($h = 6.625 \times 10^{-34}$ J-s) and f is the photon frequency. No radiated photon can have more energy than the electron that

Relative intensity

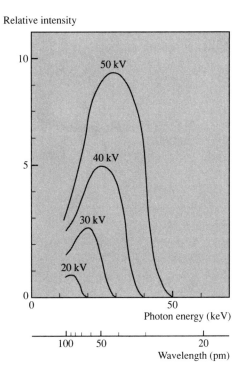

Photon energy (keV)

Wavelength (pm)

FIGURE 15.4
The effect of the anode voltage on the emission spectrum from an x-ray tube. From B. Jacobson and J. G. Webster, *Medicine and Clinical Engineering*, Prentice-Hall. ©1977. p. 405. (Reprinted by permission of Prentice-Hall)

produces it in collision. Therefore, in Figure 15.4, the photon bremsstrahlung energies do not exceed eV_A and are limited by the anode voltage.

EXAMPLE 15.2 For a 40-kV anode voltage, find the maximum photon energy of the radiated x-ray.

SOLUTION The maximum energy in the electron of the beam is eV. So the maximum electron energy $= 1.602 \times 10^{-19} \, (40 \times 10^3)$.

$$E_{P\text{max}} = 6.408 \times 10^{-15} \quad \text{(in J)}$$

X-ray photons have a frequency given by

$$f = c/\lambda \quad \quad \quad \textbf{(15.4)}$$

where c is the speed of light (3×10^8 m/s) and λ is the wavelength of the radiation in meters.

EXAMPLE 15.3 In the previous example, find the shortest wavelength contained in the x-ray beam.

SOLUTION   Combining Equations (15.3) and (15.4) yields

$$E_{P\text{max}} = \frac{hc}{\lambda_{\text{min}}}$$

or

$$\lambda_{\text{min}} = \frac{6.625(10^{-34})3(10^{8})}{6.408(10^{-15})}$$

$$= 0.3101 \times 10^{-10} \text{ m } (0.31 \text{ Å})$$

X-Ray Absorption

Medical x-ray imaging is done by applying x-rays to the surface of the body and measuring how much passes through. That is, the amount of x-rays absorbed by the body is measured by taking the difference of the input and output radiation energies. X-ray absorption is the basic mechanism for discrimination between organs in a body under x-ray observation. Bone tissue, for example, absorbs more x-ray than muscle, and therefore can be easily distinguished from it. Exactly how much x-ray is absorbed by different tissues is determined by Lambert's law. He observed that with x-rays, equal thicknesses of material absorb equal proportions of radiation $\mathfrak{I}$. In other words, the fraction of x-ray energy absorbed is proportional to the thickness of the material absorbing it. Lambert's law is stated mathematically as

$$\frac{d\mathfrak{I}}{\mathfrak{I}} = -\mu\rho \, ds \qquad \textbf{(15.5)}$$

where ρ is the medium density (g/cm^3), s is the distance through the material, and μ is a proportionality constant called the *mass attenuation coefficient*. The units of μ are cm^2/g. The symbol $d\mathfrak{I}$ represents the differential change in the x-ray intensity, and ds is the differential change in distance. Solution of Equation (15.5) as given in Box 2 yields the formula

$$\mathfrak{I} = \mathfrak{I}_0 e^{-\mu\rho s} \qquad \text{(in W/m}^2\text{)} \qquad \textbf{(15.6)}$$

where $\mathfrak{I}_0$ is the x-ray intensity incident on the tissue, and $\mathfrak{I}$ is the intensity of x-rays that emerge from the tissue of thickness s.

Box 2

CALCULUS FOR CLARITY

To prove that Equation (15.6) is a solution of Equation (15.5), simply differentiate both sides of Equation (15.6). This gives

$$\frac{d\mathcal{I}}{ds} = \mathcal{I}_0(-\mu\rho)e^{-\mu\rho s}$$

$$= -\mu\rho\mathcal{I}$$

Rearranging the terms yields

$$\frac{d\mathcal{I}}{\mathcal{I}} = -\mu\rho\, ds$$

which gives back Equation (15.5) and proves the statement.

Values for μ in units of cm^2/g are given in Figure 15.5, illustrating the relative values for bone and muscle. Also, typical densities of biological tissues are included in Table 15.2. It is apparent that to study bone a physician should use a low anode voltage, say 60 kV, so that it is easy to distinguish it from muscle. On the other hand, if the physician wishes to blank out the bone to distinguish underlying muscle tissue from fat, he or she should use a high anode voltage, say 200 kV. It is apparent from Table 15.2 that the densities of the soft tissues are not widely different. Fur-

TABLE 15.2
Density of Common
Biological Materials

Material	Density (g/cm³)
Air	0.0013
Water	1.0
Muscle	1.06
Fat	0.91
Bone	1.85

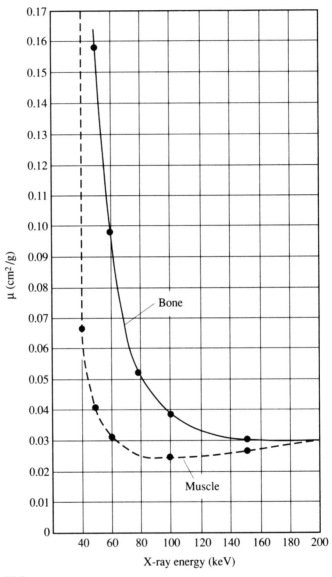

FIGURE 15.5
The mass attenuation coefficient versus the x-ray photon energy.

thermore, the μ values are nearly equal. Therefore, it is difficult to get large values of contrast between soft tissues using x-ray.

EXAMPLE 15.4   Suppose the incident x-ray intensity on water is 1 W/cm^2. Compute the intensity that emerges from a container of water 2 cm thick.

The photon energy is 20 keV, and the corresponding mass attenuation is 0.523 cm^2/g.

SOLUTION

$$\mathcal{I}_{H_2O} = 1 \ W/cm^2 e^{-(0.523 \ cm^2/g)(1 \ g/cm^3)(2 \ cm)}$$

$$= e^{-2(0.523)} = 0.3513 \ W/cm^2$$

EXAMPLE 15.5 Suppose the incident x-ray on bone is 1 W/cm^2. Compare the energy emerging from bone with a density of 1.2 g/cm^3 having the dimensions of Example 15.4, with the result 0.3513 W/cm^2 for $\mathcal{I}_{H_2O}$. At 20 kV, the mass attenuation constant for bone is 2.51 cm^2/g.

SOLUTION

$$\mathcal{I}_B = 1 \ e^{-(2.51)(1.2)(2)} = 0.0024 \ W/cm^2$$

Notice that the ratio of

$$\frac{\mathcal{I}_B}{\mathcal{I}_{H_2O}} = \frac{0.0024}{0.3513} = 0.0068 \ (-21.7 \ dB)$$

and that this is a power ratio.

Obviously the x-ray intensity emitted from water is far greater than that emitted from bone. This means that the bone absorbs more x-ray energy than water. Furthermore, this difference in x-ray intensities on film will produce an image having good contrast properties.

Tissue Contrast

The contrast in the image on film made by two tissues is defined in terms of the relative intensities of the x-rays that reach the film. $\mathcal{I}_1$ is the intensity of x-rays emitted from tissue 1 and $\mathcal{I}_2$ is the intensity of x-rays emitted from tissue 2. The contrast between the two tissues is then defined by the equation

$$C_{12} = 10 \log \frac{\mathcal{I}_1}{\mathcal{I}_2} \quad \text{(in dB)} \quad (15.7)$$

Here the multiplier 10 is used because the ratio $\mathcal{I}_1$ to $\mathcal{I}_2$ is a power ratio. Applying Equation (15.6) then yields

$$C_{12} = 10 \log \frac{\mathcal{I}_0 e^{-\mu_1 \rho_1 s_1}}{\mathcal{I}_0 e^{-\mu_2 \rho_2 s_2}}$$

where s_1 is the thickness of tissue 1 and s_2 is the thickness of tissue 2. Manipulation of this equation yields

$$C_{12} = 10(\log e)(\mu_2\rho_2 s_2 - \mu_1\rho_1 s_1)$$

or

$$C_{12} = 4.3429(\mu_2\rho_2 s_2 - \mu_1\rho_1 s_1) \text{ dB} \qquad (15.8)$$

From this equation we conclude that the contrast between two tissues depends on their mass attenuation coefficient, density, and thickness. In fact, C_{12} increases with differences between these parameters.

15.2 X-RAY EQUIPMENT BLOCK DIAGRAM

The basic components that must be part of any medical diagnostic x-ray unit are shown in Figure 15.6. In general, the purpose of these components is to create an x-ray image of high density, high contrast, and high sharp-

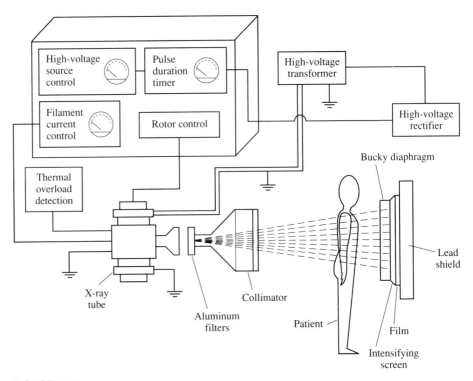

FIGURE 15.6
A block diagram of an x-ray machine.

ness on film or other imaging device. This must be done while minimizing the dose of ionizing radiation given to the patient. The *density*, or darkness, of the image is proportional to the amount of x-rays that penetrate the film, and would increase in proportion to x-ray tube beam current, for example. *Contrast* is a measure of the darkness of a desired image compared to its surroundings, and it is basically determined by the relative attenuation of the object. This factor is often directly affected by x-ray beam voltage. *Sharpness*, or clarity of the edges, is reduced in an image by blurring due to distortions in the x-ray beam as it passes from the x-ray tube to the patient.

A high-voltage source from 20 to 200 kV is necessary in order to produce x-rays at the x-ray tube anode. However, the duration of time the high voltage is applied to the tube must be carefully limited, in order that the patient does not receive an excessive dose, the film does not become overexposed, and the x-ray tube does not overheat. Since the x-ray tube is operated in its thermally limited mode, the x-ray intensity in watts per square meter is adjusted by the x-ray tube filament current. As a protection against overheating, the temperature of the tube anode is monitored with a temperature detector. If it exceeds a specified value, a thermal overload will be detected, and the high-voltage supply will be turned off automatically. This will eliminate the source of heat and cause the x-ray tube to turn off. Most x-ray tube anodes are rotated by induction-motor action in order to limit the beam power on any one spot and to help cool the anode. The voltage level from the high-voltage source in Figure 15.6 is amplified passively by a high-voltage transformer to the 20–200-kV level. It is then rectified and passed through the x-ray tube, which will pass conventional current in only one direction, from anode to cathode. X-rays produced by the tube anode are either absorbed in lead or collimated through the x-ray tube opening. Since most of the power in the medical x-ray is bremsstrahlung radiation, it contains a broad range of frequencies. The x-rays at unwanted frequencies only increase the patient dose and decrease image contrast. Aluminum filters cut to an appropriate thickness absorb lower x-ray frequencies and reduce these negative effects. The intensity of low-frequency, or soft, x-rays incident on the patient is reduced by use of an aluminum filter. Soft x-rays do not contribute significantly to diagnostic data in many procedures, but they do increase the overall dose. Thus the aluminum serves an important function. Another means of reducing patient dose is to confine the x-rays to the region of interest on the body. An external collimator between the patient and the filters serves this function by limiting the mass of the body exposed to x-rays.

X-rays inside the patient create x-ray scattering, which tends to blur the images. To absorb the scattered x-rays and eliminate the subsequent blurring, the radiologist uses a lead grid called a *Bucky diaphragm*, which is tapered to pass the x-rays incident on the patient. Radiation following these x-ray paths strikes the film and leaves an image as desired, while the scattered x-rays are absorbed by the Bucky.

The X-Ray Tube

An x-ray tube is an expensive wearing element in medical radiological equipment, costing thousands of dollars and requiring replacement as often as twice a year in many x-ray machines. The wearing mechanism is the tungsten of the cathode, which boils off to produce the electron beam. The approximately 1% efficiency of the tube means that 99% of the electron beam energy must be dissipated as heat. This heat flow through the anode, caused by the electron beam striking it, raises its temperature to destructive levels if it is not limited. Rotating the anode at speeds ranging from 3,600 to 10,000 rpm, with an electric motor armature, as illustrated in Figure 15.7, spreads the heat over a larger mass and allows it to be dissipated by radiation. A cutaway view of an x-ray tube in Figure 15.7(a) shows the rotating anode (1), which would normally be directly in line with the cathode (2). An x-ray tube is shown in its mounting, including the stator used to rotate the anode, in Figure 15.7(b).

For any tube, the amount of heat that can be dissipated is fixed. This means that the joules of heat energy that can be absorbed by the anode of a given tube over a given time period are also fixed. Since the energy absorbed by the anode is proportional to the product of the anode voltage V_A, the beam current I_B, and the exposure time T_D, a set of curves called the *x-ray tube rating chart* must be consulted to find the maximum exposure time for a given tube V_A or I_B. An example curve is given in Figure 15.8 for a hypothetical tube.

EXAMPLE 15.6   A physician orders 100-keV x-rays to be delivered at a beam current of 330 mA. Using the tube rating chart given in Figure 15.8, find the maximum time the tube may be turned on without overheating.

SOLUTION   The current 330 mA on the 100-kV curve of the x-ray tube rating chart intersects with the time $T_D = 0.2$ s, the maximum exposure time allowed.

The efficiency, η, of the x-ray tube is equal to the ratio of the power emitted in the x-ray beam to the power in the electron beam producing x-rays. That is, the power of the x-ray beam, P_X, is proportional to V_A^2. Also, large values of both I_B and the atomic number of the material, Z, increase the probability of a collision of the beam electron with an atom of

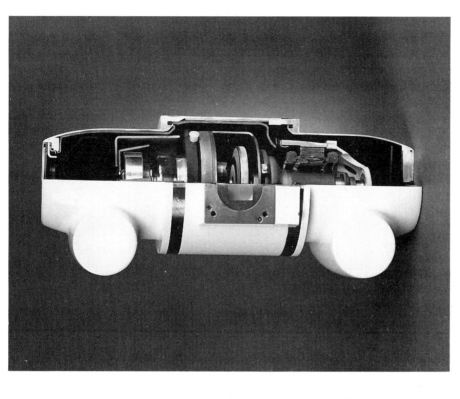

(b)

(a)

FIGURE 15.7
(a) A cutaway view of an x-ray tube. (b) An x-ray tube mounted in its casing showing the stator to rotate the anode. (Courtesy of Tubemaster, Inc.)

459

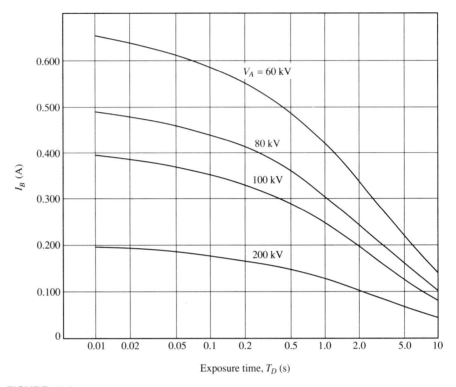

FIGURE 15.8
The tube exposure time limit at given current and anode voltage levels.

the anode material. Therefore, the power, P_X, in the x-ray beam is proportional to all of these factors, as

$$P_X = kI_B Z V_A^2$$

where k is a proportionality constant. The power in the electron beam is just $V_A I_B$. The tube efficiency, η, is defined as the ratio of P_X to the power in the electron beam. Therefore

$$\eta = \frac{kI_B Z V_A^2}{I_B V_A}$$

$$= kZV_A \tag{15.9}$$

Empirically the constant k is determined to be $k = 1.4 \times 10^{-9}$, in units of V^{-1}.

EXAMPLE 15.7 Compute the efficiency of a tungsten anode x-ray tube operating at an anode voltage of 100 kV.

SOLUTION The atomic number $Z = 74$ for tungsten. Therefore Equation (15.9) becomes

$$\eta = (1.4 \times 10^{-9})(74)(10^5) = 0.0104$$

So

$$\eta = 1.04\%$$

The anode is beveled, as shown in Figure 15.1. The bevel directs the x-rays out the side of the tube. The desired x-rays pass through a slot into a collimator arranged as shown in Figure 15.6. Some of the x-rays from the anode scatter about in the tube and are absorbed by lead shielding.

The Collimator

In order to reduce the dose of x-rays to the patient, the beam should not strike any more of the body than necessary. The necessary shaping of the x-ray beam is done with a collimator, as illustrated in Figure 15.9. The shut-

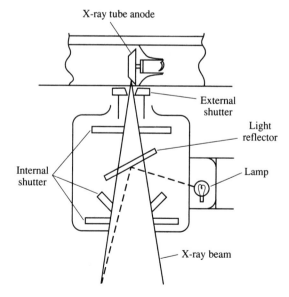

FIGURE 15.9
A collimator for directing x-rays at the patient.

ters consist of a heavy metal to absorb unwanted x-rays. A lamp and reflective mirror that make a visible pattern on the patient, so that the attendant can tell where the x-rays will strike, can be used to align the beam.

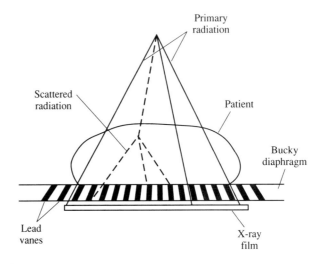

FIGURE 15.10
A Bucky grid for reducing the effects of x-ray scattering in the patient.

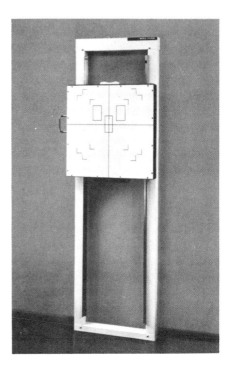

FIGURE 15.11
A vertical Bucky stand for patient-erect radiographic studies of the chest. (Courtesy of Raytheon Medical Systems)

The Bucky Grid

After x-rays enter a patient, some rays are deflected off their straight-line course by close encounters with atoms. This is called *scattering*, and it causes a smearing of the image at the edges and deteriorates image sharpness. The sharpness of the image is recovered by use of a Bucky grid, illustrated in Figure 15.10. Here slots are arranged in lead so that rays traveling in straight lines from the x-ray tube through the patient will strike the film, whereas scattered radiation will strike the lead lining the slots and be absorbed. Since some x-rays are lost by this process, the density of the image will be diminished and slots themselves will block some of the film and reduce the image resolution. The Bucky grid is part of the vertical Bucky stand illustrated in Figure 15.11.

The X-Ray Detector

The x-rays now pass into a film sensitive to both x-rays and light, such as silver bromide. Since the film is relatively insensitive to x-ray, a phosphor coating, such as shown in Figure 15.12, is used to produce light when hit by x-rays. The amount of x-rays captured is increased by placing a material with a high atomic number, called a Hi-Z screen, above the phosphor. This introduces secondary radiation by the scattering process. Although this scattering would tend to decrease the image sharpness, the effect is minimal because the high-Z screen is immediately adjacent to the phosphor, and the deflected x-rays travel only a small distance.

A special-purpose x-ray machine for radiographic studies of the female breast, called a mammograph, is shown in Figure 15.13. The patient stands

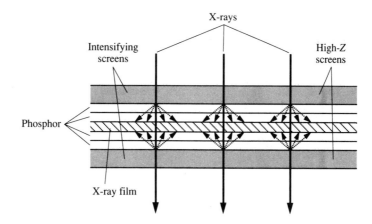

FIGURE 15.12
An image-intensifying film.

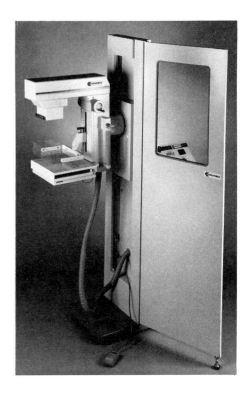

FIGURE 15.13
A mammograph for detection of female
breast tumors. (Courtesy of Kramex)

to the left of the shield, and the attendant stands behind it to operate the
controls.

The Power Supply

The power supply for an x-ray machine plays a crucial and active role in
x-ray production. The radiation is turned on and off in the power supply.
It is used to control the x-ray energy and consequently the image contrast,
as well as the beam current and consequently the image density. Thermal
overload from the x-ray tube anode creates signals that turn the power supply off as appropriate. The power supply must be large to handle several
kilowatts of power and several hundred kilovolt levels. At such high voltages, safety precautions are necessary. The voltage breakdown of air at sea
level is 75 kV/in. Therefore, at x-ray voltages, a conductor, such as a technician's hand, within several inches of a high-voltage terminal can draw a
deadly arc of voltage. As a safety precaution when working on x-ray power
supplies, a technician should turn off all power supplies, if possible, and
the capacitors should be discharged before components are touched.

A simplified x-ray block diagram for a single-phase power supply is
shown in Figure 15.14. The kV to the x-ray tube are controlled by adjust-

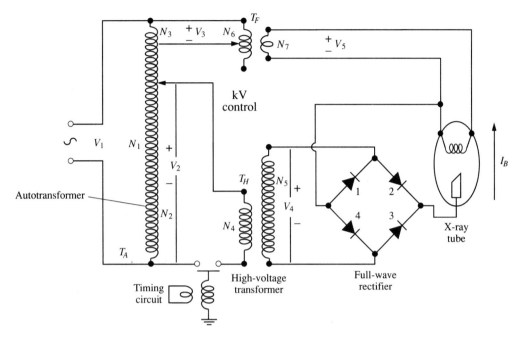

FIGURE 15.14
A single-phase high-voltage power supply.

ing N_2 on the low-voltage autotransformer varactor T_A. The low voltage prevents arcing of the transformer wiper arm. High voltage of about 100 kV is then produced by a fixed high-voltage transformer, T_H. The filament heater is controlled by a step-down transformer T_F. Adjusting the turns ratio N_6 sets the mA, beam current, of the x-ray tube by increasing the heat to the filament and boiling off more electrons for the thermally limited current.

Considering the transformers T_A, T_F, and T_H to be ideal, the following voltage relationships hold:

$$V_2 = \frac{N_2}{N_1} V_1$$

$$V_3 = \frac{N_3}{N_1} V_1$$

$$V_5 = \frac{N_7}{N_6} V_3$$

$$V_4 = \frac{N_5}{N_4} V_2$$

The full-wave rectifier in Figure 15.14 has diodes 2 and 4 conducting when the voltage drop V_4 is positive, producing a positive tube current I_B. When V_4 is negative, diodes 1 and 3 conduct, and the others are off, again producing I_B in the same direction.

The single-phase power supply described above is limited in its efficient power-handling capability. High-power equipment often uses a three-phase power source. The crucial change in the power supply for three phases is in the high-voltage transformer, illustrated in Figure 15.15. In a three-phase voltage system, V_{AB}, V_{BC}, and V_{CA} are the same magnitude and are dis-

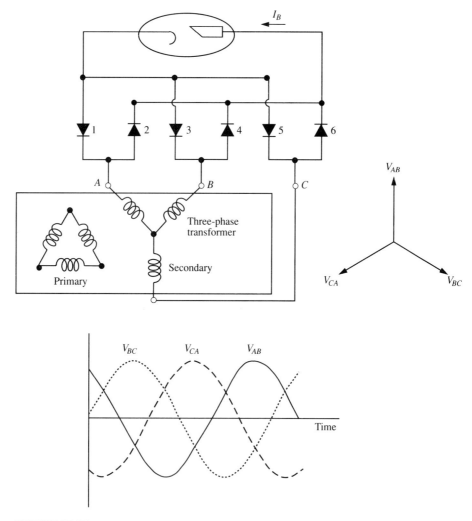

FIGURE 15.15
A three-phase x-ray tube power supply.

placed in phase by 120° from each other, as illustrated in the figure. The current I_B is always in the same positive direction, and is determined at any instant in time by the voltage V_{AB}, V_{BC}, or V_{CA}, whichever has the highest absolute value. To verify that I_B is always positive, you may trace the current through the circuit and verify the following table:

Voltage polarity		Diodes on
V_{AB}	Pos	2,3
	Neg	1,4
V_{BC}	Pos	4,5
	Neg	3,6
V_{CA}	Pos	1,6
	Neg	2,5

For example, when V_{AB} is positive, diodes 2 and 3 conduct, provided also that V_{AB} is greater than both V_{BC} and V_{CA} at the instant considered.

15.3 FLUOROSCOPIC SYSTEM

In various medical procedures, physicians view an x-ray image instantly so they can monitor movements of organs and other objects put into the body.

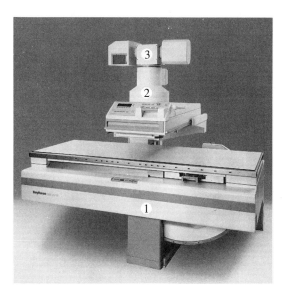

FIGURE 15.16
An x-ray with (1) an under-table tube, (2) an image intensifier unit, and (3) a camera. (Courtesy of Raytheon Medical Systems, Medical Equipment Division)

In a cardiac catheterization procedure, the physician may wish to watch the catheter as it is moved through the veins into the heart ventricle. Or when a kidney stone is being pulverized with ultrasonic waves, it may be monitored using x-rays. Such instantaneous fluoroscopic pictures are called *real-time images*, such as we see on live television broadcasts.

The basic components of the fluoroscopic unit in Figure 15.16 (p. 467) are the x-ray tube (1), fed by a high-voltage supply and control unit under the table. The patient is placed on the table top. A lead shield protects the operator from radiation. An image intensifier (2) amplifies the image and converts the x-ray into light. A television camera (3) then picks up the im-

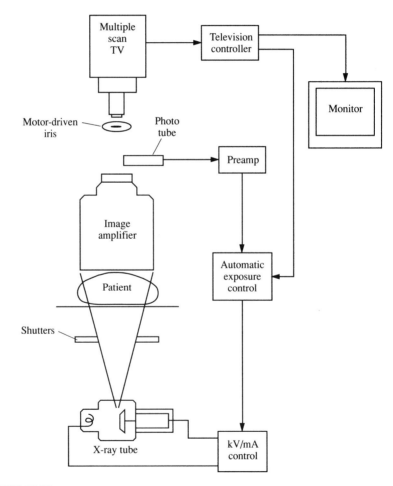

FIGURE 15.17
A typical digital fluoroscopic system.

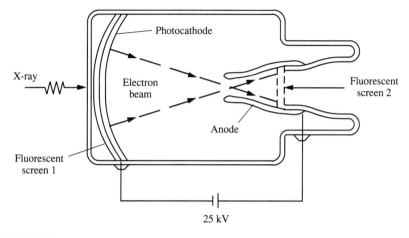

FIGURE 15.18
An image intensifier.

age and transfers it to a television monitor for viewing by the radiologist or operator. A block diagram of a typical digital fluoroscopic system appears in Figure 15.17. In this system, information about the image density is fed to an automatic exposure control so that if the image begins to fade, the beam current on the x-ray tube will automatically increase.

The unique component of a fluoroscopic system is the image intensifier, shown in Figure 15.18. The x-rays strike a fluorescent screen, producing light. The light then strikes the photocathode, which produces electrons. The electrons are accelerated by a 25-kV potential and are focused on the fluorescent screen, which produces increased light and a denser image. This light image can then be photographed or picked up with a television camera.

The fluorescent screens consist of many 2–3-μm phosphor crystals that emit light when bombarded by high-energy particles. For example, a medium-short persistence of blue color is produced by ZnS:Ag(Ni) crystals.

If light photons with sufficient energy strike a photocathode, electrons are emitted, known as photoelectrons. Common photocathode materials consist of alloys of cesium and tin.

15.4 X-RAY CT SCANNERS

The invention of the computer tomography (CT) scanner in 1970 was made possible by a previously established mathematical insight and by the development of the dedicated minicomputer. The mathematical basis for producing an image of the cross section of the body is that if one measures the total attenuation along rows and columns of a matrix, one can compute the attenuation of the matrix elements at the intersections of the rows and columns. The number of mathematical operations necessary to yield clinically applicable and accurate images is so large that a computer is essential to do them. This is the main reason why the CT scanner is a primary example of a medical instrument for which the computer is an indispensable component.

Figure 15.19 illustrates the block diagram of a typical CT scanner. The timing, anode voltage kV, and beam current mA are controlled by a dedicated microcomputer through a control bus. The high-voltage d.c. power supply drives an x-ray tube that can be mechanically rotated along the circumference of a gantry. The x-rays pass through the patient, who is lying in a tube through the center of the gantry, and impinge upon several of as many as 1000 detectors fixed in place around the circumference of the gantry. The microcomputer senses the position of the tube and samples the out-

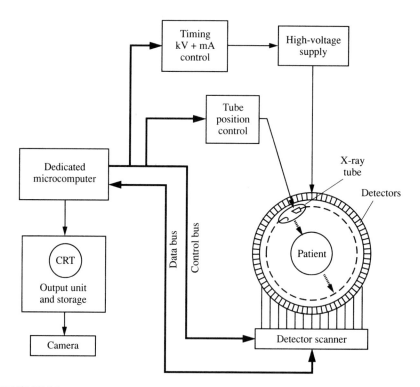

FIGURE 15.19
A block diagram for a CT scanner.

put of the detector along a diameter line opposite the tube. A calculation based on data from a complete scan of the tube is made by the computer. The output unit then produces a visual image of a transverse plane cross section of the patient. The output may then be displayed on a cathode-ray tube and/or photographed with a camera to produce a hard-copy record.

The detectors may consist of ionization chambers, filled with a gas such as xenon, sealed at both ends, and having two conductors forming a capacitor on the sides. A high d.c. voltage is applied to the capacitor. An x-ray entering the chamber ionizes a xenon atom, causing it to migrate to the capacitor plate, and causing a current in the high-voltage lead. This current is proportional to the radiation and is fed to the computer as data for computing the image.

A simplified example calculation called *Back Projection Reconstruction* will now be presented in order to illustrate how the attenuation values along the surface of a transverse slice can be computed from knowledge of externally measured attenuation factors. A detailed rationale for the steps is not presented, but the specific illustration demonstrates the manner of analysis involved in the calculations.

Suppose the actual attenuation values, normalized to zero, are

$$\begin{bmatrix} 0 & 2 \\ 3 & 4 \end{bmatrix}$$

Each number in the matrix represents the attenuation of the space where it is located. For example, here the "2" is a measure of the attenuation in the upper right-hand corner of the matrix. The attenuation values are measured from the outside as those seen along the rows, 2 and 7. Using these as the first estimate, we have attenuation numbers

$$\begin{bmatrix} 2 & 2 \\ 7 & 7 \end{bmatrix}$$

1st Estimate

The second estimate is obtained from the values measured along the columns, giving the sums, 3 and 6:

$$\begin{bmatrix} 3 & 6 \\ 3 & 6 \end{bmatrix}$$

Adding this to the first estimate yields a second estimate:

$$\begin{bmatrix} 5 & 8 \\ 10 & 13 \end{bmatrix}$$

2nd Estimate

A third estimate results from values measured along the northeast diagonal:

$$\begin{bmatrix} 0 & 5 \\ 5 & 4 \end{bmatrix}$$

Adding this to the second estimate yields a third estimate:

$$\begin{bmatrix} 5 & 13 \\ 15 & 17 \end{bmatrix}$$

3rd Estimate

The fourth estimate results from measurements of total attenuation along the northwest diagonal:

$$\begin{bmatrix} 4 & 2 \\ 3 & 4 \end{bmatrix}$$

Adding this to the third estimate gives

$$\begin{bmatrix} 9 & 15 \\ 18 & 21 \end{bmatrix}$$

4th Estimate

Now we normalize this to zero by subtracting 9 from each element:

$$\begin{bmatrix} 0 & 6 \\ 9 & 12 \end{bmatrix}$$

Then we divide by 3 to yield

$$\begin{bmatrix} 0 & 2 \\ 3 & 4 \end{bmatrix}$$

Final Image

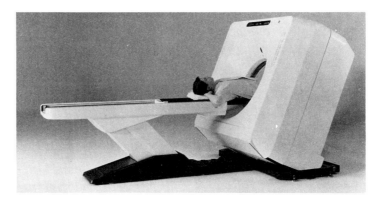

FIGURE 15.20
A CT scanner with a table for placing the patient under the x-ray tube and detectors.
(Courtesy of GE Medical Systems, Inc.)

The final matrix is the same as the first one. The numbers in the matrix correspond to the attenuations of locations on a tissue slice, having the same spatial relationship as the matrix numbers.

Thus the final image has the same attenuation values as the actual transverse slice, but the values were obtained from external measurements of attenuation alone. The CT scan x-ray is used to measure these values externally; the computer finds the matrix values. The illustration is for a 2×2 matrix that could be done by hand. The computer is needed to calculate larger, more accurate matrices.

Advanced models of the CT scanner create images at an angle other than $90°$ to the body axis. This is done by tilting the gantry at an angle, as illustrated in Figure 15.20.

15.5 NUCLEAR MEDICINE IMAGING

In order to produce images of body organs and structures, radioactive nuclear medicines such as radioisotopes and radiopharmaceuticals are injected. These medicines are typically absorbed by the organs and emit radiation that can be detected and localized. Information about the size, tissue structure, and biochemical activity of the organs can be deduced and can lead to the diagnosis of disease. It is important that the half-life of the nuclear medicines is short, so as to reduce the radiation dose given to the patient.

In this section, instrumentation and components that detect, measure, and localize radioactive medicines are described.

TABLE 15.3
Example Radionuclides

Isotope	Half-life	Typical radiation	Typical target organs
Phosphorus 32 (^{32}P)	14.3 days	Beta	Liver
Chromium 51 (^{51}Cr)	27.8 days	Gamma	Red blood cells; urinary
Barium 131 (^{131}Ba)	11.6 days	Gamma	Intestinal
Iodine 131 (^{131}I)	8.1 days	Gamma	Thyroid; blood
Technetium 99m (^{99m}Tc)	6.0 hr	Gamma	Brain; lung

Radioisotopes and Radiopharmaceuticals

Early nuclear scientists at the turn of the century discovered three types of radiation emitted spontaneously from matter. These were arbitrarily called alpha, α, beta, β, and gamma, γ, rays. Alpha rays are positively charged helium nuclei that do not penetrate tissue very well and so are not very useful in nuclear medicine.

Beta rays consist of negatively charged electrons and, like alpha rays, are particle radiation. Gamma rays are electromagnetic radiation, with energy levels above those of medical x-rays. Example radionuclides that produce clinically significant amounts of beta and gamma rays are listed in Table 15.3.

Because of the low tissue-penetrating capability of beta radiation, most procedures using it are done *in vitro*, that is, in a glass tube. *In vivo* procedures, on the other hand, are done on the tissue directly. These radiation procedures are frequently done using the high tissue-penetrating characteristic of gamma radiation. The central element of nuclear medicine imaging equipment is the detector, which can localize radiation and measure the dose.

Radiation Detectors

The most simple and basic radiation detector for x-rays and gamma rays, as well as for alpha and beta rays, consists of a parallel plate capacitor in air, connected through an ammeter to a battery, as shown in Figure 15.21. The radiation will produce either positive or negative ions in the air, helium, or argon gas between the capacitor plates. The ions will be attracted by the voltage on the capacitor plates and will cause a current in the ammeter. The current has units of coulombs per second (C/s) and roentgens have units of coulombs per kilogram (C/kg). Therefore, the ammeter can be calibrated

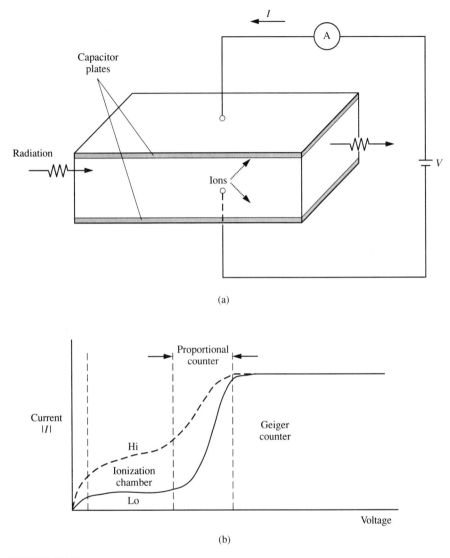

FIGURE 15.21
A basic ionization chamber.

to read roentgens per second (R/s) of radiation. Depending upon the voltage level applied to the capacitor plates, the unit serves different functions, as indicated in Figure 15.21(b).

For low voltages of about 100 V/cm, every ion produced between the plates will be conducted to the plate and produce the same current regardless of changes in the applied voltage V. This is the *ionization chamber* mode of operation, in which the current *I* is proportional to the radiation intensity. Large radiation follows the Hi curve and small radiation follows the Lo curve. As voltage *V* is increased, the ions have secondary collisions and produce more ions, amplifying the current due to the radiation in proportion to the radiation intensity. This is called the *proportional counter* mode. If the voltage is increased so high that any radiation pulse causes all atoms in the chamber to ionize by a general avalanche effect, the chamber is operating as a *Geiger counter*. In the Geiger counter mode each ionizing event causes the same-value pulse output. The radiation intensity is measured by counting the number of pulses per second.

Personnel exposed to radiation need to know their accumulated dose so they can keep their level below the Occupational Safety and Health Administration (OSHA) restriction of 5 rads per year. A measurement of one rad of radiation means the body has absorbed 0.01 joules per kilogram (J/kg) of x-ray radiation. Convenient pocket-size radiation detectors are available to make this measurement. In Figure 15.22, a charged-capacitor-type radiation monitor is shown.

To operate the capacitor radiation monitor, the charging plug is moved against the center conductor and a high voltage is applied. Then the charging plug is moved away. The center conductor will hold its charge, being insulated by high-quality insulators. The outside conductor is a conductive plastic that passes radiation, which ionizes the space between the two conductors. These ions cause a current that lowers the charge on the center conductor. After exposure to radiation, the charging plug is put in contact with the center conductor, and the voltage is read. The change in voltage is then a measure of the radiation exposure since it was charged. (See Figure 15.23.)

Another common personal radiation detector is a film badge. Ionization radiation causes a darkening of the silver halide in the photographic

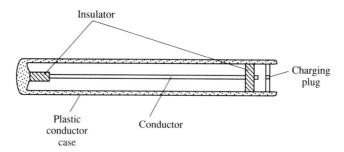

FIGURE 15.22
A capacitor radiation monitor.

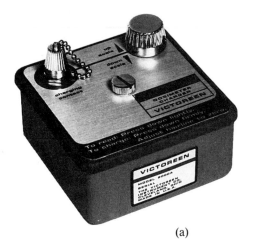

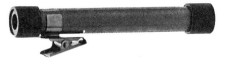

(b)

(a)

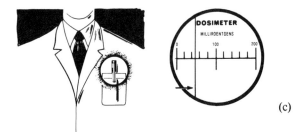

(c)

FIGURE 15.23
(a) A dosimeter charger, (b) a pocket dosimeter, and (c) a film badge. (Courtesy of Nuclear Associates, Division of Victoreen, Inc.)

emulsion. A photoelectric densitometer may then be used to measure the radiation exposure of the film.

The detectors we have discussed tend to be insensitive because, being gas or film, they do not capture all of the radiation incident upon them. Crystal scintillation tends to be more sensitive and, because it takes place in a solid which absorbs more radiation, is widely used in electronic imagers.

Crystals of sodium iodide (NaI), laced with traces of thallium, produce light when irradiated by x-ray or gamma-ray photons. A photodetector may then be used to measure the light intensity. NaI crystal detectors are used in nuclear medicine systems, and, in particular, in conjunction with a photomultiplier tube.

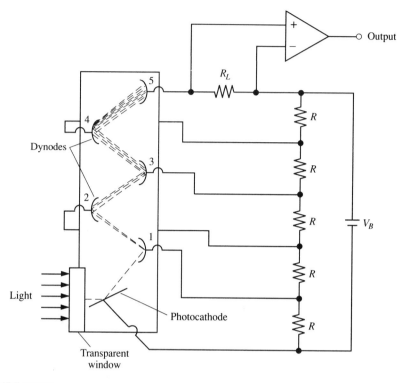

FIGURE 15.24
A photomultiplier tube circuit.

The Photomultiplier Tube

A photomultiplier tube consists of a photocathode that produces electrons when light impinges on it. Then a set of plates amplify the electron beam by a process of secondary emission, as illustrated in Figure 15.24.

A photocathode consists of an opaque substrate coated with a cesium lead compound. Typical sensitivities run from 3 to 150 microamps per lumen (μA/lm). The supply voltage, V_B, causes equal voltage drops across successive dynodes, or plates, numbered 1, 2, 3, 4, 5, and so on. These voltages accelerate the electrons from the photocathode, causing secondary emission from each dynode, such that the beam current increases successively from dynode 1 to dynode 5. The output current through R_L is thus amplified and may be detected with a differential amplifier.

Gamma-Ray Camera

A gamma-ray camera, sometimes called an Anger Scintillation Camera after its inventor Hal O. Anger, is used to localize and measure the gamma rays from a patient who has been injected with a radionuclide. The block diagram in Figure 15.25 illustrates a patient under a gamma-ray scanner.

If, for example, a radiopharmaceutical such as barium 131 (^{131}Ba) is taken into the intestine, the camera head would be placed over the patient's

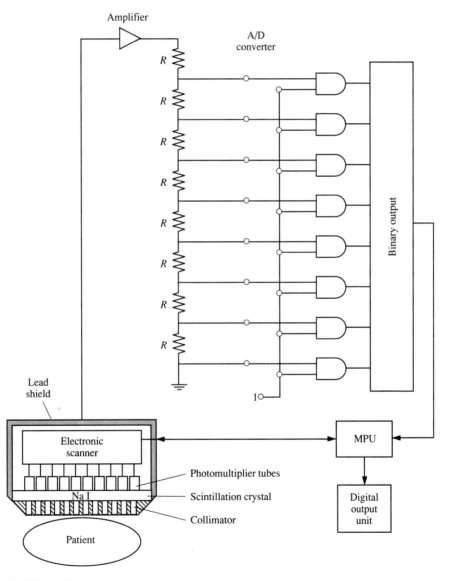

FIGURE 15.25
A gamma-ray camera circuit.

abdomen. Radiation from the ^{131}Ba isotope is passed through a pinhole collimator to eliminate scattering effects, and directed into a large (15-inch diameter) sodium iodide (NaI) scintillation crystal optically coupled to an array of 14 photomultiplier tubes. The light flashes from the crystal create a current in the photomultipliers. Each photomultiplier is successively scanned. The photomultiplier puts out a corresponding pulse of current. The pulse height is measured by the A/D converter shown in Figure 15.25. Larger pulses will turn on more of the AND gate outputs, producing a binary number output that can be processed by a microprocessor that correlates it with the position of the photomultiplier in the camera head. A digital output unit may produce a dot-matrix printout showing the large concentrations of radiopharmaceutical as an increased density of dots on an *x-y* plot. The data may also be displayed on a cathode-ray tube on which the *x-y* position is fixed, as on an oscilloscope, and the intensity of the image would correspond to the radiation intensity on the appropriate position.

A gamma camera, with an attendant behind a shield to protect her from radiation, is illustrated in Figure 15.26.

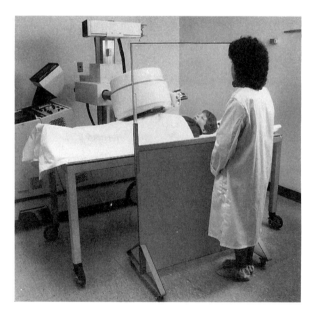

FIGURE 15.26
A patient being scanned with a gamma camera, being observed by an attendant from behind a protective shield. (Courtesy of Nuclear Associates, a Division of Victoreen, Inc.)

15.6 RADIATION DOSE

One of the side effects of x-radiation or nuclear medicine is the dose absorbed by the patient and those using the x-ray machinery. The dose can be computed from a knowledge of the x-ray beam current, anode voltage, and radiation pattern. It is most important to carefully define the units of ionizing radiation as follows:

Quantity	Name	Units	Conversion
Activity	Becquerel (Bq)	s^{-1}	1 curie (Ci) = $3.7(10^{10})$ Bq
Exposure	roentgen (R)	C/kg	1 R = 2.58×10^{-4} C/kg
Dose	rad	J/kg	1 rad = 0.01 J/kg

To correlate the various types of ionizing radiation, we define roentgen equivalent man (rem): the dosage of ionizing radiation that will have the same biological effect as one roentgen of x- or gamma radiation.

EXAMPLE 15.8   The x-radiation incident on a 50-kg man is 0.5 W/m^2, and the radiation intensity that emerges from him is 0.05 W/m^2. How many rads does he receive during a 50-ms exposure over a body surface of 0.5 m^2?

SOLUTION   The joules of energy absorbed are

$$(0.5 - 0.05)\,(\text{W/m}^2)\,(0.5\ \text{m}^2)\,(0.05\ \text{s}) = 0.0113\ \text{J}$$

The dose, D, is

$$D = (0.0113\ \text{J}/50.00\ \text{kg}) = 2.26 \times 10^{-4}\ \text{J/kg}$$

$$= (2.26 \times 10^{-4}\ \text{J/kg})\,[1\ \text{rad}/(0.01\ \text{J/kg})] = 2.26 \times 10^{-2}\ \text{rad}$$

The dose is therefore 22.6 mrad.

To compute the dose of radiation left in a volume of tissue, refer to Figure 15.27, which depicts a tissue with density ρ. The dose equals the joules per kilogram of x-ray left in the tissue. To derive a formula for dose we first find the power loss in the tissue, then we compute the energy loss in joules and divide by the tissue mass in kilograms:

$$\text{Power in tissue} = \mathcal{I}_0 A - \mathcal{I}_0 A e^{-\mu \rho s}$$

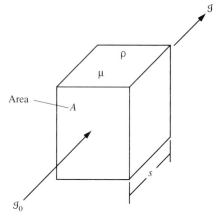

FIGURE 15.27
A geometric model for dose calculations.

For an x-ray pulse of duration T_D seconds,

$$\text{Energy in the tissue} = \Im_0 A T_D (1 - e^{-\mu\rho s})$$

Since the tissue mass $= As\rho$, we have

$$\text{Dose} = \frac{\Im_0 T_D (1 - e^{-\mu\rho s})}{\rho s}$$

EXAMPLE 15.9   A 1000-cm³ volume of muscle tissue is radiated with an x-ray of 2 W/m². The path length of the x-rays is 10 cm. The x-rays are delivered at 100 kV for a duration of 50 ms. Compute the dose of the x-ray.

SOLUTION   Find μ in Figure 15.5, and ρ from Table 15.2, then

$$\text{Dose} = \frac{\dfrac{2\ \text{W}}{\text{m}^2}(1 - e^{-0.0252\ \text{cm}^{-1}(10\ \text{cm})})50(10^{-3})\text{s}}{\dfrac{1\ \text{g}}{\text{cm}^3}\dfrac{\text{kg}}{1000\ \text{g}}\left(\dfrac{100\ \text{cm}}{\text{m}}\right)^3(0.1\ \text{m})}$$

$$= 0.000223\ \frac{\text{J}}{\text{kg}}\frac{\text{rad}}{0.01\ \text{J/kg}} = 0.0223\ \text{rad}$$

$$= 22.3\ \text{mrad}$$

The dosage from ionizing radiation is cumulative because the probability of cell damage increases as more x-rays pass through the body. Government regulations require that occupationally induced x-rays, which are absorbed by the whole body, should not exceed a cumulative dose (CD) of

$$CD = 5(n - 18) \text{ rad} \qquad (15.10)$$

where n is the worker's age in years. A one-year exposure should not exceed 5 rad. In medical application to patients, physicians may decide to exceed these limits when they feel the risk to the patient from disease exceeds the risk of x-ray exposure.

The number of rads of dose absorbed from a given exposure to radiation depends upon the material as well as the photon energy level. Figure 15.28 gives data on the ratio of rads/roentgen (rad/R) for bone and muscle. Rads nearly equal roentgens in the soft tissue of the body. Since soft tissue makes up most of the body, we can say that in humans the dose in rads is approximately equal to the exposure in roentgens.

Government regulations on the allowed x-ray dose have become more stringent as long-term effects have become apparent. In 1900, the permissible whole-body dose was 10 rem per day. This is now reduced by nearly one thousand times, to 5 rem per year! The reason for these regulations is summarized by the description of the effects of ionizing radiation on humans, given in Figure 15.29.

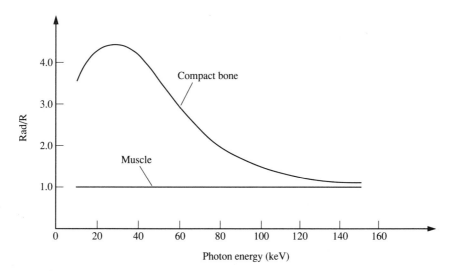

FIGURE 15.28
The relationship of an absorbed dose to exposure in body tissues over the diagnostic energy range.

0.03 rem:
Average dose from chest x-ray.

0.2 rem:
Average annual dose for New York area residents
from environmental and medical sources.

0.5 rem:
Exposure limit set by Nuclear Regulatory Commission
for pregnant workers in the nuclear industry
throughout pregnancy.

1 rem:
Average dose from lumbo-sacral spine x-ray.

1-5 rem:
Federal guidelines call for action to protect public
if it is anticipated that a nuclear accident would
result in a dose of this size.

5 rem:
Annual exposure limit for most nuclear workers.

10 rem:
30-year cancer incidence rises by about 1,193
cases per million in persons exposed to this level,
in addition to 170,000 fatal cancers that would be
expected without the exposure.

10-25 rem:
Small, short-term changes in the blood of some of
those exposed.

25 rem:
Limit for most emergency workers.

25-50 rem:
Nearly all those exposed show low white and
red blood cell counts in 24 hours.

50-100 rem:
Nausea within 12 hours for 5 percent of those
exposed.

75 rem:
Limit for emergency workers in lifesaving
activities.

100-200 rem:
Vomiting in 5 to 50 percent of those exposed
within three hours; hair loss in up to 10 percent
of population, in 5 to 10 days.

225 rem:
Death within 60 days for 5 percent of those
exposed, without medical care.

400 rem:
Death within 60 days for 50 percent of those
exposed, without medical care.

500-600 rem:
Death within 60 days for 90 percent of those
exposed, without medical care.

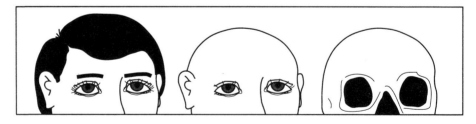

FIGURE 15.29
The effects of ionizing radiation on human beings. From Office of Radiation and Nuclear
Safety, Rensselaer Polytechnic Institute; Nuclear Regulatory Commission Committee on
the Biological Effects of Ionizing Radiation. (Used by permission of Robert Ryan)

Since x-ray is a carcinogen, it is essential to reduce dose levels due to
stray x-rays to less than 5 rads per year. This is usually done with shielding by a massive material such as lead, iron, or concrete. Since the dose in
rads is proportional to the x-ray intensity in watts per meter squared

(W/m^2), it follows directly from Equation (15.6) that the dose out of a shield D_{OUT} is related to the dose into the shield, D_{IN}, in rads, by

$$D_{OUT} = D_{IN}e^{-\mu\rho s} \qquad (15.11)$$

where s is the thickness of the shield.

EXAMPLE 15.10 At a photon energy of 200 keV, the mass attenuation coefficient = 2.65 cm²/g. What thickness of lead (density ρ of 11.3 g/cm³) is needed to reduce the dose to 5% of its initial value?

SOLUTION

$$\frac{D_{OUT}}{D_{IN}} = e^{-2.65(11.3)s} = 0.05$$

Solving this for s gives $s = 0.1$ cm $= 1$ mm.

Anyone who has worn a lead shield during x-ray procedures has probably wondered if a lighter material is available to shield x-rays. Unfortunately, material less dense than lead must be thicker, keeping the weight about the same.

The thickness of lead required for radiation protection may be deduced from Table 15.4.

TABLE 15.4
**Thickness of Lead Required
to Reduce Useful Beam to 5%**

Potential (kV)	Required lead thickness (mm)
60	0.1
100	0.16
140	0.70
200	1.0
250	1.7
400	2.3

Source: *Medical X-Ray and Gamma-Ray Protection for Energies up to 10 MeV.* (NCRP Report #33) National Council on Radiation Protection and Measurements (Feb. 1968).

Table 15.4 can be used to compute the percentage reduction in beam intensity for several thicknesses of lead. For example, at 60 kV, 0.1 mm of lead is required to reduce the beam to 0.05 times its original value. A second 0.1 mm layer will reduce it by 0.05 again, yielding 0.0025 times its original value.

EXAMPLE 15.11   Use Table 15.4 to determine the thickness of lead required to reduce a useful beam to 0.1 percent of its useful value, at 100 kV.

SOLUTION   The number of thickness, n, is the power to which 0.05 (5%) must be raised to obtain 0.1 percent:

$$(0.05)^n = 0.001$$

Take the natural logarithm of both sides:

$$\ln(0.05)^n = \ln 0.001$$

$$n = \frac{\ln(0.001)}{\ln(0.05)} = 2.3$$

Each thickness of lead from Table 15.4 is 0.16 mm. Thus the total thickness of lead required is $(0.16)(2.3) = 0.36$ mm.

When iron is substituted for lead, the thickness requirement increases by an order of magnitude, more than tenfold. Table 15.5 gives the number of times the thickness of iron must be greater than the thickness of lead.

When concrete (density 2.35 g/cm^2) is substituted for lead it must be roughly one hundred times as thick, as indicated in Table 15.6.

TABLE 15.5
Iron Equivalents (mm) of Lead at Different
X-Ray Tube Potentials

Lead thickness (mm)	Tube potential			
	150 kV	**200 kV**	**300 kV**	**400 kV**
1	11	12	12	11
2	25	27	20	18
3	37	40	28	23
4	50	55	35	28

Source: National Bureau of Standards Handbook #50.

TABLE 15.6
Concrete Equivalents (mm) of Lead at Different
X-Ray Tube Potentials

Lead thickness (mm)	Tube potential			
	150 kV	200 kV	300 kV	400 kV
1	80	75	56	47
2	150	140	89	70
3	220	200	117	94
4	280	260	140	112

Source: National Bureau of Standards Handbook #50.

REFERENCES

Brown, J. G. *X-rays and Their Applications*. New York: Plenum Press, 1966.

Bureau of Radiological Health and Training Institute Environmental Control Administration. *Radiological Health Handbook 20852.10.6.3*. U.S. Department of Health, Education and Welfare, 1970.

Feinberg, B. N. *Applied Clinical Engineering*. Englewood Cliffs, NJ: Prentice-Hall, 1986.

Jacobson, B., and Webster, J. G. *Medicine and Clinical Engineering*. Englewood Cliffs, NJ: Prentice-Hall, 1977.

Macovski, A. *Medical Imaging Systems*. Englewood Cliffs, NJ: Prentice-Hall, 1983.

Millman, J., and Seely, S. *Electronics*. 2nd ed. New York: McGraw-Hill, 1951.

EXERCISES

1. An x-ray tube is designed so that no cathode space charge exists at medical x-ray energies (above 20 keV). The cathode material is thoriated tungsten. Compute the beam current as a function of cathode temperature when the cathode area is 1 cm^2. Compare the computed current, I_B, with the same calculation on a tungsten cathode of the same area.

2. An x-ray tube having a cathode with a 1 cm^2 area must be able to handle up to 12 A with no space charge at an x-ray energy level as low as 20 keV. Calculate the maximum distance between the cathode and anode that will ensure that the thermally limited current is flowing.

3. Calculate the maximum photon energy of x-rays radiated from an anode having 90 kV applied. Express the answer in joules.

4. Compute the wavelength of the x-rays in Exercise 3.

5. The beam current in a tungsten anode x-ray tube is 5 mA, and the anode voltage is 100 kV. The efficiency of the tube is 1.04%. Suppose all of the x-ray energy is evenly distributed over a 1 m² area. Find the intensity $\mathcal{I}$ of the x-rays in units of watts per square meter (W/m²).

6. Suppose x-rays such as those produced in Exercise 5 are passed through muscle 2 cm thick. Calculate the intensity of the x-rays that emerge from the muscle.

7. Repeat Exercise 6 if the tissue is changed to bone.

8. A beam of x-ray is incident on muscle tissue at an intensity of 10 W/m². Make a plot of the intensity as a function of the distance through the material for energy levels corresponding to the following anode voltages:
   (a) 200 kV
   (b) 100 kV
   (c) 20 kV
   Draw all the curves on the same axis for better comparison.

9. Repeat Exercise 8, but change the muscle to bone. Compare the two plots. Which absorbs the most x-rays, bone or muscle?

10. Repeat Exercise 8, but change the muscle to air, assuming the mass attenuation coefficient for air is approximately equal to that of muscle.

11. Calculate the contrast between bone and muscle tissues that are both 3 cm thick as a function of the x-ray energy level, E_P, in units of electron-volts. Let E_P range from 20 to 150 keV.

12. Explain how adjusting the anode voltage on an x-ray will help you see beneath bone.

13. A diagnostic x-ray delivers a dose of 50 mrad to patients who are being screened at a rate of 1 per minute. If the machine is used for 10 hours per day, 300 days per year, what dose could an unprotected operator receive each year? What would be the physiological effect of such a dose?

14. (a) How thick should a lead shield be so that the maximum dose that the operator could receive is 5 rad per year in the situation described in Exercise 13. For medical x-rays given here, assume the mass attenuation coefficient of lead to be approximately 1 cm²/g at an energy of 0.1 MeV for the x-ray. The density of lead is 11.35 g/cm³.
   (b) How thick should an iron shield be to reduce this dose to 5 rad/yr?
   (c) How thick should a concrete shield be to reduce the dose to 5 rad/yr?

15. An x-ray tube whose characteristics are illustrated in Figure 15.8 produces 80-keV x-rays. The beam current is 300 mA. What is the maximum continuous time this tube is allowed to remain on?

16

Ultrasonic Equipment

16.1 THERAPEUTIC AND DIAGNOSTIC EQUIPMENT

Ultrasonic equipment serves a variety of functions in medicine. It is used for imaging internal organs noninvasively. It is used to apply massage and deep-heat therapy to muscle tissue. And it is used to measure blood flow and blood pressure noninvasively.

The principle of *imaging*, or making pictures of internal organs, is that of ultrasonic wave reflection. Ultrasonic waves reflect from the boundaries of two tissues, just as waves reflect from an object in water. Because the amount of reflection differs in different tissues, it is possible to distinguish between materials and make images of them using ultrasonics.

The quality that makes ultrasonic waves therapeutic is that they cause tissue matter to vibrate and heat up. It is the heat that has therapeutic effects. For use as therapy, it is necessary to couple relatively high power (up to approximately 5 W/cm^2) into the tissue.

Blood pressure and blood flow are measured by application of the *Doppler effect*. This effect is the increase in frequency of a sound reflected by a body approaching the source of the sound. To observe this effect, sing a steady tone, then move your hand rapidly toward your mouth. You will hear the increase in the pitch due to the motion of your hand.

Therapeutic Ultrasonic Equipment

Therapeutic ultrasonic equipment consists of a sinusoidal voltage generator driving a piezoelectric crystal pressed against the body tissue, as illustrated in Figure 16.1. The sinusoidal voltage generator in the figure produces

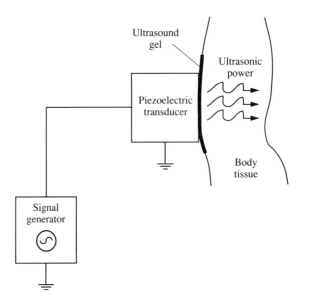

FIGURE 16.1
Therapeutic ultrasonic equipment.

a voltage to be applied to the crystal transducer. The requirement of the generator is that it generate a voltage high enough to produce between 1 and 10 W on the transducer in the frequency range from 1 to 10 MHz. The piezoelectric effect causes the crystal to change its size and shape slightly when the electric field intensity changes, as driven by the voltage generator. The electric forces on the crystal atoms cause the atoms to move. Since the applied voltage is sinusoidal, it sets up sinusoidal vibrations in the crystal that are called *ultrasound*. To get these sound waves into the tissue efficiently, it is necessary to match the impedance of the transducer to the impedance of the tissue, because of the maximum power transfer theorem. The acoustic impedance, or impedance to sound waves, is higher in the transducer than in body tissue, such as muscle. That is, the transducer, being ceramic, is hard, while the muscle is relatively soft. The acoustic impedance of materials often increases as a function of increased hardness.

The impedance is matched by filling all of the voids between the tissue surface, and filling the transducer with a gel. If this gel is not properly applied, the transducer can be damaged and skin burns can occur because too much energy will stay in the transducer and overheat it.

Besides resulting from overheating, failures can also arise from breakage. The crystals are relatively brittle, and the metal adhesives may dry out or come loose. If epoxy is used in the construction, it also may deteriorate, or break.

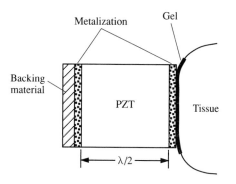

FIGURE 16.2
A PZT ultrasonic transducer.

Piezoelectric Transducers

The piezoelectric crystal used for ultrasound occurs naturally as quartz. Practical transducers are constructed of ammonium dihydrogen phosphate (ADP) or lead zirconate titanate (PZT). ADP dissolves in water, but it can be used in high-power applications. PZT is a commonly used transducer made from ceramic.

The crystal is cut to one half wavelength, $\lambda/2$, at the frequency of the ultrasonic signal. This causes it to resonate at that frequency and give its maximum power output. In order to get the electric field throughout the crystal, the two ends perpendicular to the half wavelength axis are metalized. This forms a parallel plate capacitor, as illustrated in Figure 16.2. These are wired to the voltage generator, and the structure is covered with electrical insulation. In order to direct the energy out of one surface of the crystal, a backing material is applied to the surface opposite the tissue. This reflects ultrasonics; therefore, waves travel out of only one surface of the transducer. The impedance matching of the crystal may be adjusted by fixing a container of oil between the crystal and the tissue contact surface. The acoustic impedance of oil can be adjusted by changing its viscosity, that is, by diluting it. In other words, just as you can match the impedance of an amplifier to that of an antenna by adjusting the turns in a transformer connecting them, so you can impedance-match an ultrasonic transducer to skin by adjusting the viscosity of oil at the interface.

Ultrasonic Imaging Equipment

The voltage generator in ultrasonic imaging devices hits the piezoelectric transducer with a short pulse and causes it to oscillate at its resonant frequency. It is also possible to use a pulse-modulated generator to drive the piezoelectric crystal. The pulse generated would be long compared to the period of the 1 to 10 MHz ultrasonic oscillation. It would be short, however, compared to the acoustic transmission time in the tissue. Sound velocity in the body averages about 1540 m/s. Therefore, 1 mm in distance requires 0.65 μs on the average.

The pulse of ultrasonic energy travels into the tissue. It is reflected from tissue boundaries, causing echoes. By the time the echoes reach the transducer, the pulse generator has turned off, and the echo creates an oscillation in the transducer again. The echo is like that of a drum beat reverberating off a wall, except the drum operates at a lower, audible frequency.

The electronic signal from the transducer induced by the ultrasonic echo would go into the limiter in Figure 16.3. The function of the limiter is to protect the receiver from the transmitted pulse. The small echo, from 40 to 100 dB below the transmitted pulse, is passed by the limiter. However, the transmitter pulse is severely clipped off to provide the protection.

The receiver is a conventional radio frequency (RF) unit operating in the 1 to 10 MHz range. It contains a detector circuit that filters out the ultrasonic frequencies and delivers the pulse to the output. The reflected pulse then appears on the display unit.

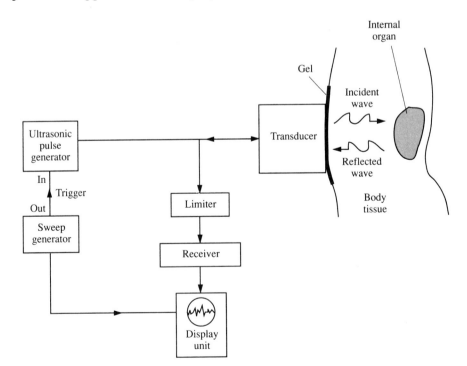

FIGURE 16.3
A block diagram of ultrasonic imaging equipment.

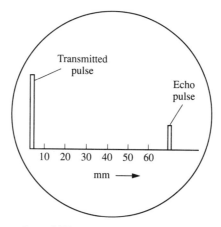

1 μs = 0.77 mm tissue thickness, round trip

FIGURE 16.4
An A-mode display.

The Display Unit

A simple image display can be made from a conventional oscilloscope. This is called an *A-mode display*. A trigger from the pulse generator initiates the horizontal sweep when the pulse is transmitted. The beam then travels along the horizontal axis shown in Figure 16.4. The horizontal scale is calibrated approximately according to the speed of sound in most body tissue. Based on the 1540 m/s average speed, it takes 1 μs for ultrasound to pass through 1.54 mm of tissue one way. On the A-scope it makes a round trip. Therefore 1 μs on the A-scope horizontal display is equivalent to 0.77 mm of tissue thickness. Controls at the receiver may be set so that the receiver gain increases in proportion to the distance along the sweep. This tends to make the echoes equal in size and compensates for tissue attenuation of the ultrasound echo.

Scanning-Type Displays

The A-mode display gives information about the distance between tissue boundaries. For example, it may be used to measure organ thickness. In order to add a dimension, and give breadth information, scanning-type displays are used.

A *B-mode display* may be generated by pivoting the transducer on an axis, causing it to rotate through an arc. The rotational speed, being mechanical, is slow compared with the time required for each sweep. The transmitted pulse appears at the origin in Figure 16.5. The depth is propor-

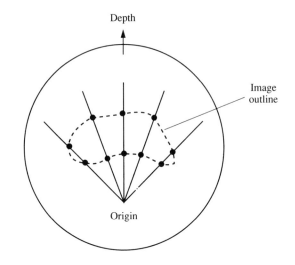

FIGURE 16.5
A B-mode display.

tional to the distance along each radial line. Ultrasonic echoes appear as an intensity-modulated dot, as indicated in the figure. The result is an outline of the body tissue in two dimensions.

A B-mode display may also be generated with a phased array transducer, illustrated with an ultrasonic imager in Figure 16.6. A phased array transducer consists of a set of piezoelectric transducers placed along a line. Each transducer is pulsed successively in time. Depending upon the time between the firing of each transducer, constructive interference of the transmitted wave will occur along a particular radial line. The direction of the radial line is varied by changing the firing time between successive transducers in the display.

The phased array transducer can be scanned faster than the rotating transducer, because the control pulses are electronic and travel at the speed of light. In a practical application, a linear phased array may be useful for getting images of the heart from a site between the ribs, for example.

A single transducer is used to generate an *M-mode display* (Figure 16.7), where the M stands for motion, because it measures the motion of the tissue. As with the B-mode display, the intensity of the reflections from the tissue is recorded as an intensity of the spot on the CRT. The horizontal axis of the CRT is slowly scanned so that if the tissue is moving, as in the case of a heart valve, the new position will be recorded on successive scans. From the scan rate, usually on the order of seconds per scan, it is possible to calculate the rate of motion of the tissue.

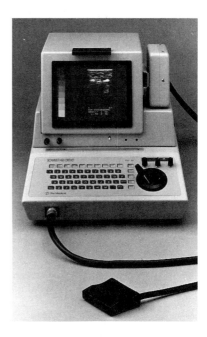

FIGURE 16.6
An ultrasound imager with a phased array transducer. (Courtesy of PIE Medical)

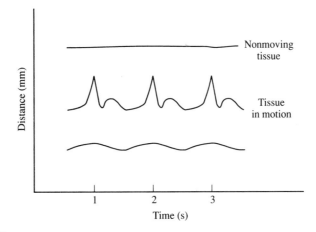

FIGURE 16.7
An M-mode display.

Several transducer shapes are illustrated in Figure 16.8(a). The flat single transducer matches the impedance of the skull in brain midline studies. A rounded transducer can be placed near the apex of the heart for heart valve studies. In Figure 16.8(b), a trans-anal transducer suitable for insertion into the colon is shown.

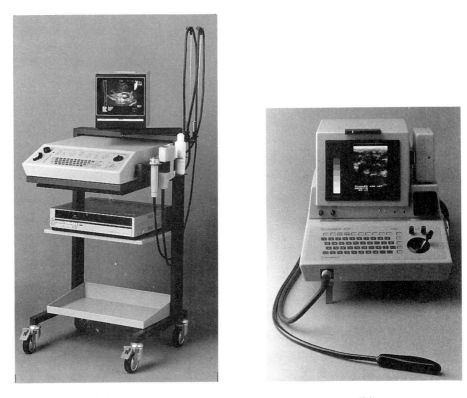

(a)   (b)

FIGURE 16.8
An ultrasonic imager (a) with transducers in their holsters, (b) showing a trans-anal trans-ducer attached to a patient cable. (Courtesy of PIE Medical)

16.2 ULTRASONIC WAVES

Ultrasonic equipment is used to generate and measure ultrasonic waves. To understand the equipment and its operation, it is necessary to understand ultrasonic wave mechanics. Ultrasonic waves are similar to the pressure and flow waves discussed in Chapter 11. A pressure difference, p, across two points in matter, whether air, tissue, or metal, causes a displacement of the atoms, giving them a velocity, v. The atoms do not move very far because they are bound by elastic forces. However, the energy of one atom is transferred to other atoms, and it propagates through the matter at its own velocity, c.

There exists an analogy of ultrasonic waves to voltage waves: ultrasonic pressure, p, is analogous to voltage, and the particle velocity, v, of ultrasonic waves is analogous to current for reasons similar to those discussed in Chapter 11. Furthermore, the acoustic impedance is analogous to the impedance of an electrical circuit. Therefore, your knowledge of electrical circuits will help you to understand ultrasonics.

An ultrasonic wave is a traveling pressure wave. If you were to drop a rock into a smooth lake, waves would propagate out from the point of impact. We have all observed how these waves travel. The force that causes the undulation of the water that we observe is a pressure wave. A mathematical expression that describes it is

$$p = P_0 e^{-\alpha x} \cos(\beta x - \omega t) \tag{16.1}$$

This is the mathematical expression for a traveling sinusoidal wave. In this equation, p is pressure, β is the phase constant, x is position, $\omega = 2\pi f$ is the radian frequency, t is time, and α is an attenuation constant. For clarity of presentation, and because it is not of primary importance in ultrasonic imaging, we will restrict ourselves to the case that $\alpha = 0$, the lossless case. The description of the traveling wave is then taken as

$$p = P_0 \cos(\beta x - \omega t) \tag{16.2}$$

where P_0 is the magnitude of the pressure wave. The traveling-wave behavior of Equation (16.2) is illustrated in Example 16.1.

EXAMPLE 16.1   (a) Plot the following pressure wave equation for the case

$$p = P_0 \cos(\beta x - \omega t)$$

where $\beta = 1$ rad/m, $f = 1$ Hz, and $P_0 = 10$ N/m^2.
(b) Is this a forward-traveling wave or a backward-traveling wave?

SOLUTION   See Figure 16.9. Note that in the successive graphs taken at $t = 0$, $\frac{1}{8}$, and $\frac{1}{4}$ seconds, the crest of the wave has moved in position to the right. Therefore we conclude that this is a forward-traveling wave.

The crest velocity is derived from dx/dt when the pressure, p, is constant in Equation (16.2). That is,

$$\beta x - \omega t = \text{constant}$$

Differentiating both sides gives

$$\beta \frac{dx}{dt} - \omega = 0$$

Plot Equation (16.2) for $t = 0$, 1/8, and 1/4 s.

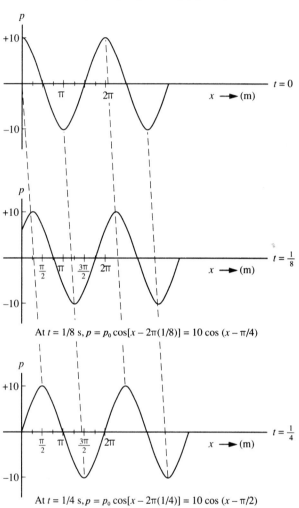

At $t = 1/8$ s, $p = p_0 \cos[x - 2\pi(1/8)] = 10 \cos(x - \pi/4)$

At $t = 1/4$ s, $p = p_0 \cos[x - 2\pi(1/4)] = 10 \cos(x - \pi/2)$

This is a forward-traveling wave.

FIGURE 16.9
A plot of a forward-traveling wave.

Therefore, defining the crest velocity $c = dx/dt$ yields

$$c = \frac{\omega}{\beta}$$ **(16.3)**

The wavelength, λ, is the distance between wave crests at any time t. For example, at $t = 0$, Equation (16.2) shows that

$$\lambda = \frac{2\pi}{\beta} \tag{16.4}$$

Then, combining Equations (16.3) and (16.4) gives

$$c = \lambda f \tag{16.5}$$

The wave in Figure 16.9 travels in the positive x-direction. Changing the sign in the argument reverses the direction of the wave. That is,

$$p = P_0 \cos(\beta x + \omega t)$$

travels in the negative x-direction and is called a backward-traveling wave.

Because the wave crest travels through the medium, we call it a propagating wave. The propagating pressure wave causes a displacement of the particles of matter through which it travels. A mathematical expression describing the velocity, v, is

$$v = V_0 \cos(\beta x - \omega t) \tag{16.6}$$

Since Equation (16.6) has the same form as Equation (16.2), plotting it will show that it too is a propagating wave. It is analogous to the current in an electric wave, which is the velocity of charges. In a water wave caused by a splash, it represents the velocity of the water making the wave.

Completing the analogy, we can define the impedance of a forward-traveling wave as the *characteristic impedance, Z_0*. That is,

$$Z_0 = \frac{p}{v} = \frac{P_0 \cos(\beta x - \omega t)}{V_0 \cos(\beta x - \omega t)}$$

and canceling the cosine functions,

$$Z_0 = \frac{P_0}{V_0} \tag{16.7}$$

In general, the characteristic impedance is defined as the wave impedance of a single wave traveling in one direction. It can also be shown that the characteristic impedance is a physical property of the medium supporting the traveling wave, and is given by

$$Z_0 = \rho c \qquad (16.8)$$

where ρ is the material density in kg/m^3, and c is the velocity of sound in the medium in m/s. The units of Z_0 are then

$$\left(\frac{kg}{m^3}\right)\frac{m}{s} = \left(\frac{kg}{m^2 s}\right)$$

Wave Reflections

The key principle of operation for ultrasonic imaging equipment, as well as for most other ultrasonic equipment other than therapeutic massagers, is the principle of traveling wave reflection, commonly known in the audio spectrum as echo. Tissues are distinguished from one another by their relative reflected wave intensities. It is important to understand what property of the tissue influences reflection so that the proper uses and limitations of the equipment can be appreciated. We shall see that tissue density is the most distinctive feature in the ultrasonic spectrum. Although an exact analysis of reflections in biological tissue is very complex, to understand the principle and limitations of ultrasonic imaging, it is sufficient to consider only two tissues.

When a wave impinges on the boundary of two tissues, some of the wave is reflected back. For example, if the wave is traveling in tissue 1 with a characteristic impedance $Z_{01} = \rho_1 c_1$ and strikes a medium having a characteristic impedance $Z_{02} = \rho_2 c_2$, the pressure wave is reflected back. The situation is illustrated in Figure 16.10, in which the dimension x is taken as

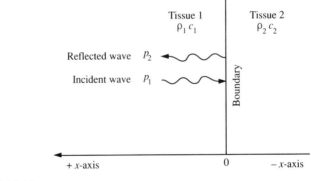

FIGURE 16.10
Waves reflected from a boundary.

positive going toward the left, and $x = 0$ is the boundary between the two tissues. The wave incident on the boundary travels in the negative x-direction and has the formula

$$p_1 = P_{01} \cos(\beta_1 x + \omega t)$$

and the reflected wave is some fraction R of that as

$$p_2 = RP_{01} \cos(\beta_1 x - \omega t)$$

The minus sign on the ωt indicates the wave travels in the positive x-direction. R is called the *reflection coefficient* and is defined as

$$R = \frac{\text{pressure magnitude reflected at the boundary } x = 0}{\text{pressure magnitude incident on the boundary at } x = 0} \qquad \textbf{(16.9)}$$

The pressure in tissue 1 is the sum $p_1 + p_2$, or

$$p = P_{01}[\cos(\beta_1 x + \omega t) + R \cos(\beta_1 x - \omega t)] \qquad \textbf{(16.10)}$$

Each of these pressures causes a velocity, and the velocity of the reflected wave is in a direction opposite to that of the incident wave, accounting for the minus sign preceding the R in the following equation for particle velocity:

$$v = V_{01}[\cos(\beta_1 x + \omega t) - R \cos(\beta_1 x - \omega t)] \qquad \textbf{(16.11)}$$

Because of the analogy already mentioned that pressure plays the role of voltage and particle velocity plays the role of current, the *wave impedance* Z is defined as

$$Z = \frac{p}{v} \qquad \textbf{(16.12)}$$

That is, wave impedance equals the pressure divided by the velocity of the wave composed of the sum of all incident and reflected waves. Notice that Z is equal to the characteristic impedance of Equation (16.7) only when there are no reflected waves and $R = 0$ in Equations (16.10) and (16.11).

A means of measuring the reflection coefficient is derived by considering the wave impedance at the boundary. First set $x = 0$ in Equations (16.10) and (16.11). Insert these into Equation (16.12) to yield

$$Z(0) = \frac{P_{01}[\cos(\omega t) + R \cos(-\omega t)]}{V_{01}[\cos(\omega t) - R \cos(-\omega t)]}$$

Here the cosines cancel because $\cos(\omega t) = \cos(-\omega t)$. Also, using Equation (16.7) we have

$$Z(0) = Z_{01} \frac{1 + R}{1 - R}$$

where Z_{01} is the characteristic impedance of tissue 1. In addition, because there are no reflected waves to the right of the boundary, we note that $Z(0) = Z_{02}$, the characteristic impedance of tissue 2. Therefore we have

$$\frac{Z_{02}}{Z_{01}} = \frac{1 + R}{1 - R} \qquad (16.13)$$

This is solved for the reflection coefficient as

$$R = \frac{Z_{02} - Z_{01}}{Z_{02} + Z_{01}} \qquad (16.14a)$$

Now, using Equation (16.8),

$$R = \frac{\rho_2 c_2 - \rho_1 c_1}{\rho_2 c_2 + \rho_1 c_1} \qquad (16.14b)$$

This equation shows that the reflection coefficient can be calculated from the physical properties of the tissue, namely its density ρ and speed of sound c.

The data necessary to compute the reflection coefficient, R, in common biological tissues is given in Table 16.1.

TABLE 16.1
Physical Parameters of Tissues

Material	Density, ρ (g/cm³)	Speed of sound, c (m/s)
Air	0.001	331
Bone	1.85	3360
Muscle	1.06	1570
Fat	0.93	1480
Blood	1	1560

EXAMPLE 16.2   Use Table 16.1 to compute the characteristic impedance of muscle tissue, Z_{OM}.

SOLUTION   From Equation (16.8),

$$Z_{OM} = \left(1.06\frac{\text{g}}{\text{cm}^3}\right)\left(\frac{\text{kg}}{1000 \text{ g}}\right)\left(\frac{100 \text{ cm}}{\text{m}}\right)^3\left(1570\frac{\text{m}}{\text{s}}\right)$$

$$= 1.66 \times 10^6 \text{ kg/m}^2\text{s}$$

Analysis of a Typical Ultrasonic Reflection

The typical ultrasonic equipment used for diagnosis propagates a pulse of ultrasonics into a tissue, turns off the transmitter, and waits for the reflection. Because of this, the incident and reflected curve can be treated separately.

EXAMPLE 16.3   A short pulse of ultrasonic energy is applied to muscle and reflected from an underlying bone. The density and velocity of propagation of sound in each of these tissues are indicated in Figure 16.11. The pressure of the incident wave is 0.1 N/m² in magnitude. Compute the magnitude of the pressure of the reflected wave.

SOLUTION   The reflection coefficient R is equal to the ratio of the magnitude of the reflected wave, P_{02}, to the incident wave, P_{01}. $R = P_{02}/P_{01}$ as indicated in Equation (16.9). To compute R we need Equation (16.14). Here, applying Equation (16.8) to tissue 1,

$$Z_{01} = (1.06)(1570)(100^3)(1/1000)$$

$$= 1.66 \times 10^6 \text{ kg/m}^2\text{s}$$

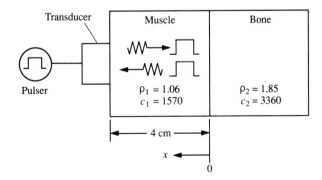

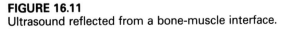

FIGURE 16.11
Ultrasound reflected from a bone-muscle interface.

and in tissue 2,

$$Z_{02} = (1.85)(3360)(100^3)(1/1000)$$

$$= 6.22 \times 10^6 \text{ kg/m}^2\text{s}$$

From Equation (16.14a), then, the reflection coefficient is

$$R = \frac{6.22(10^6) - 1.66(10^6)}{1.66(10^6) + 6.22(10^6)} = 0.578$$

Thus the pressure of the reflected wave P_{02} is

$$P_{02} = RP_{01} = 0.578(0.1) = 0.0578 \text{ N/m}^2$$

Ultrasonic Power

Consistent with the analog of pressure for voltage and velocity for current, the power density, $\mathcal{P}$, of an ultrasonic wave is given by

$$\mathcal{P} = PV$$

where P is the root-mean-square (rms) value of pressure and V the rms value of velocity. The power density is also given by

$$\mathcal{P} = \frac{P^2}{Z_0} \tag{16.15}$$

Using Equation (16.7) for the characteristic impedance Z_{01}, we have

$$\mathcal{P}_1 = \frac{P_{01}{}^2}{Z_{01}}$$

This is the power in the incident wave in tissue 1. Likewise, the reflected power in tissue 1 is

$$\mathcal{P}_2 = \frac{(RP_{01})^2}{Z_{01}}$$

Thus we see that the ratio of the reflected power density to the incident power is equal to the square of the reflection coefficient. Or

$$\frac{\mathcal{P}_2}{\mathcal{P}_1} = R^2 \tag{16.16}$$

That is, the *power reflection coefficient* equals the square of the pressure reflection coefficient, R^2.

For an engineer or service professional, it is important to understand ultrasonic power, since that is the quantity that causes harmful side effects. Although ultrasonic radiation does not have a lasting cumulative effect as x-ray does, and it does not cause cancer as x-ray can, high-power ultrasonics in excess of 1 W/cm² can cause injury to patients from overheating and can cause mechanical tissue damage due to cavitation. Fortunately, diagnostic ultrasound uses power well below the danger level. However, therapeutic ultrasound for muscle massage and the like may cause high-power side effects.

Attenuation in Ultrasonic Waves

In order to know how deep into the tissue the power penetrates in therapeutic ultrasound equipment, attenuation factors have been measured as given in Table 16.2.

Typical ultrasonic frequencies range from 1 to 5 MHz. From Table 16.2, we see that attenuation at 1 MHz for muscle is 1.3 dB/cm, and at 5 MHz it is 6.5 dB/cm. The operating technician may use this fact to selectively heat surface muscle by choosing a frequency that would distribute the power relatively evenly over the muscle. Note that attenuation of 3 dB absorbs half the power available.

**TABLE 16.2
Attenuation Factors in
Biological Tissues**

Tissue	Attenuation factor (dB/cm/MHz)
Fat	0.63
Muscle	1.3
Bone	20
Lung	41

16.3 ULTRASONIC BLOOD FLOW EQUIPMENT

Ultrasonic equipment is often used to measure the velocity of objects such as a stream of blood, a moving heart valve, or the motion of an artery in response to a pressure pulse. Blood flow is monitored either by observing frequency shift due to the Doppler effect, or by observing shifts in the transit time of waves going first upstream, then downstream through the blood. An analysis of the Doppler effect is considered first.

An Analysis of the Doppler Effect

The Doppler effect is simply what someone moving away from a source of sound, such as a whistle, experiences. That person will hear a pitch lower than the pitch heard by a person standing still. And likewise, someone moving toward the whistle will hear a higher pitch. The situation is illustrated in Figure 16.12. The sound waves produce compressions in air separated by

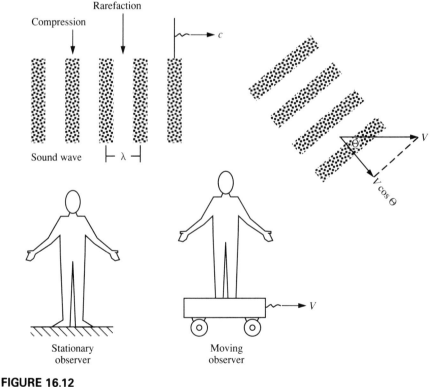

FIGURE 16.12
The Doppler effect.

a wavelength λ. The stationary observer hears a frequency given by Equation (16.5),

$$f = c/\lambda$$

The crest velocity observed by the person on the platform traveling at a velocity V, however, will be $c - V$. Furthermore, the wavelength of the sound, unaffected by the platform, remains the same. Therefore, the person hears a frequency f_p of

$$f_p = \frac{c - V}{\lambda}$$

Taking the ratio of these two equations gives

$$\frac{f_p}{f} = 1 - \frac{V}{c}$$

or

$$f_p = \left(1 - \frac{V}{c}\right)f$$

If the platform moves at an angle Θ with respect to the sound wave, the platform projected velocity is $V \cos \Theta$, so that

$$f_p = \left(1 - \frac{V}{c} \cos \Theta\right)f \qquad (16.17)$$

The echo frequency of the ultrasound reflected from the moving platform, f_s, heard by the stationary observer, will be affected by the velocity $2V \cos \Theta$, because the change in the path length is that due to the incident wave plus the reflected wave, so that

$$f_s = \left(1 - \frac{2V}{c} \cos \Theta\right)f \qquad (16.18)$$

Much of the ultrasonic equipment used in medicine responds to the difference between the signal frequency f and the echo frequency, called

$$\Delta f = f - f_s$$

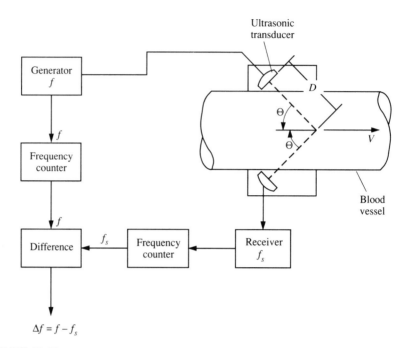

FIGURE 16.13
An ultrasonic blood flow meter.

Then, from Equation (16.18),

$$\Delta f = f - f\left(1 - \frac{2V}{c}\cos\Theta\right)$$

or

$$\Delta f = \frac{2V}{c}f\cos\Theta \qquad\qquad (16.19)$$

The difference frequency can be measured by the circuit in Figure 16.13, and the flow velocity V is computed from

$$V = \frac{\Delta f c}{2f\cos\Theta} \qquad\qquad (16.20)$$

where Δf is the difference frequency, f is the generator frequency, Θ is the angle of the transducer as specified, c is the velocity of sound in blood or the fluid, and V is the fluid velocity in m/s.

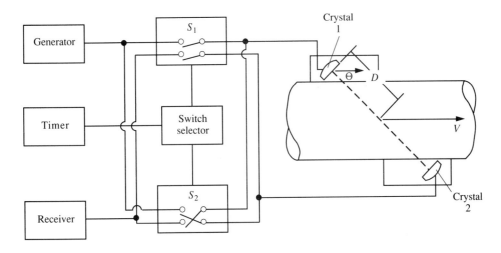

FIGURE 16.14
Blood flow measurement by transit time difference.

An Analysis of Transit Time

Another measurement that can be made electronically to deduce the flow rate V is the transit time. In Figure 16.14, the distance D the sound travels is related to the downstream transit time T_D as follows:

$$D = T_D(V \cos \Theta + c)$$

In the downstream direction the velocity of the sound is increased by the velocity of the stream that carries it. This decreases the downstream transit time. The transit time upstream T_U, however, is increased so that

$$D = T_U(c - V \cos \Theta)$$

The difference in transit time is then $\Delta T = T_U - T_D$, or

$$\Delta T = \frac{-D}{c + V \cos \Theta} + \frac{D}{c - V \cos \Theta}$$

$$= \frac{-(cD - VD \cos \Theta) + Dc + VD \cos \Theta}{c^2 - (V \cos \Theta)^2}$$

For small values of V we have $V^2 \ll c^2$, so

$$\Delta T = \frac{2VD \cos \Theta}{c^2}$$

The flow velocity V is then

$$V = \frac{\Delta T c^2}{2D \cos \Theta} \tag{16.21}$$

where ΔT is the difference between upstream and downstream transit time, Θ is the angle of the transducer, c is the speed of sound in the fluid. A circuit for measuring the transit time difference ΔT is given in Figure 16.14. The switch selector first closes S_1 and opens S_2. This connects the generator to crystal 1 and the receiver to crystal 2, and the upstream transit time is measured. Subsequently, the switch selector opens S_1 and closes S_2. This connects the generator to crystal 2 and the receiver to crystal 1 and measures the downstream transit time.

The difference ΔT between these two times is then measured, and the blood velocity, V, is then read out according to Equation (16.21).

REFERENCES

Feinberg, B. "Medical Ultrasound Systems." Chapter 9 in *Applied Clinical Engineering*. Englewood Cliffs, NJ: Prentice-Hall, 1986.

Goldstein, A. "Ultrasonic Imaging." In *Encyclopedia of Medical Instrumentation*, Vol. 4, edited by J. G. Webster. New York: John Wiley & Sons, 1988.

Kraus, J. D., and Carver, K. R. *Electromagnetics,* 2nd ed. New York: McGraw-Hill, 1973.

Peura, R. A. "Principles of Ultrasound." Chapter 9 in *Biomedical Engineering and Instrumentation*, edited by J. D. Bronzino. Boston: Prindle, Weber & Schmidt, 1986.

Wells, P. N. T. *Biomedical Ultrasonics*. London: Academic Press, 1977.

EXERCISES

1. An ultrasonic signal has a velocity of 1500 m/s at 2 MHz.

   (a) Compute the wavelength.
   (b) Compute the phase constant, β, in units of m^{-1}.

2. An ultrasonic wave is propagating into bone tissue at a frequency of 3 MHz.

   (a) Compute the wavelength of the wave.
   (b) Compute the phase constant, β.
   (c) Compute the period, T.

3. An ultrasonic wave in bone at 2 MHz measures a pressure of 2 N/m^2 at $t = 0$ and $x = 0$, in Figure 16.9.

(a) Write the equation for the wave in the form $p = P_0 \cos(\omega t + \beta x)$.

(b) Plot this wave as a function of x when $t = 0$ s.

4. (a) Plot the wave in Exercise 3 as a function of position when $t = T/8$ seconds, where T is the period of the wave.

(b) Determine the direction of propagation for this wave by comparison with Exercise 3.

5. An ultrasonic wave is incident upon a muscle-to-bone boundary. The incident power is 1 W/cm^2.

(a) Compute the pressure of the incident wave in rms units.

(b) Compute the pressure of the reflected wave in rms units.

(c) Compute the reflected power in watts.

6. An ultrasonic wave has a power of 2 W/cm^2 in bone.

(a) Compute the pressure wave magnitude in rms units.

(b) Compute the rms velocity wave magnitude of the bone atoms caused by the pressure wave.

7. Compute the reflection coefficient at the boundary of fat and bone.

8. If 3 W/cm^2 of power is incident upon a fat-to-bone boundary, how much power is reflected back toward the ultrasonic transducer?

*9. A piezoelectric crystal has a characteristic impedance of 24×10^6 kg/m^{2}s. An impedance-matching transformer one quarter wavelength long matches this impedance to bone. Compute the characteristic impedance, Z_T, of this transformer.

APPENDIXES

A. Computer Programs

B. Laplace Transforms

C. Medical Terminology

Computer Programs

The odd-numbered programs listed here are written for the Hewlett-Packard HP-15C hand-held programmable calculator. They can be run on the HP-11C calculator where indicated in the program description if the key-strokes gπ are replaced by fπ. These are keystroke programs that calculate equations and follow flow diagrams in the text, as indicated in the program descriptions.

BASIC language, IBM version A4.00 programs following these flow diagrams are listed as the even-numbered programs so that other types of computers can be used by the student if desired.

PROGRAM A-1   Calculator HP-11C, HP-15C
PROGRAM DESCRIPTION: Computes Equation (4.1). Flow diagram is in
                    Figure 4.5.
REGISTERS: R_s-STO 1 R_d-STO 2 C_d-STO 3
INITIAL DATA: Key f into the x-register. Key in g DEG.

STEP	KEY	STEP	KEY	STEP	KEY	STEP	KEY
001	f LBL B	002	2	003	X		
004	gπ	005	X	006	RCL 3	007	X
008	RCL 2	009	X	010	ENTER	011	1
012	g$\rightarrow$P	013	STO 4	014	x$\rightleftharpoons$y	015	STO 5
016	RCL 5	017	CHS	018	ENTER	019	RCL 4
020	1/x	021	RCL 2	022	X	023	f$\rightarrow$R
024	RCL 1	025	+	026	STO 6	027	x$\rightleftharpoons$y
028	ENTER	029	RCL 6	030	g$\rightarrow$P	031	g RTN

OUTCOME: x-register contains $|Z|$, y-register contains θ.

PROGRAM A-2   BASIC

```
10 PI=3.141592654#
20 REM APPENDIX A-2 COMPUTES EQUATIONS (4.6), (4.7), (4.8)
30 INPUT"ENTER TEMP:";T
40 BETA=4000
50 RTO=10
55 VA=10
60 TO=310
70 R1=4
80 R2=1000
90 R3=1000
140 E=2.718282
220 RT=RTO*E^(BETA*((1/T)-(1/TO)))
230 RP=RTO*((BETA-2*TO)/(BETA+2*TO))
240 RTP=RP*RT/(RP+RT)
250 VO=VA*((R1/(R1+RTP))-(R2/(R2+R3)))
260 PRINT"VO = ";VO
270 GOTO 30
Ok
RUN
ENTER TEMP:? 306
VO = -.3059948
```

PROGRAM A-3   CALCULATOR: HP-11C, HP-15C
PROGRAM DESCRIPTION: Program for Example 4.11. Flow diagram in Figure
                     4.23.
REGISTERS: R_1-STO 1 R_2-STO 2 R_3-STO 3 R_x-STO 4 G-STO 5 1-STO 6
           V_a-STO 7
INITIAL DATA: Key Δl into the x-register.

STEP	KEY	STEP	KEY	STEP	KEY	STEP	KEY
001	f LBL A	002	RCL 5	003	X		
004	RCL 4	005	X	006	RCL 6	007	÷
008	RCL 4	009	+	010	RCL 1	011	+
012	1/x	013	RCL 1	014	X	015	RCL 2
016	RCL 3	017	+	018	1/x	019	RCL 2
020	X	021	−	022	RCL 7	023	X
024	g RTN						

OUTCOME: x-register contains V_{OUT}.

PROGRAM A-4   BASIC

```
10 PI = 3.141592654#
20 REM APPENDIX A-4 COMPUTES EQ. 5.18
```

```
30 INPUT "ENTER V1: ";V1
40 INPUT "ENTER ALPHA: "; AL
50 V2=1
60 RF=700
70 RI=300
80 VO=(V1*-(RF/RI))+(AL*V2*(1+(RF/RI)))
90 PRINT "VO=";VO
100 GOTO 30
Ok
RUN
ENTER V1: ? 2
ENTER ALPHA: ? .1
VO=-4.333333
```

PROGRAM A-5   CALCULATOR: HP-11C, HP-15C
PROGRAM DESCRIPTION: A program for the CMRR by Equation (5.26).
REGISTERS: α-STO 3 R_f-STO 4 R_i-STO 5 CMRR-STO 7
INITIAL DATA: Key α into the x-register.

STEP	KEY	STEP	KEY	STEP	KEY	STEP	KEY
001	f LBL B	002	STO 3	003	RCL 5		
004	RCL 4	005	÷	006	1	007	+
008	RCL 3	009	X	010	1	011	–
012	g ABS	013	STO 7	014	1/x	015	g LOG
016	2	017	0	018	X	019	g RTN

OUTCOME: x-register contains CMRdB.

PROGRAM A-6   BASIC

```
10 PI=3.141592654#
20 REM APPENDIX A-6 COMPUTES EQ. 6.9
30 INPUT"ENTER FREQUENCY :";F
40 W=2*PI*F
50 RO=7000000!
60 R3=30000
70 R4=20000
80 CS=2E-12
90 VS=120
95 RF=7000000!
100 X=(RF/R3)+(RF/R4)+1:Y=W*RO*CS:GOSUB 350
110 M1=MAG:A1=ANGLE
120 X=.0001:Y=W*RO*CS*VS:GOSUB 350
130 M2=MAG:A2=ANGLE
140 VCM=M2/M1 : TH=A2-A1
```

```
150 PRINT"VCM= ";VCM;" ANGLE= ";TH
160 GOTO 30
350 REM
360 ANGLE=ATN(Y/X)
370 MAG=X/COS(ANGLE): MAG=ABS(MAG)
380 ANGLE=ANGLE*180/PI
390 RETURN
Ok
RUN
ENTER FREQUENCY :? 60
VCM= 1.083761E-03 ANGLE= 89.99042
```

PROGRAM A-7   CALCULATOR: HP-11C, HP-15C
PROGRAM DESCRIPTION: Program for Equation (6.27).
REGISTERS: V_1-STO 0 R_1-STO 1 R_2-STO 2 R_f-STO 3 R_i-STO 4 α_1-STO 5
         α_2-STO 6 V_{BB}-STO 8
INITIAL DATA: Key V_1 into the x-register.

STEP	KEY	STEP	KEY	STEP	KEY	STEP	KEY
001	f LBL B	002	STO 0	003	RCL 6		
004	CHS	005	1	006	+	007	RCL 2
008	X	009	RCL 1	010	+	011	1/x
012	RCL 8	013	CHS	014	RCL 5	015	RCL 0
016	X	017	+	018	X	019	RCL 3
020	X	021	STO 7	022	RCL 2	023	RCL 6
024	X	025	RCL 1	026	+	027	1/x
028	RCL 8	029	RCL 5	030	RCL 0	031	X
032	+	033	X	034	RCL 3	035	X
036	RCL 7	037	+	038	RCL 0	039	RCL 5
040	X	041	RCL 3	042	X	043	RCL 4
044	÷	045	+	046	RCL 0	047	RCL 5
048	X	049	+	050	gRTN		

OUTCOME: x-register contains V_{OUT}.

PROGRAM A-8   BASIC

```
10 PI=3.141592654#
20 REM APPENDIX A-8 COMPUTES EQ. 1.8
30 INPUT"ENTER FREQUENCY :";F
40 R=100000!
50 C=.000001
60 W=2*PI*F
70 X=1:Y=-1/(W*R*C):GOSUB 350
```

```
80 M1=1/MAG:A1=-1*ANGLE
90 PRINT"GV= ";M1;" ANGLE= ";A1
100 GOTO 30
350 REM
360 ANGLE=ATN(Y/X)
370 MAG=X/COS(ANGLE): MAG=ABS(MAG)
380 ANGLE=ANGLE*180/PI
390 RETURN
Ok
RUN
ENTER FREQUENCY :? 4
GV= .9291521 ANGLE= 21.69698
```

PROGRAM A-9   CALCULATOR: HP-11C, HP-15C
PROGRAM DESCRIPTION: Computes Equation (7.4).
REGISTERS: R-STO 1 C-STO 2
INITIAL DATA: Key f into the x-register.

STEP	KEY	STEP	KEY	STEP	KEY	STEP	KEY
001	f LBL D	002	g deg	003	g CF 8		
004	STO 0	005	2	006	X	007	gπ
008	X	009	RCL 2	010	X	011	RCL 1
012	X	013	ENTER	014	1	015	g$\rightarrow$P
016	1/x	017	STO 3	018	x⇌y	019	CHS
020	STO 4	021	g RTN					

OUTCOME: x-register contains angle θ, y-register contains $|G_v|$.

PROGRAM A-10   BASIC

```
10 PI=3.141592654#
20 REM APPENDIX A-10 COMPUTES EQ. 7.6
30 INPUT"ENTER FREQUENCY :";F
40 R1=5000
50 C1=.000001
60 R2=100000!
70 C2=.000001
80 W=2*PI*F
90 X=1:Y=W*R1*C1:GOSUB 350
100 M1=1/MAG:A1=-ANGLE
110 X=1:Y=-1/(W*C2*R2):GOSUB 350
120 M2=1/MAG:A2=-ANGLE
130 GV=M1*M2
140 THETA=A1+A2
```

```
145 IF GV<0 THEN GV=-GV
150 GVDB=20*(LOG(GV)/LOG(10))
160 PRINT"GV =";GV;" ANGLE=";THETA
170 PRINT"GV (DB)=";GVDB
180 GOTO 30
350 REM
360 ANGLE=ATN(Y/X)
370 MAG=X/COS(ANGLE): MAG=ABS(MAG)
380 ANGLE=ANGLE*180/PI
390 RETURN
Ok
RUN
ENTER FREQUENCY :? 20
GV = .8440648 ANGLE=-27.59204
GV (DB)=-1.472485
```

PROGRAM A-11   CALCULATOR: HP-11C, HP-15C
PROGRAM DESCRIPTION: Calculates Equation (7.10). Flow diagram in Figure 7.15.
REGISTERS: R-STO 1 C_1-STO 2 C_2-STO 3
INITIAL DATA: Key f into the x-register.

STEP	KEY	STEP	KEY	STEP	KEY	STEP	KEY
001	f LBL A	002	g DEG	003	g CF 8		
004	2	005	X	006	gπ	007	X
008	RCL 1	009	X	010	STO 0	011	RCL 3
012	X	013	ENTER	014	1	015	g→P
016	STO 4	017	x⇌y	018	STO 5	019	RCL 0
020	RCL 2	021	X	022	ENTER	023	2
024	g→P	025	RCL 4	026	X	027	x⇌y
028	RCL 5	029	+	030	x⇌y	031	f→R
032	1	033	–	034	STO 4	035	x⇌y
036	RCL 0	037	RCL 2	C38	X	039	–
040	ENTER	041	RCL 4	042	g→P	043	1/x
044	x⇌y	045	CHS	046	g RTN		

OUTCOME: x-register contains θ, y-register contains $|A_v|$.

PROGRAM A-12   BASIC

```
10 PI=3.141592654#
20 REM APPENDIX A-12 COMPUTES EQ. 7.12
30 INPUT"ENTER FREQUENCY :";F
40 R1=9300
```

```
50 R2=18600
60 C=2E-09
70 Z=1/(2*PI*F*R2*C)
80 X=1:Y=-Z:GOSUB 350
90 M1=MAG:A1=ANGLE
100 Z=1/(2*PI*F*R1*C)
110 X=2:Y=-Z:GOSUB 350
120 M1=M1*MAG:A1=A1+ANGLE
130 ANGLE=A1:MAG=M1:GOSUB 300
150 X=X-1:Y=Y+(1/(2*PI*F*R1*C))
160 GOSUB 350
170 M1=MAG:A1=ANGLE
180 M1=1/M1:A1=A1*-1
185 M1=M1
190 PRINT"GV= ";M1;" ANGLE= ";A1
200 GOTO 30
300 ANGLE=PI*ANGLE/180
310 X=MAG*COS(ANGLE)
320 Y=MAG*SIN(ANGLE)
330 ANGLE=ANGLE*180/PI
340 RETURN
350 REM
360 ANGLE=ATN(Y/X)
370 MAG=X/COS(ANGLE): MAG=ABS(MAG)
380 ANGLE=ANGLE*180/PI
390 RETURN
Ok
RUN
ENTER FREQUENCY :? 6050
GV = -0.707 ANGLE= -89.99314
```

PROGRAM A-13   CALCULATOR: HP-11C, HP-15C
PROGRAM DESCRIPTION: Computes Equation (7.14), third-order, low-pass
                     filter gain. Flow diagram in Figure 7.21.
REGISTERS: R-STO 1 C_1-STO 2 C_2-STO 3 C_3-STO 7
INITIAL DATA: Key f into the x-register.

STEP	KEY	STEP	KEY	STEP	KEY	STEP	KEY
001	f LBL A	002	g DEG	003	2		
004	X	005	gπ	006	X	007	RCL 1
008	X	009	STO 0	010	RCL 3	011	X
012	ENTER	013	1	014	g$\rightarrow$P	015	STO 4
016	x$\rightleftarrows$y	017	STO 5	018	RCL 0	019	RCL 2
020	X	021	ENTER	022	2	023	g$\rightarrow$P

024 RCL 4	025 X	026 x ⇌ y	027 RCL 5
028 +	029 x ⇌ y	030 f → R	031 1
032 −	033 STO 4	034 x ⇌ y	035 RCL 0
036 RCL 2	037 X	038 −	039 ENTER
040 RCL 4	041 g → P	042 1/x	043 STO 4
044 x ⇌ y	045 CHS	046 STO 5	047 RCL 0
048 RCL 7	049 X	050 ENTER	051 1
052 g → P	053 1/x	054 RCL 4	055 X
056 x ⇌ y	057 CHS	058 RCL 5	059 +
060 g RTN			

OUTCOME: x-register contains θ, y-register contains $|A_v|$.

PROGRAM A-14   BASIC

```
10 PI=3.141592654#
20 REM APPENDIX A-14 COMPUTES EQ. 7.16
30 INPUT"ENTER FREQUENCY :";F
40 R=2652.6
50 C=.000001
60 W=2*PI*F
70 X=1:Y=W*R*C:GOSUB 350
80 M1=MAG*MAG:A1=ANGLE*2
90 MAG=M1:ANGLE=A1:GOSUB 300
100 X1=X:Y1=Y
110 Y1=Y1+W*R*C
120 X=X1:Y=Y1:GOSUB 350
130 M1=1/MAG:A1=ANGLE*-1
140 M2=W*R*C:A2=90
150 M3=M1*M2:A3=A2+A1
160 MAG=M3:ANGLE=A3:GOSUB 300
170 X1=X-(1/3):Y1=Y
180 X=X1:Y=Y1:GOSUB 350
190 M1=MAG:A1=ANGLE
200 PRINT"GV= ";M1;" ANGLE= ";A1
210 GOTO 30
300 ANGLE=PI*ANGLE/180
310 X=MAG*COS(ANGLE)
320 Y=MAG*SIN(ANGLE)
330 ANGLE=ANGLE*180/PI
340 RETURN
350 REM
360 ANGLE=ATN(Y/X)
370 MAG=X/COS(ANGLE): MAG=ABS(MAG)
```

```
380 ANGLE=ANGLE*180/PI
390 RETURN
Ok
RUN
ENTER FREQUENCY :? 30
GV = -.1490699 ANGLE= -63.43
```

PROGRAM A-15   CALCULATOR: HP-11C, HP-15C
PROGRAM DESCRIPTION: Computes Equations (8.14) and (8.15).
REGISTERS: R-STO 1 L-STO 2 C-STO 3 V_P-STO 4
INITIAL DATA: Key t into the x-register.

STEP	KEY	STEP	KEY	STEP	KEY	STEP	KEY
000		001	f LBL .4	002	STO 0	003	g RAD
004	RCL 1	005	2	006	÷	007	RCL 2
008	÷	009	STO 5	010	RCL 2	011	1/x
012	RCL 3	013	÷	014	RCL 5	015	g x^2
016	−	017	$\sqrt{x}$	018	STO 6	019	RCL 0
020	X	021	SIN	022	RCL 5	023	RCL 0
024	X	025	CHS	026	e^x	027	X
028	RCL 4	029	RCL 1	030	X	031	X
032	RCL 2	033	÷	034	RCL 6	035	÷
036	g RTN						

OUTCOME: x-register reads v_R.

PROGRAM A-16   BASIC

```
10 REM APPENDIX A-16 COMPUTES EQ. 8.16, 8.17, 8.18
20 INPUT"ENTER TIME :";T
30 R=180
40 L=.1
50 C=.000016
60 V=5000
70 AL=R/(2*L)+SQR(((R/(2*L))^2)-(1/(L*C)))
80 Y=R/(2*L)-SQR(((R/(2*L))^2)-(1/(L*C)))
160 Z=R*V/L
170 Z1=(EXP(-AL*T)-EXP(-Y*T))/(Y-AL)
180 ANS=Z*Z1
190 PRINT"VR= ";ANS
200 GOTO 20
Ok
RUN
ENTER TIME :? .003
VR= 2361.707
```

PROGRAM A-17   CALCULATOR: HP-11C, HP-15C
PROGRAM DESCRIPTION: Computes Equation (9.8).
REGISTERS: R_1-STO 1 R_2-STO 2 R_P-STO 3 V_B-STO 4 V_{OUT}-STO 5
INITIAL DATA: Key α into the x-register.

STEP	KEY	STEP	KEY	STEP	KEY	STEP	KEY
000		001	f LBL A	002	STO 0	003	CHS
004	1	005	+	006	RCL 0	007	X
008	RCL 3	009	X	010	RCL 2	011	X
012	RCL 0	013	CHS	014	1	015	+
016	RCL 0	017	X	018	RCL 3	019	X
020	RCL 1	021	+	022	RCL 1	023	RCL 2
024	+	025	X	026	STO 6	027	÷
028	CHS	029	1	030	+	031	1/x
032	STO 7	033	RCL 1	034	RCL 2	035	X
036	RCL 4	037	X	038	RCL 0	039	CHS
040	2	041	X	042	1	043	+
044	X	045	RCL 6	046	÷	047	CHS
048	RCL 1	049	RCL 5	050	X	051	RCL 1
052	RCL 2	053	+	054	÷	055	+
056	RCL 7	057	X	058	g RTN		

OUTCOME: Read V_R in the x-register.

PROGRAM A-18   BASIC

```
10 PI=3.141592654#
20 REM APPENDIX A-18 COMPUTES EQ. 11.12
30 INPUT"ENTER FREQUENCY :";F
40 RC=1.1347E+11
50 LC=3.008E+09
60 CC=7.04E-16
70 CD=2.04E-15
80 W=2*PI*F
90 X=0:Y=W*(CD+CC):GOSUB 350
100 M1=1/MAG:A1=-ANGLE
110 X=RC:Y=(W*LC-(1/(W*(CD+CC)))):GOSUB 350
120 M2=MAG:A2=ANGLE
130 GP=M1/M2:A=A1-A2
140 GP=20*(LOG(GP)/LOG(10))
170 PRINT"GP= ";GP;" ANGLE= ";A
180 GOTO 30
300 ANGLE=PI*ANGLE/180
310 X=MAG*COS(ANGLE)
320 Y=MAG*SIN(ANGLE)
```

```
330 ANGLE=ANGLE*180/PI
340 RETURN
350 IF X=0 THEN X=9.9E-14
360 ANGLE=ATN(Y/X)
370 MAG=X/COS(ANGLE)
375 IF MAG<0 THEN MAG=-MAG
380 ANGLE=ANGLE*180/PI
390 RETURN
Ok
RUN
ENTER FREQUENCY :? 90
GP= -4.3612 ANGLE= -170.2194
```

PROGRAM A-19   CALCULATOR: HP-15C
PROGRAM DESCRIPTION: Computes Equation (11.17).
REGISTERS: R_H-STO 1 R_{EQ}-STO 2 C_{EQ}-STO 3 L_{EQ}-STO 4
INITIAL DATA: Key f into the x-register.

STEP	KEY	STEP	KEY	STEP	KEY	STEP	KEY
001	f LBL A	002	STO 0	003	RCL 1		
004	ENTER	005	RCL 0	006	RCL 3	007	X
008	gπ	009	X	010	2	011	X
012	1/x	013	CHS	014	f I	015	1/x
016	0	017	ENTER	018	RCL 0	019	RCL 3
020	X	021	gπ	022	X	023	2
024	X	025	1/x	026	RCL 1	027	X
028	CHS	029	f I	030	X	031	STO 5
032	f Re≧Im	033	STO 6	034	RCL 2	035	ENTER
036	RCL 0	037	RCL 4	038	X	039	gπ
040	X	041	2	042	X	043	f I
044	RCL 5	045	ENTER	046	RCL 6	047	f I
048	+	049	1/x	050	RCL 5	051	ENTER
052	RCL 6	053	f I	054	X	055	f Re≧Im
056	ENTER	057	f Re≧Im	058	g 5 8	059	g→P
060	g LOG	061	2	062	0	063	X
064	g RTN						

OUTCOME: Read $|P_{MEAS}/P_{ACT}|$ in x-register, θ in y-register.

B

Laplace Transforms

B.1 THE LAPLACE METHOD

In the Laplace method, electrical circuits are formed of sources and impedances in a manner similar to that used in phasor domain analysis of sinusoidal steady-state circuits. The sources are called *step sources* in the Laplace domain, and the impedances are called *Laplace domain impedances*.

The Step Source

The source is defined as a voltage source turned on and off by a switch in Figure B.1 at $t = 0$. The source in terms of the Laplace variable is a constant value V_{OUT}/s. This equivalent Laplace domain source operates like an ideal source in circuit analysis and has an internal impedance of zero. Several sample plots of voltage $V_{aa'}$ as a function of time are given in Fig-

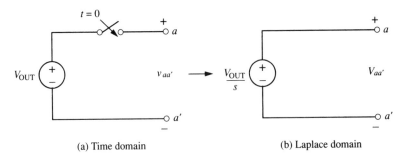

(a) Time domain   (b) Laplace domain

FIGURE B.1
Laplace equivalent step-voltage source.

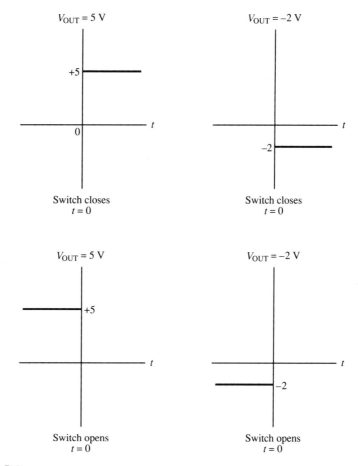

FIGURE B.2
The source voltage as a function of time for various values of V_{OUT}.

ure B.2. When the switch closes at $t = 0$, the voltage is initially zero and then steps up to V_{OUT}. On the other hand, when the switch opens at $t = 0$, the voltage at nodes aa' is initially V_{OUT} and then jumps to zero. Figure B.1(b) is called the Laplace equivalent circuit of a switch in series with a constant voltage source.

Laplace Equivalent Impedances

The circuit impedances to a step function are in the same form as the phasor impedance, except the $j\omega$ is replaced by the Laplace variable s, and account is made of the current or voltage that exists at the instant before the switch of the source is thrown. For a capacitor, C, the voltage at the time the switch is thrown remains constant and has the same value the instant before and the instant after the switching.

The Laplace domain equivalent, shown in Figure B.3, consists of a capacitor of impedance $1/sC$ in series with a voltage source in the polarity shown, of value v_0/s. In the Laplace domain, the voltage, V, is a function of the Laplace variable s, as is the Laplace domain current I. These are related by the equation

$$V = \frac{I}{sC} + \frac{v_0}{s} \qquad \text{(B.1)}$$

where v_0 is the initial voltage on the capacitor before the switch is thrown.

The equivalent circuit for the inductor takes into account the initial current through the inductor, i_0. The current i_0 remains constant during the transient while the switch is thrown. The Laplace domain equivalent in Figure B.4 consists of an inductor of impedance sL in series with a voltage source of value Li_0 in the polarity shown. The Laplace domain voltage V and current I are functions of the Laplace variable s and are related by the equation

$$V = sLI - Li_0 \qquad \text{(B.2)}$$

It is important to maintain the relative polarities of V and I as indicated in Figure B.4.

The Laplace domain equivalent of a resistor is illustrated in Figure B.5. The resistor R presents a Laplace domain impedance of value R. The variables V and I are functions of the Laplace variable s and are related by the equation

$$V = IR \qquad \text{(B.3)}$$

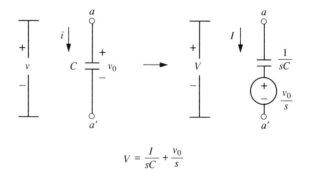

$$V = \frac{I}{sC} + \frac{v_0}{s}$$

FIGURE B.3
The Laplace equivalent of a capacitor.

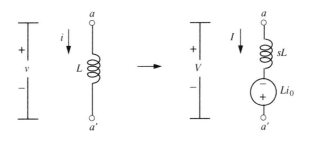

$$V = sLI - Li_0$$

FIGURE B.4
Laplace equivalent circuit of an inductor.

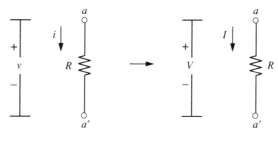

$$V = IR$$

FIGURE B.5
Laplace equivalent circuit of a resistor.

Circuit Analysis of Laplace Equivalent Elements

Kirchhoff's current law (KCL) and voltage law (KVL) apply to the preceding Laplace equivalent elements when arranged in circuits of branches and nodes. Therefore, the analysis methods, including the principle of superposition, voltage division, and current division, and the rules for combining series and parallel elements, apply to circuit elements arranged as Laplace equivalents. The Ohm's law relationships and voltage sources are given in Equations (B.1), (B.2), and (B.3). The Laplace equivalent of a constant source V_{OUT} and a switch is given in Figure B.1 as V_{OUT}/s.

EXAMPLE B.1 At $t = 0$, the switch is thrown on a capacitor initially charged to 10 V as in Figure B.6(a). Find the Laplace voltage V_R as a function of the Laplace variable s after the switch is thrown.

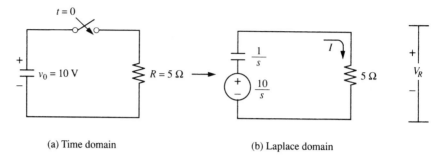

(a) Time domain   (b) Laplace domain

FIGURE B.6
The time domain and Laplace domain circuits for a capacitor discharging into a resistor.

SOLUTION Applying KVL and Ohm's law to the Laplace circuit given in Figure B.6(b),

$$V_R = \frac{10}{s} - \frac{I}{s}$$

and

$$I = \frac{V_R}{5}$$

These two equations yield

$$V_R = \frac{10}{s} - \frac{V_R}{sR}$$

Then

$$V_R\left(1 + \frac{1}{sR}\right) = \frac{10}{s}$$

Or, since $R = 5\ \Omega$,

$$V_R = \frac{10}{s + 0.2}$$

Here the voltage across the resistor is given as a function of the Laplace variable s. To find the voltage as a function of time, it is necessary to use Laplace transform tables.

TABLE B.1
Selected Laplace Transforms

$F(s)$	$f(t)$ for $t > 0$
(1) $\dfrac{K}{s + \alpha}$	$e^{-\alpha t} K$
(2) $\dfrac{K}{(s + \alpha)(s + \gamma)}$	$\dfrac{e^{-\alpha t} - e^{-\gamma t}}{\gamma - \alpha} K$
(3) $\dfrac{K}{(s + \alpha)(s + \beta)(s + \gamma)}$	$\dfrac{Ke^{-\alpha t}}{(\beta - \alpha)(\gamma - \alpha)} + \dfrac{Ke^{-\beta t}}{(\alpha - \beta)(\gamma - \beta)} + \dfrac{Ke^{-\gamma t}}{(\alpha - \gamma)(\beta - \gamma)}$
(4) $\dfrac{K}{(s + \alpha)^2 + \omega^2}$	$\dfrac{K}{\omega} e^{-\alpha t} \sin \omega t$

Laplace Transform Tables

In order to find the function of time corresponding to the voltage or current given as a function of the Laplace variable s, tables of transforms have been developed. Such a table, Table B.1, is here made up of two columns headed by $f(t)$ for the function of time corresponding to the Laplace function $F(s)$. Tables are available that are complete enough that most engineering functions can be found by consulting them. Sometimes it is necessary to rearrange the terms in $F(s)$ algebraically to match the unknown constants. Of course, if the appropriate Laplace transform is not found in the table, you could refer to the Laplace transform definition and perform the integration indicated, but that is beyond the scope of this text and will not be necessary in the cases treated.

EXAMPLE B.2   Use the Laplace transform table to determine the voltage across the resistor V_R as a function of time in Example B.1.

SOLUTION   The appropriate Laplace transform pair from Table B.1 is Transform (1). There,

$$F(s) = \frac{K}{s + \alpha}$$

and

$$f(t) = Ke^{-\alpha t}$$

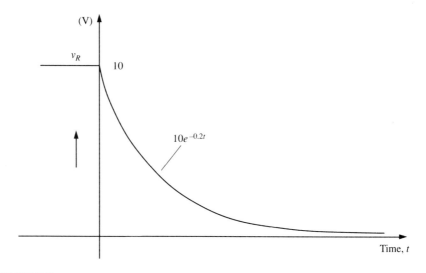

FIGURE B.7
A discharging capacitor.

An equivalent transform pair is obtained by multiplying both sides of the pair by the same constant, in this case $K = 10$. That is, if

$$F(s) = \frac{10}{s + \alpha}$$

then

$$f(t) = 10e^{-\alpha t}$$

The constant α in this case is 0.2. Using the transform,

$$v_R = 10e^{-0.2t}$$

A plot of the step response of the capacitor is given in Figure B.7.

RC Circuit Step Response

The input impedance of modern electronic circuits can very often be represented by a resistance in series with the input lead and a shunting capacitor to ground, as illustrated in Figure B.8. Such circuits are commonly of metal-oxide-semiconductor (MOS) construction. The input wire is connected to a metalization on a silicon dioxide (glass) insulator grown on top of the active semiconductor, as the name MOS implies. The metal-oxide semiconductor naturally forms a capacitance often connected to ground. Since this type of circuit is widely used in digital applications, it is important to understand its step response. The reason for this is that a digital signal is a sequence of steps between the 1 and 0 states.

We first consider the charging case. In Figure B.8, the switch is moved from position 1 to position 2 at $t = 0$. The capacitor will have some initial voltage at $t = 0$, V_I, and will charge up until v_C reads V_F, called the final voltage because the capacitor will maintain this voltage indefinitely, for the given switch setting.

The Laplace method can be used to find the charging equation for Figure B.8 for $t > 0$. The Laplace domain equivalent circuit appears in Figure B.9. Our goal is to compute the Laplace domain voltage V_C as a function of s. The Laplace tables will then be consulted to find the charging capacitor voltage, v_C, as a function of time, t.

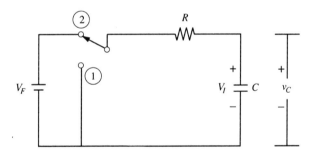

FIGURE B.8
Circuit for charging a capacitor.

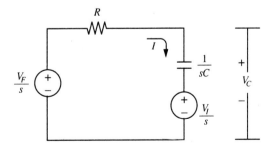

FIGURE B.9
Laplace equivalent of a charging capacitor.

First, in Figure B.9, Ohm's law is used to compute the current, I:

$$I = \frac{\dfrac{V_F}{s} - \dfrac{V_I}{s}}{R + \dfrac{1}{sC}}$$

Multiplying top and bottom by s/R yields

$$I = \frac{1}{R}\left(\frac{V_F - V_I}{s + \dfrac{1}{RC}}\right)$$

Then KVL yields

$$V_C = \frac{I}{sC} + \frac{V_I}{s}$$

$$= \frac{V_I}{s} + \frac{1}{sRC}\left(\frac{V_F - V_I}{s + \dfrac{1}{RC}}\right)$$

or

$$V_C = \frac{V_I}{s} + \frac{V_F - V_I}{RC}\left(\frac{1}{s\left(s + \dfrac{1}{RC}\right)}\right) \tag{B.4}$$

The Laplace table can be used to transform each term of Equation (B.4) to the time domain individually. For the first term, Transform (1) of Table B.1 is used. Each side of the transform is multiplied by V_I and α is taken as 0. The function of time is then

$$V_I e^{-0t} = V_I$$

The second term of Equation (B.4) is written in the time domain by means of Transform (2) in Table B.1. Here, $\alpha = 0$ and $\gamma = 1/RC$. Both sides of the transform are multiplied by the constant $(V_F - V_I)/RC$. Therefore, the second term is

$$\frac{V_F - V_I}{RC} (RC)(1 - e^{-t/RC})$$

The time domain equation for v_C is the sum of the equations for each term of Equation (B.4). Therefore

$$v_C = V_I + (V_F - V_I)(1 - e^{-t/RC})$$

Rearranging these terms gives the familiar form of the charging equation,

$$v_C = V_F + (V_I - V_F)e^{-t/RC} \qquad \text{(B.5)}$$

This equation is widely used and is valuable to memorize. It is helpful in this task to check the equation against Figure B.8. Notice that when $t = 0$, $v_C = V_I$, the initial voltage. Also, note that when t becomes large, $t \gg RC$, the capacitor voltage v_C approaches V_F, the final value. This check will help you keep the signs correct in Equation (B.5).

Next we consider the discharging case. In Figure B.8, the switch is moved from position 2 to position 1 at $t = 0$. The capacitor will have some initial voltage V_I at $t = 0$ and will discharge to zero.

The Laplace method can be used to find the discharging equation for Figure B.8 for $t > 0$. The Laplace domain equivalent circuit appears in Figure B.10. Our goal is to compute the Laplace domain voltage V_C as a function of the Laplace variable s. Again, the Laplace tables will be consulted to find the discharging capacitor voltage v_C as a function of t.

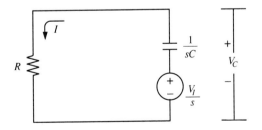

FIGURE B.10
Laplace equivalent for discharging a capacitor.

To find V_C in Figure B.10, apply Ohm's law to write

$$\frac{V_I}{s} = I\left(\frac{1}{sC} + R\right)$$

Solve this for I, to yield

$$I = \frac{V_I}{R\left(s + \dfrac{1}{RC}\right)}$$

Then notice in Figure B.10 that

$$V_C = IR$$

The two previous equations are solved for V_C by eliminating I, so that

$$V_C = \frac{V_I}{\left(s + \dfrac{1}{RC}\right)}$$

This is V_C in the Laplace domain. To find the time domain equivalent, use the Laplace transform in Table B.1, Transform (1). Both sides of that transform are multiplied by the constant V_I and α is taken as $1/RC$. Therefore, the time domain equivalent of V_C is

$$v_C = V_I e^{-t/RC} \tag{B.6}$$

This equation describes the discharge of a capacitor through a resistor R. The initial voltage, V_I, decays to zero. The time required for the discharge is measured in time constants.

Definition: One *time constant*, τ_C, equals the time required for the voltage v_C across the capacitor to fall to $1/e$ times its initial value ($e = 2.7182\ldots$). From Equation (B.6) we see that

$$\tau_C = RC \quad \text{(in s)} \tag{B.7}$$

As a rule, a charging (or discharging) transient is considered complete after five time constants.

C

Medical Terminology
by Marcia Aston

C.1 COMMON PREFIXES

A medical term has several basic components, one of which is a prefix. Prefixes always precede word roots. The root is the foundation of a word or its element. For example, the element or word root "gastr-" means stomach. By putting another element in front of the word root, the meaning of the root word is altered, becoming more specific, for example. Thus, by adding the element "epi-" (meaning "above") as a prefix to the word "gastric" ("pertaining to the stomach"), the new medical term "epigastric," meaning "pertaining to the region above the stomach," is formed.

The following alphabetical list includes fifty of the most common prefixes used in medical terminology and their meanings.

Prefix	Meaning	Prefix	Meaning
a-, an-	not, without	de-	down, lack of
ab-	away from	dia-	through, complete
ad-	toward	dys-	bad, painful, difficult
ana-	up, apart	ec-, ecto-	out, outside
ante-	before, forward	en-, endo-	in, within
anti-	against	epi-	above, upon, on
auto-	self	eu-	good, well
bi-	two	ex-	away from, out
brady-	slow	hemi-	half
cata-	down	hyper-	excessive, beyond
con-	with, together	hypo-	deficient, under
contra-	against, opposite	in-	not, in

Prefix	Meaning	Prefix	Meaning
infra-	below, inferior	poly-	many
inter-	between	post-	after, behind
macro-	large	pre-, pro-	before, in front of
mal-	bad	pseudo-	false
meso-	middle	re-	back
meta-	change, beyond	retro-	behind, back
micro-	small	semi-	half
pan-	all	sub-	under
para-	near, beside, abnormal	supra-	above
		syn-, sym-	together, with
per-	through	tachy-	fast
peri-	surrounding	trans-	across
polio-	gray matter of brain or spinal cord	ultra-	beyond, excess

C.2 COMMON SUFFIXES

Suffixes are a basic component of medical words. Suffixes are always at the endings of words, following prefixes and word roots or elements. They often describe the condition of a part of the body or an action involving a body part. For instance, in the word "cardiogram," cardi-" (meaning "heart") is the root word and "-gram" (meaning "record") is the suffix.

The following alphabetical list includes fifty of the most commonly used medical suffixes and their meanings.

Suffix	Meaning	Suffix	Meaning
-algia	pain	-graphy	process of recording
-cele	hernia	-itis	inflammation
-centesis	surgical puncture	-logy	study of
-clysis	irrigation, washing	-lysis	destruction, breakdown
-coccus	berry-shaped bacteria		
-cyte	cell	-malacia	softening
-dynia	pain	-megaly	enlargement
-ectasis	stretching, dilation	-oma	tumor
-ectomy	removal, excision	-opsy	to view
-emesis	vomiting	-osis	condition (usually abnormal)
-emia	blood condition		
-genesis	condition of, forming	-pathy	disease
-gram	record of	-penia	deficiency
-graph	instrument for recording	-pepsia	digestion

Suffix	Meaning	Suffix	Meaning
-pexy	fixation, putting in place	-sclerosis	hardening
-phagia	eating, swallowing	-scope	instrument for examination
-phobia	fear	-spasm	a sudden, violent involuntary muscular contraction
-plasia	development, formation		
-plasty	surgical repair	-stalsis	contraction
-poiesis	formation	-stasis	stopping, controlling
-ptosis	drooping, sagging	-stenosis	tightening, stricture
-ptysis	spitting	-stomy	new opening
-rrhagia,		-therapy	treatment
rrhage	bursting forth of blood	-tome	cutting instrument
		-tomy	incision, section
-rrhaphy	suture	-tresia	opening
-rrhea	flow, discharge	-trophy	nourishment, development
-rrhexis	rupture		

C.3 THE TERMINOLOGY OF GENERAL ANATOMY

The following terms pertain to the body as a whole.

Body Cavities. Some of the important viscera (internal organs) are found in the following body cavities.

Cavity	Organs
Cranial	Brain
Thoracic	Lungs, heart, trachea, aorta
Abdominal	Stomach, intestines, spleen, gallbladder, liver, pancreas
Pelvic	Urinary bladder, urethra, ureters, uterus, vagina
Spinal	Spinal cord nerves

The cranial and spinal cavities are called *dorsal* because of their location on the back portion of the body. The thoracic, abdominal, and pelvic cavities are considered ventral because of their location on the front or belly side of the body.

The thoracic and abdominal cavities are separated by a muscular partition called the diaphragm.

The abdomen is also divided into six anatomical regions. These divisions are used in describing anatomically the regions in which organs and structures are found:

Hypochondriac – two upper lateral regions beneath the ribs.
Epigastric – region of the stomach.
Lumbar – two middle lateral regions.
Umbilical – region of the navel or umbilicus.
Hypogastric – lower middle region below the umbilicus.
Iliac or Inguinal – Two lower lateral regions.

Anatomical Divisions of the Back

Cervical	Neck region
	7 cervical vertebrae
Thoracic	Chest
	12 thoracic vertebrae
Lumbar	Loin or flank
	5 lumbar vertebrae
Sacral	Sacrum
	5 fused bones
Coccygeal	Coccyx (tailbone)
	4 fused pieces

The spinal column (vertebrae) is made of bone tissue; the spinal cord (nerves running through the column) is made up of nerve tissue. Between each pair of vertebrae is found a piece of cartilage called a disk, which acts as a shock absorber.

Positional and Directional Terms

Afferent – Leading toward a structure.
Efferent – Leading away from a structure.
Anterior (ventral) – The front of the body.
Posterior (dorsal) – The back of the body.
Central – Pertaining to the center.
Deep – Away from the surface.
Superficial – Near the surface.
Distal – Away from the beginning of a structure.
Proximal – Pertaining to the beginning of a structure.
Inferior (caudal) – Away from the head.
Superior (cephalic) – Pertaining to the head.
Lateral – Pertaining to the side.
Medial – Pertaining to the middle.
Supine – Lying on the back.
Prone – Lying on the belly.

Planes of the Body

Frontal – Vertical plane dividing the body into anterior and posterior portions.

Sagittal – Vertical plane that divides the body lengthwise into right and left halves.

Transverse – The plane that runs across the body horizontally, dividing the body into upper and lower portions.

C.4 TERMINOLOGY OF CIRCULATION

There are three main types of blood vessels in the body:

1. *Arteries* are large blood vessels that lead oxygenated blood away from the heart to all parts of the body.
2. *Capillaries* are very thin-walled vessels that carry oxygenated blood from arteries to the cells of the body.
3. *Veins*, which have thinner walls than arteries, conduct the waste-filled blood from the tissues back towards the heart.

The heart pumps blood through two systems of circulation. In *pulmonary circulation*, blood circulates between the heart and the lungs. Nonoxygenated blood circulates from the *right atrium* (upper chamber of the heart) into the *right ventricle* (lower chamber) into the *pulmonary artery* and from there to the lungs. Here the oxygen-deficient blood is reoxygenated and expels carbon dioxide. The newly oxygenated blood then flows into the *pulmonary vein*, back to the left side of the heart (*left atrium* and *left ventricle*), from which it is pumped into the *aorta* and out into the body through the *systemic circulation*.

Two highly important arteries are the *coronary arteries*, which branch off from the *aorta* above the heart. A *myocardial infarction* (heart attack) may occur if these arteries are blocked by a blood clot.

There are two phases to the heartbeat. *Diastole* occurs when the walls of the heart chambers relax and blood flows into the heart through the veins. *Systole* occurs next as the heart chamber walls contract to pump blood into the pulmonary artery and the aorta. The cardiac cycle of relaxation and filling, then contracting and pumping, takes about 0.9 s and occurs between 70 and 80 times a minute. The heart pumps about two and a half ounces of blood with each contraction; that is to say, about five quarts a minute or 75 gallons an hour.

C.5 TERMINOLOGY OF RESPIRATION

There are actually two processes involved in respiration: *external respiration*, in which oxygen is inhaled into the lungs from the outside environment; and *internal respiration*, the exchange of the gases oxygen and carbon dioxide at the tissue cell level.

In the process of respiration, air (oxygen) is inspired (inhaled) through the nose, *pharynx* (throat), *larynx* (voice box), and *trachea* (windpipe). The trachea divides into two *bronchi* (branches), each of which leads into a lung. The bronchi branch into *bronchioles*, at the end of which are air sacs called *alveoli*. The gases oxygen and carbon dioxide are exchanged between the alveoli and the capillaries. The alveoli then carry the waste carbon dioxide back through the lungs to be *expired* (exhaled).

The lungs are divided into *lobes*; the right lung is divided into three lobes, the left lung into only two. The *apex* is the upper part of the lung, the *hilum* is the midline area (for the entrance and exit of blood vessels, nerves, and bronchial tubes), and the *base* is the lower area. The lungs are lined with a smooth membrane called the *pleura* in an airless sac called the *pleural cavity*.

Between the lungs is the *mediastinum*, a thick wall enclosing the heart, aorta, esophagus, and bronchial tubes.

C.6 TERMINOLOGY OF THE NERVOUS SYSTEM

There are two major classifications of the nervous system, the *central nervous system* and the *peripheral nervous system*. The central nervous system is made up of the brain and the spinal cord, each covered by three protective membranes called the *meninges*. The outermost of the three membranes, the *dura mater*, is a tough, resilient membrane. The second layer surrounding the brain and spinal cord is the *arachnoid membrane*, so called because of its weblike structure. The third layer of the meninges, that closest to the brain and spinal cord, is the *pia mater*, a soft, delicate layer that provides the brain with a rich blood supply. The brain is also called the *encephalon* and consists of three parts, the *cerebrum*, the *cerebellum*, and the *brain stem*. The outer layer of the brain is called the *cerebral cortex*, the center of intellectual functions. The cerebellum regulates the coordination of muscular movements and is the center for balance. In the brain stem, the *thalamus* is a relay station for sensory impulses. The *hypothalamus* controls body temperature and centers for appetite, thirst, sleep, feelings, and sexual drive. The *medulla oblongata* connects the spinal cord with the rest of the brain and contains important centers for regulating internal body activities such as respiration, heartbeat, and the dilation of the blood vessels. In the brain is a system of cavities called *ventricles* in which *cerebrospinal fluid* is generated. This fluid surrounds both brain and spinal cord and helps to protect them from stresses.

The peripheral nervous system is made up of *motor* and *sensory nerve fibers*, and these peripheral nerves branch and lead to all of the organs of the body. The motor nerve fibers control muscles and glands, while sensory fibers carry information about various parts of the body to the central nervous system. The motor pathways move outward from the brain and spinal cord and are called *efferent*. The sensory pathways, moving inward toward the brain and spinal cord, are called *afferent*.

The functions of the body that are not voluntarily controlled (by a conscious act of the will) are regulated by the *autonomic nervous system*. Examples of these functions are circulation, digestion, excretion, and glandular functions. The autonomic nervous system is made up of two motor systems that work in opposition to each other, the *sympathetic* and *parasympathetic* systems. Thus, if the nerve impulses are stimulated by the sympathetic nervous system — for example, if the heart rate increases — the parasympathetic system will bring about a state of equilibrium (*homeostasis*) by slowing down the heart rate.

C.7 TERMINOLOGY OF SENSORY ORGANS

The sensory organs receive information from the environment and pass it on to the brain. The major sensory organs are the eye and the ear; other sensors include the skin, taste buds, and olfactory organs.

The visual sense comes to the brain through the eye, whose wall is composed of three layers. The *sclera*, the outermost layer, includes the transparent *cornea*. The middle layer, the *choroid*, is a membrane merging with the *iris*, the colored part of the eye surrounding the pupil. Behind the iris is the *crystalline lens*, whose *ciliary muscles* adjust its shape and thickness. These changes in the shape of the lens aid in the refraction, or bending, of light rays. This refractive power is called *accommodation*. The innermost layer is the *retina*, the sensitive nerve layer of the eye.

As light energy in the form of waves travels through the eye, it is refracted, or bent, by the cornea, the lens, and various eye fluids, so that it focuses on the retina's *receptor cells* called *rods and cones*. The perception of color depends on the cone cells, while rod cells function better in dim light. The rods and cones are connected to the *optic nerve*, fibers from which lead to the brain.

In the ear, sound waves are received by the external ear (*auditory canal*) and are transmitted to the eardrum (*tympanic membrane*), then through the middle ear by means of three small bones called the *malleus*, the *incus*, and the *stapes*. The membrane called the *oval window* separates the middle from the inner ear. The inner ear, also called the *labyrinth*, leads to the *cochlea*, filled with special fluids called *perilymph* and *endolymph* through which the vibrations travel. The *receptors* located in the cochlea relay the sound waves to *auditory nerve fibers*, which end in the *auditory center* of the brain.

Another important function of the ear is the maintenance of the pressure of air in the middle ear to the pressure of air in the outside environment. This is done by means of the *eustachian tube*, which communicates with the pharynx.

The sense of balance is located in the inner ear (three *semicircular canals* filled with *lymph*). Sensitive *hair cells* fluctuate in response to head movements, thus sending nerve impulses to the brain to ensure that equilibrium is maintained.

Somatic sensors react to touch, pressure, warmth, cold, and pain. *Touch receptors* are most closely spaced on fingertips, lips, and the tip of the tongue. *Pressure receptors* are located in the subcutaneous and deeper senses. Temperature senses (*heat and cold receptors*) have separate nerve fiber connections. Thus, a warm object will stimulate only the heat receptors, while a cool object will affect only cold terminals.

Pain sensors are known as *free nerve endings* (branching of nerve fiber). They protect the body from damage so there is little *adaptation* (adjustment) with continued stimulation.

The *olfactory* organ is located in the upper part of the nasal cavity, where its primary purpose is the interpretation of smell, which is closely related to the sense of taste.

The sense of taste involves receptors in the tongue (tip, border, and base) known as *taste buds*. There are four basic tastes: sweet, sour, bitter, and salty. Taste perception is limited to dissolved substances.

Index

A-mode display, 493
A-stable multivibrator, 304
a.c. current gain, 34
a.c. equivalent circuit, 139
A/D converter, 480
accumulator, 400
acoustic impedance, 490
action potential, 44, 55
active electrode resistance, 316
address bus, 398, 402
adhesive disposable electrodes, 323
Agsten, G. T., 337
aiming light, 334
air bubbles, 128
airway resistance, 372
alarm, 70
algebraic equations, 21
alpha rays, 474
alphanumeric labels, 409
alphanumerics, 399
aluminum filters, 457
Amarasingham, R., 278
ammonium dihydrogen phosphate, 491
amplifiers, 135–158
analog to digital converter, 407
anatomical regions, 539

Anbar, M., 393
anesthesia delivery equipment, 78
anesthetic exhaust, 79
anesthetic machines, 77
anesthetics, 69
    nonflammable, 313
Anger Scintillation Camera, 478
antistatic sheets, 81
    spray, 85
aortic valve, 341
argon laser, 335
arithmetic logic unit, 399
arterial pressure measurement, 344
arterial systolic pressure (SYST), 344
artificial blood circulators, 75
artificial heart, 15, 75, 283
artificial heart valves, 283
artificial kidney, 16
ASCII code, 403
Association for the Advancement of
    Medical Instrumentation, 73, 86
asystole, 409
atomic weights, 39
atrioventricular node (AV), 45, 46,
    177, 283
atrium, 341
attenuation, 505

audio spectrum, 500
Auth, D. C., 337
automatic machine diagnosis, 180

B-mode display, 493
Babbs, C. F., 278
Back Projection Reconstruction, 471
bacterial filter, 377
Bahill, A. T., 56
Baker, L. E., 128
balloon pump, 17
balloon-tipped catheter, 17, 351
band-pass filter, 237
barium platinocyanide, 9
base resistance, 34
basic language, 515
battery, rechargeable, 183
battery-operated devices, 185
bedside monitors, 410
Bender, G. T., 443
Berger, Hans, 11
beta radiation, 474
beta waves, 230
bicep brachii, 52
binary number system, 396
binaural, differential stethoscope, 7
biofeedback, 5
biopotential, 37, 42–49
biopotential amplifier, 135–170
biopotential electrodes, 40
biopotential laws, 37–41
bipolar connection, 227
bipolar electrode, 288
bipolar junction transistor (BJT), 32
bit, 396
Bliss, W. R., 18
block diagram x-ray, 456
blood cell counter, 437–442
blood flow, 17
blood gas analyzer, 425
blood partial pressure, 371
blood pressure, 16, 341
blood proteins, 431
blood serum pH, $^PCO_2$, $^PO_2$, 428
Bode plots, 234

body cavities, 539
body planes, 541
body plethysmograph, 389–392
body resistance, 317
Boltzmann's constant, 42, 43
Bourland, J. D., 278
Bovie, 313
bowel gas, 323
bradycardia, 179, 283
brain waves, 223, 230
breathing, 374
    patient-initiated, 374
bremsstrahlung radiation, 449
bronchitis, 372
Bronzino, J. D., 34, 309, 417
Brown, J. G., 487
Brown, J. H. V., 56
Brown, J. M., 56, 86, 255, 377
bubbles, 128
Bucky grid, 458, 463
buffer, 152, 240
buffer amplifier, 152
building wiring, 61
bundle branch, 45
Bunsen, 433
Bunsen burner, 433
Butterworth filter, 241, 245

calculus, 208, 223
calibration, 89
calomel electrode, 443
Cammann, George P., 7
cancer, 445
capacitive coupling, 64
capacitive reactance, 22
capacitor radiation monitor, 535
carcinogen, 484
cardioversion, 264, 267
Carr, J., 56, 86, 255, 377
Carver, K. R., 511
catheter, 341–355
    bubble, 364
    components, physical formulas, 359
    frequency response, 360
    leak, 364

measurements, 355–367
pinch, 363
troubleshooting tips, 367
tuning, 363
catheterized heart, 74
catheterized patient, 67
cathode material coefficient, 447
cathode-ray tube, 201, 445
cathode rays, 9
cavitation, 505
cell vaporization, 49
depolarized, 44
spherical model, 49
central processing unit, 398
central station monitor, 405–413
centrifuge, 10
cerebral ventricle, 355
characteristic impedance, 499, 500
characteristic radiation, 449
Chardack, William, 15, 283
charge distribution, 90
chart recorders, 11
chassis, 62
chassis-to-ground leakage, 72
chemical electrodes, 42, 423–429
chest lead connection, 191
chloride membrane electrode, 423
chlorine, 42
chloroform, 81
circuit analysis, 23, 529
circuit board, 85, 405
circuit-board swapping, 85
circuit branch, 23
circulation, 341–348, 541
Citron, P., 309
Clark electrode, 427
Clark, Barney, 15, 283
Clark, J. W., 56
clinical engineering, 72
clinical laboratory, 10
coagulation mode, 315
Cobbold, R. S. C., 128
coherent, 333
collector resistance, 34, 138
collimator, 457, 461

collodion cement, 225
color code, 61
colorimeter, 431–437
common prefixes, 537
common-mode (CM) reduction amplifier, 216
common-mode interference, 137
common-mode rejection ratio (CMRR), 158–164, 198, 227
common-mode voltage, 137, 160, 190
reduction, 198
comparator, 294
complementary metal-oxide semiconductor, 284
complex numbers, 22
compliance, 356, 357, 360
component level
testing, 416
troubleshooting, 89, 127, 416
computer, on a chip, 395
computer processing unit, 399
computer programs, 515
computer tomography (CT), 18
conductive
clothing, 80
floor, 80
footwear, 81
constantan, 117
contrast, 446, 455
control bus, 398
control system, 371
controlled-gain differential amplifier, 154
cordohmeter, 87
Cormack, Allan, 18
Craib, A. R., 255
cranial cavities, 539
Creamer, M., 11
critical areas, 74
critical care, 60
critical care units, 410
Cromwell, L., 368
crossover compensation, 209
Cruikshank, William, 10

crystal scintillation, 477
CT scanner, 395, 469–473
current division, 29
current gain, 30
  transistor, 328
Cushing, Harvey, 313
cyclopropane, 79, 81
cyclotron, 14

Dalziel, C. F., 56
d.c. current gain, 32
d.c. defibrillator, 15
defibrillation, 53
defibrillator, 45, 261–278
  a.c., 261
  amplifier, 183
  analyzer, 277
  battery pack, 278
  block diagram, 263
  capacitor, 267
  d.c., 261
  discharge buttons, 265
  electrodes, 277
  energy delivery, 267
  Lown, 267, 271
  paddles, 277
  pulse, 262
  troubleshooting, 277
  voltage, overdamped, 275
  voltage, underdamped, 273
  voltage, waveform, 270
Demarre, D. A., 217
depolarization, 341
DeVries, William C., 15, 283
diagnosis, 3
diagnostic circuitry, 263
diagnostic equipment, 371, 489
diastole, 45, 342
Dickson, J. F., 56
dielectric constant, 49
diethyl ether, 81
diff amp, 135–143
  buffer amplifier, 157
  chip, 255

differential amplifier, 89, 135, 227,
    384, 439
  ideal, 144
  inverting mode, 140
  noninverting mode, 140
  symbol, 140
differential capacitor, 121
differential equations, 21
differential gain, 140
differential capacitive transducer,
    121–126
diffraction gratings, 431
diffusion, 39
diffusion coefficient, 40
digital circuits, 4
digital logic, 396
digital pulse oscillator, 284, 294
direct pressure measurement, 348
diseases, diagnosed, 231
displays, 185
Dobson, Matthew, 9
Doppler effect, 489
dosimetry, 79
dot matrix, 185
double insulation, 64, 74
drift current, 40
drift equation, 39
driven patient leads, 74
dual-in-line packages, 163
duty cycle, 322

ECG, 4, 11, 177–198, 341
  augmented lead connections, 185
  block diagram, 180
  calibration switch, 180
  chest lead, 193
  clinical variables, 177
  distinctive features, 179
  driven-right-leg system, 201
  fetus, 184
  hard-copy display, 185
  operator error, 195
  R-wave, 264
  sources of interference, 182

standard connection, 185
stress testing, 184
T-wave, 264
ectopic, 261
ectopic beats, 53, 180
EEG, 4, 11, 223–233
  audio, 232
  block diagram, 227
  electrodes, 223
  frequency bands, 230
  stimulus-evoked responses, 233
  troubleshooting, 231, 254
  visual, 232
Egan, D. F., 393
Eggert, A. A., 443
Einstein relationship, 39–40
Einthoven, Willem, 11
Einthoven triangle, 188
electrical circuits, 21
  hazards, 59–68
  safety analyzer, 72
  shock, 49–59
electrocardiogram, 20, 38, 46, 177, 185
electrocardiograph (*see also* ECG), 4,
    11, 177–198, 341
electrocorticographic electrode, 225
electrodes, 89–100
  active blade-type, 315
  adhesive, 318
  bipolar, 316
  capacitance, 96
  cutting, 313
  equivalent circuit, 93
  gel, 60, 263, 318
  ground-plate, 316
  hemostat, 315
  impedance, 320
  invasive, 90
  needle, 231
  noninvasive, 90
  patient-plate, 314
  pregelled, 216, 318
  resistance, 96
  return, 318

rigid metal, 323
suction, 90
surface, 90
transducer, 89–100
electrode-heart resistance, 284
electrode-lead cable, 90
electrode-muscle contact, 289
electrode-skin resistance, 267
electroencephalogram, 38, 135
electroencephalograph (*see* EEG)
electroencephalography, 396
electrolyte, 39
electrolyte gel, 90
electromyogram, 135
electromyographic potentials, 158
electronic circuits, 19–33
electron-volt, 450
electrooculogram, 38
electroretinogram, 38
electrosurgical analyzer, 330
electrosurgical knives, 5
electrosurgical unit (ESU), 13,
    313–323
  analyzer, 322
  block diagram, 321
  coag modes, 322
  cut modes, 322
  cutting mode, 315
  pencil electrode, 323
  power amplifier, 327
  service manual, 331
  troubleshooting, 330
elevated chassis voltage, 67
elevated voltage, 67
emergency power systems, 75
emitter resistance, 34, 138
emphysema, 372
endocardial lead, 288
energy interruptions, 73
enflurane, 78
engineering analysis, 20
engineering design, 20
environmental effects, 428
epicardial lead, 288

epilepsy, 232
epoxy, 490
equipment, block diagram, 85
    diagnostic checks, 417
    disassembling, 86
    equipment under test, 72
    history, 85
    records, 417
    repair records, 83
    safety program, 72
    schematic, 85
    self-testing procedures, 85
    service manual, 82, 85
error message, 85, 415
esophageal lead, 195
ether, 79
ethyl chloride, 81
ethylene, 81
ethylene oxide, 81
evoked response, 255
excited state, 333
explosion, 59
explosive gas, 80
extended self-test, 392
external pacemakers, 77
external pressure transducer, 363
eyeglasses, 336

Fahrenheit, Gabriel D., 6
Federal Drug Administration, 73
feedback control, 4
feedback transform, 5
Feinberg, B. N., 86, 278, 487, 511
Ferdinand II, 6
fetal monitor, 216
fibrillation, 261
    atrial, 180
    ventricular, 180
Fick's law, 39
film badge detector, 476
filter, 233–255
    band-reject, 251
    bandwidth, 235
    first order, 236
    gain, 234

order, *n*, 235
quality, *Q*, 235
resonant frequency, 235
roll-off, 234, 235
third-order, 247
fire, 59
flag register, 401
flame, due to sparks, 79
flame photometer, 431, 433–437
flameproof clothing, 82
flammable anesthetics, 14
    environment, 69
    substances, 81
flexible power cords, 81
floating world, 406
flow rate, 509
Floyd, T. L., 164, 255, 337
fluid inertance, 356
fluid systems, 20
fluid-electrical analogy, 358
fluorescent screen, 469
fluorocarbons, 78
fluoroscope, 351
fluoroscopic unit, 467–469
Food, Drug and Cosmetic Act, 73
foot-treadle switch, 81
Freeman, J. J., 86

Gage, Andrew, 283
Galileo, 6
Galioto, F. M., 309
Galvani, Luigi, 37
gamma-ray camera, 14, 478
gamma rays, 474
gantry, 470
Ganz, W., 17, 351, 368
Garcia, Manuel, 9
gauge factor, 113
gauge pressure, 347
Geddes, L. A., 128, 368
Geiger Counter, 476
gel, transducer, 490
general anatomy, 539
Gerhard, G. C., 337
glass electrode, 443

glass filters, 433
glass magnifiers, 8
Goldman's equation, 42, 423, 424
Goldstein, A., 511
Gowers, William, 10
Greatbatch, Wilson, 15, 283
ground fault interrupter, 68
ground wire, 61, 64
grounded world, 406
Guyton, A. C., 56, 368

haemacytometer, 10
half-cell potential, 93, 94
halothane, 78, 81
hand-held calculator, 22
Hayt, W. H., 278
hazardous situations, 62
hearing for diagnosis, 6
heart, 49
    pumping cycle, 341
    ventricle, 355
heart fibrillation, 59
heart sound, 342
heat sink, 164, 327
heat-sensitive paper, 185
Helmholtz, Hermann von, 8
hematocrit, 10, 437
hemodialysis, 16
hemodynamics, 346
hemoglobin, 371, 430, 438
Hewlett-Packard 78534 monitor, 405
Hewlett-Packard HP-15C calculator,
    515
high-frequency effects, 53
high-input-impedance buffer, 152
high-pass filter, 244
high-pressure gas release, 77
Hilburn, J. L., 165
history of medical equipment, 5–19
Holter monitor, 184, 216, 396
Holter, Norman, 184
hospital, 59
hospital air, 380
hot spots, 81
hot wire, 61

Hounsfield, Geoffrey, 18
Houry, O. H., 18
Hunsinger, D. L., 393
hydrodynamics, 346
Hymen, Albert S., 283
hyperbaric chambers, 81
hypodermic needles, 5
hysteresis voltage, 296

ideal current source, 21
ideal filter, 233
ideal voltage source, 21
image intensifier, 469
image quality, 446
imaging, 489
    ultrasonic equipment, 491
impedance, 22
impedance matching, 4, 201
implantable batteries, 287
inductive coupling, 64
inductive reactance, 22
inductive transducers, 126–127
inertance, 356
infection, 77
infectious agents, 73
input impedance, 204, 532
inspections of equipment, 74
instrument sterilization, 78
instrumentation amplifiers,
    troubleshooting, 163
insurance, 73
integrated circuits, 32, 201
integrator, 385
intensive care units, 75, 410
interconnecting cables, 83
interference, 251
    power-line, 159
interference factors, 89
interstitial fluid, 50
intra-aortic, 17
invasive units, 5
involuntary contraction, 51
ion valence, 40
ionic current, 40
ionization chambers, 471

ionizing radiation, 19
iron lung, 14
isolation transformer, 69, 80

Jacobson, B., 337, 487
Jarvik, Robert K., 15, 283
Javitt, J., 417
Johnson, D. E., 165
Johnson, J. R., 165
Joint Commission on Accreditation
    of Healthcare Organizations, 73

Kemmerly, J. E., 278
keystroke program, 22, 515
kidney dialysis machines, 75
Kirchhoff, 433
Kirchhoff's current law (KCL), 24,
    529
Kirchhoff's voltage law (KVL), 24
Kolft, W. J., 17
Kondraski, G. V., 255
Korotkoff sounds, 344
Kraus, J. D., 511

Laennec, Rene T. H., 7
Lambert's law, 453
Langmuir-Childs law, 447
Laplace domain, 272, 526, 528
Laplace domain impedances, 526
Laplace equivalent elements, 529
Laplace equivalent impedances, 272,
    527
Laplace equivalents, 529
Laplace method, 270, 526–531
Laplace transform table, 273, 531
Laplace variable, 528
large-scale integrated circuit, 294
laser, 5, 333–337
    action, 333
    beam, 336
    beam manipulator, 333
    CO_2, 333
    gas, 333
    spot diameter, 334

surgery, 313
surgical devices, 333
Lawson, J., 17
lead zirconate titanate, 491
leakage current, 64, 72, 74, 322
leakage current specifications, 75
Leeming, M. N., 86
left ventricle, 45
lens, 8
let-go current, 51, 52, 54
Lewis, R., 309
light-emitting diodes, 71, 430
light pump, 336
Lillehei, C. Walton, 15
line isolation monitor, 69
linear variable differential trans-
    former, 126
liquid crystal display, 185
Lisnerski, K. J., 393
lithium, 433
lithium-iodine cells, 286
load pick-up time, 75
lobes of the brain, 223
local building codes, 73
low-frequency currents, 55
low-pass filter, 241
Lown, Bernard, 15, 262, 278
lung capacity, 390
lysing, 438

M-mode display, 494
machine diagnosis, 4
machine language, 396–398
Macovski, A., 487
macroshock, 53, 59, 181
    hazards, 62
McWane, J. W., 309
magnetic resonance imagers (MRI),
    11, 395
magnetism, 73
maintenance manual, 216, 414
maintenance personnel, 89
Malvino, A. P., 165, 309
manufacturer's service manual, 410

mass attenuation coefficient, 454
material constant, 109
Maurizi, J. J., 393
maximum power transfer, 206
mean cell hemoglobin concentration, 438
mean cell volume, 438
measuring instrument, 4
mechanical devices, 20
medical applications, 121
medical battery-powered instruments, 136
medical device amendments, 73
medical instrument transducers, 89
medical instrumentation, 3–5, 19
medical suffixes, 538
medical terminology, 537
membrane potential, 38
memory, 4
memory chip, 402
memory location, 399
mercury cells, 286
mercury timer, 442
metal fatigue, 67
metal-oxide semiconductor, 532
metal-to-electrolyte interface, 96
meter movement, 4
methane, 323
methoxyflurane, 78
Michaels, D., 217
microprocessor, 4, 19, 332, 395, 398–404
    block diagram, 398
    input unit, 399
    output unit, 399
microprocessor-based equipment, 392, 395
    monitor, 405–410
microshock, 37, 55, 60, 181
    hazards, 64
Millman, J., 487
minicomputer, 18
Mirowski, M., 278

mitral valve, 341
mobility, 40
modules, 83
mole, 39
monitor, 3, 4
monochromatic light, 333
monostable multivibrator, 304
montage, 227
MRI, van-mounted, 19
multivibrator, positive-edge triggered, 306
muscle, smooth, 45
muscle contraction, 44, 45, 184
myocardial depolarization, 261
myocardial infarction, 178

n-type transistor, 32
narrow-band-reject filter, 251
nasopharyngeal electrode, 225
National Fire Protection Association, 73, 86
Nd:YAG laser, 336
nebulizer, 377
negative side effects, 505
Nernst equation, 43, 52, 423
nervous system, 542
Neuman, J., 278
Neuman, M. R., 128, 217, 309
neural stimulators, 231
neutral fault, 67
neutral wire, 61
Newton, Isaac, 8
nitrous oxide, 78
nodes, 21
noise, 89
nonflammable anesthetics, 14
nonsterile area, 77
Norman, R. A., 443
notch filter, 227
notch frequency, 252
npn transistors, 32
nuclear batteries, 286
nuclear medicine, 14, 473–487
nuclear medicine imaging, 478–480

Occupational Safety and Health Administration, 73, 476
occupationally induced x-rays, 483
Ohm's law, 22
ohmmeter, 164
Olson, W. H., 86
operating room, 77, 79
operational amplifier (op amp), 143–151
  output impedance, 146
  in tandem, 149
  voltage and current sources, 147
operator technique, 267
ophthalmoscope, 8
optical coupling, 332
optical fibers, 336
optical methods of cell counting, 442
organs, 539
orifice resistance, 440
oscillator, square-wave period, 303
output impedance, 144, 208
oxygen, 69
oxygen-enriched air, 379
oxygen-rich atmosphere, 77
oxygen safety, 77
oxygen saturation (SaO$_2$), 429
oxygen system valves, 77
oxygen tents, 77
oxyhemoglobin saturation, percentage, 430

P-R interval, 57, 177
p-type transistor, 32
P-wave, 46, 47
pacemaker, 15, 45, 136, 283–293
pacemaker
  asynchronous, 291
  batteries, 286
  cable, 55
  circuit, 307
  demand, 291
  digital pulse oscillator, 283
  electrode, 288
  P-wave synchronous, 291
  programmable, 291

R-wave inhibited, 291
R-wave synchronous, 291
paddles, defibrillator, 262
  anterior-anterior, 262
  anterior-posterior, 262
palpation, 341
paper chart recorder, 201
partial pressure of carbon dioxide (^{P}CO$_2$), 426
partial pressure of oxygen (^{P}O$_2$), 81, 426
particle velocity, 501
patient leads, 160, 413
patient transducer, 413
patient-care instruments, 405
^{P}CO$_2$ electrode, 426
pediatric patients, 263
periodic inspection, 67
permeability, 42
Perron, E., 86
Perry, M., 255
Peura, R. A., 128, 368, 511
Pfeiffer, E. A., 368
pH, 424, 426
  electrode, 424
  measurement, 5
  meters, 424
pH-sensitive glass, 424
phase distortion, 240
phased array transducer, 494
phasor, 21, 23
  domain, 23, 386
  impedance, 527
  source, 23
  theory, 359
Phillips, M. L., 393
phosphor crystals, 469
photocathode, 469
photodetector diodes, 430
photometer, 431–437
photomultiplier tube, 478
physiological parameters, 3
physiological potentials, 20
physiological stability, 4
Pierce, William, 283

piezoelectric crystal, 489
platelets, 437
plethysmograph, 113, 389, 372
pn-junction semiconductor, 32
pneumatic equipment, 435
  instruments, 14
  systems, 20
pneumotachograph, 383
  volume, 386
pnp transistors, 32
^{P}O$_2$ electrode, 427
polar form, 27
polarization potential, 95, 96
polarographic electrode, 428
polypropylene membrane, 427
portable equipment, 81
positive feedback, 295
positive-pressure respirator, 14
potassium, 42, 433
potentiometer, 381
power amplifier, 327
  crossover distortion, 202
  efficiency, 205
  push-pull, 201
power bus, 61
power cord, 66
  leakage, 74
power outages, 75
power receptacle, 69, 71
power reflection coefficient, 505
power supplies, 211
power supply, 183, 216
  isolated, 183
  regulation, 214
  smooth output voltage, 214
power system, 74
power transistor chip, 327
pregelled electrodes, 195
premature ventricular contraction,
  180
pressure, 344
  average, 344
  central venous (CVP), 351, 346
  diastolic, 350
  hydrostatic, 349

  left atrium (LAP), 354
  mean arterial (MEAN), 344, 350
  measurements, 351
  pulmonary artery wedge, 354
  right atrial (RAP), 346
  transducer, 350
  wedge, 354
pressure, diastolic (DIAS), 344
pressure chambers, 81
pressure monitor, noninvasive, 342
pressure monitoring, 341
pressure transducer, 121, 405
preventive maintenance, 82
preventive maintenance inspections,
  82
principle of superposition, 33
program counter, 401
programmable calculators, 23
programmable read only memory, 402
proportional counter mode, 476
protection devices, 68–72
pulmonary function monitoring,
  371–374
pulmonary functions, 374
pulmonary instrumentation, 396
pulmonary valve, 341
pulse rate, 179
Purkinje system, 45
push-pull amplifier, 201–215
  d.c. efficiency, 210

QRS complex, 47, 57

RC charging equation, 535
R wave, 47, 180
radiation, 59, 73
radiation detectors, 474
radiation dose, 481–487
radioisotopes, 532
radionuclides, 14, 474
radiopharmaceutical, 473, 479
random access memory, 402
read only memory, 402
receptacle tester, 70, 74
red blood cells, 10, 57, 437

reflection coefficient, 501, 502
refractory period, 45
registers, 399
regulations, 59
Reiser, Stanley Joel, 34, 393
relative dielectric constant, 50
relative refractory period, 45
resistance, 22, 340
resistance measurements, 164
resistive coupling, 64
respiration, 354, 371, 542
respirator, 75, 371, 380
respiratory paralysis, 52
respiratory system, 49
resting potential, 42
resting resistance, 115
return electrode monitor, 318
right ventricle, 45
Rochlin, G. I., 34
Roentgen, Wilhelm, 9, 445
Rollo, John, 10
Roney, P. R., 417

safety analyzer, 74
safety regulations, 72
safety program, 73–82
safety tests, 73
Santonio, Santorio, 6
scalpel, 314
scanning type displays, 493
scattering, 463
schematics, 89
Scribner, B. H., 16
Seely, S., 487
selective absorption, 335
self-test, 392, 415
semiconductor chip, 135
semiconductor diodes, 32
semiconductor thermistor, 103
sensing coil, 68
sensory organs, 543
serial distribution network, 410
serum pH, 443
sheath fluid, 442
shock hazard, 55

siemens, 50
signal processing, 4, 177
signal processor, 4
signal tracing, 85, 164
silicon, 114
silicon rubber membrane, 430
Singh, A., 417
single-phase power supply, 465
sinoatrial (SA) node, 45, 180, 283
sinusoidal oscillators, 323
skin effect, 53
skin resistance, 60, 261
small a.c. signal equivalent, 33
Smith, W., 393
sodium, 42, 433
sodium iodide, 477
solder, 86, 164
    low-temperature, 164
solid-state memory, 185
somatosensory stimuli, 232
sonar, 18
sources of ignition, 77
Spach, M. S., 217
spark gap transmitters, 13
sparks, 69
spectrophotometers, 431
spherical-tip electrode, 315
spheroidal electrode, 225
sphygmomanometer, 4, 344
spinal cavities, 539
spirometers, 372, 381
Spooner, R. B., 278
square-wave generator, 299
stack pointer, 401
static charges, 80
static sparks, 81
steam sterilization, 78
step source, 270, 526
sterile region, 77
sterilization, 77
    at low temperatures, 78
stethoscope, 7, 342
stimulus, 261
stimulus current, 50
stimulus threshold, 51

stock standard, 435
strain, 113
strain gauge, 113–122, 383
    bonded, 121
    sensitivity, 120, 134
    unbonded, 121
stray capacitance, 69, 160
stress, 116
stress tester, 216
strip chart recorder, 180
suffixes, 538
surface electrode, 42, 177, 225
    troubleshooting, 127
surface potential, 177
surgery, 3
Sutphin, S. E., 443
Swan, H. J., 17, 351, 368
Swan-Ganz® catheter, 354
system, 83
system communication controller,
    410
systole, 45, 342
Sze, S. M., 56

T-wave, 47, 179
tachycardia, 179
Tacker, W. A., 278
tactile vocoder, 5
Tadoma method, 5
tape recorder, 227
telemetric programmer, 291
television camera, 468
temperature, body, 6
temperature coefficient, 107
    negative, 100
    positive, 100
temperature regulating circuits, 427
10-20 system, 223
therapeutic equipment, 5, 371, 489
therapeutic ultrasonic equipment,
    489–491
therapy, 3, 5
thermal compensation, 425
thermal conductivity, 128
thermal overload, 464

thermal styluses, 201
thermal transducers, 100–107
thermally limited current, 447
thermistor sensitivity, 128
thermistors, 100, 355
thermometer, 6
Thevenin equivalent circuit, 129, 206
Thevenin resistance, 206
Thevenin voltage source, 147
Thompkins, W. J., 417
thoracic, abdominal pelvic cavities,
    539
thoracic volume, 391
thorax, 53
thorax resistance, 267
thoriated tungsten, 487
three-phase power supply, 466
three-prong plug, 64
three-wire equipment, 62
threshold detector, 297
time constant, 536
time domain, 386
tissue contrast, 455
tissue injury, 59
tomography computer, 469
total lung capacity, 389
toxic exposure, 59
toxic materials, 73, 287
Traister, R. J., 368
transducer, 89
transistor differential amplifier, 137
transit time, 509
transit-time difference, 510
travelling pressure wave, 497–503
tricuspid valve, 341
Triebel, W. A., 417
troubleshooting, 20, 83–86, 405
    board-level, 405, 416
    charts, 84, 416
    circuit-board swapping, 216
    equipment, 83
    microprocessor-based equipment,
        413
    module, 277
    module-level, 331

pneumatic equipment, 392
system-level, 395
techniques, 127
unit-level, 215–217
two-wire equipment, 62
two-wire plug, 64

ultrasonic
blood-flow equipment, 506–510
display unit, 493
echo, 492
equipment, 489–496
massager, 5
power, 504
waves, 489, 496–504
ultrasound, 17, 490
ultrasound scanner, 18
Underwriters' Laboratories, 73
unipolar pacemaker, 289
unit, 83
urine, 10
U-wave, 47

vacuum tubes, 135
Van Valkenburg, M. E., 278
varactor, 262
ventilating system, 79
ventilation assistance, 374
ventilator, 374–380
assist mode, 379
bellows, 377
calibration analyzer, 392
main solenoid, 379
pneumatic circuits, 475
ventricular fibrillation, 261
viscera resistance, 60
viscosity, 348
visual inspection, 413
Volta, Count Alessandro, 37
voltage division, 28
voltage drops, 25
voltage gain, 30
voltage rise, 25
voluntary regulations, 73

Washburn, Sherwood, 34
water-filled catheter, 360
wave, propagating, 499
wave crest, 499
wave impedance, 501
wave reflections, 500
wavelength, 507
wearing parts, 82
Webster, J. G., 128, 337, 368, 417, 487
Weibell, F., 368
Wells, P. N. T., 511
Wheatstone bridge, 89, 107–113, 384
sensitivity, 111
white blood cells, 437
Wilson connection, 183, 191
word root, 537
work function, 446

x-ray, 9, 445–473
absorption, 452
contrast, 456
density, 456
detector, 463
dose, 445
equipment, 445
images, 351
power supply, 464
scattering, 457
sharpness, 456
shielding, 484
x-ray tube, 9, 446–449, 458–461
anode, 457
efficiency, 458
filament, 457

Yanof, H. M., 217
Young's modulus, 116

Zeimssen, Hugo von, 10
Zener diode, 214
Zoll, Paul M., 15, 283